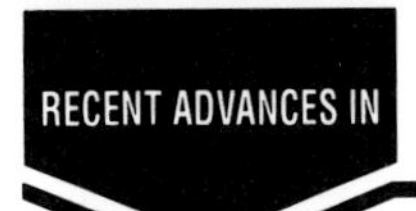

Orthopaedics

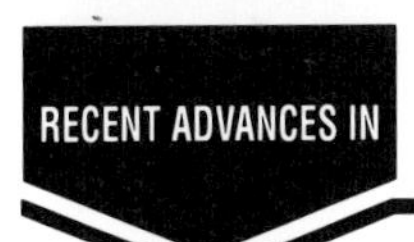

Orthopaedics

Edited by

A. Catterall MChir FRCS
Consultant Orthopaedic Surgeon, The Royal National Orthopaedic Hospital, Middlesex, UK

NUMBER SIX

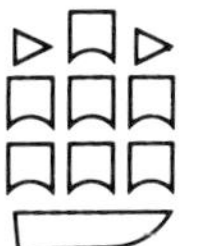

CHURCHILL LIVINGSTONE
EDINBURGH LONDON MELBOURNE NEW YORK AND TOKYO 1992

CHURCHILL LIVINGSTONE
Medical Division of Longman Group UK Limited

Distributed in the United States of America by Churchill Livingstone Inc., 650 Avenue of the Americas, New York, N.Y. 10011, and by associated companies, branches and representatives throughout the world.

First published 1992

ISBN 0-443-04386-8
ISSN 0308-4914

British Library Cataloguing in Publication Data
Recent advances in orthopaedics.
No. 6
1. Orthopedia
I. Catterall, Anthony
617′.3 RD731

Produced by Longman Singapore Publishers Pte Ltd
Printed in Singapore

Preface

The new issue of *Recent Advances in Orthopaedics* heralds the last decade of this century. It should, therefore, reflect not only current change but also the future prospects of orthopaedics in the coming decade. The future, if associated with the present financial constraints, is going to place a great strain on our practice. The planning of service needs is essential but can only be achieved by perceiving how the incidence and pattern of disease will change. The two chapters on epidemiology consider future trends in orthopaedics and accidents to provide a basis for such planning in the future.

Specialization within the field of orthopaedics continues to enlarge, and with it comes the need for sophisticated investigation. Computers with their software now provide glimpses of active pathology with the use of CT and MRI scans. This allows opinions on management not previously available. However, the language or jargon used in these investigations may be unintelligible to many of us in practice. Can this jargon be simplified? In addition we require guidance on the value of these investigations in the management of various conditions.

In the past internal fixation has been the accepted method of management for the complex fracture. External fixation was until recently considered unsatisfactory but this is now changing to assume a greater role, particularly in the management of difficult fractures with skin loss. The problem with which the clinician is faced is which frame and for how long?

In Europe and North America trauma centres have demonstrated the effectiveness of team management of the multiply injured patient. The problem, however, in the major disaster is organization and the lessons learnt from three recent disasters need to be brought to the attention of all concerned in such management in order to try and standardize, particularly the administration of these problems.

No issue of *Recent Advances* can really leave out the problems associated with hip disorders. The last issue concentrated on prosthetic design and fixation. It is, however, a conclusion of present experience that joint replacement is unreliable in the young patient. Conservative surgery should, therefore, continue to have its place but what are the indications for the various reconstructive procedures available? Does triple innominate osteotomy have the same indications as lateral shelf acetabuloplasty? The obvious answer is 'no' but the indications for these various procedures must be identified. At the other end of the spectrum, revision hip surgery for the failed joint replacement is becoming a specialty in its own right. The technical side is different and the surgeon faces the dilemmas of repeating the previous operation with the use of cement or utilizing other techniques. The magnitude of the problem is such that every orthopaedic surgeon must be able to provide satisfactory management of these cases.

The explosion in arthroscopic investigation and surgery continues. Can lessons learnt from the knee be immediately applied to the investigation and management of shoulder problems? The variability of the normal anatomy in the past resulted in a number of unnecessary procedures. The experiences of shoulder arthroscopy is providing a much better understanding of the normal and the achievements of treatment. Clarification of the treatment options is certainly needed.

In the upper limb the morbidity from injuries to the brachial plexus continues to disable young members of our society. Much has been written in the past about this but a review of the results of open surgical exploration and particularly the management of pain associated with this condition is relevant. In a similar way flexor tendon injuries are always with us. Have the techniques changed and what can be hoped for from primary repair or a secondary tendon graft?

The new issue of *Recent Advances* tries to reflect the questions that are pertinent to these discussions. It cannot in itself reflect all aspects of orthopaedics and trauma but merely highlight recent advances in the burning issues.

London 1992 A. Catterall

Contributors

Rolfe Birch MChir FRCS
Orthopaedic Surgeon, St Mary's Hospital, and Peripheral Nerve Injury Unit, Royal National Orthopaedic Hospital, London, UK; Civilian Consultant, Royal Navy

John P. Bull CBE MA MD FRCP
Formerly Director of the MRC Industrial Injuries and Burns Research Unit, Birmingham Accident Hospital, UK

A. Catterall MChir FRCS
Consultant Orthopaedic Surgeon, Royal National Orthopaedic Hospital, Stanmore, Middlesex, UK

S. A. Copeland MB BS FRCS
Consultant Orthopaedic Surgeon, The Royal Berkshire Hospital, Reading, Berkshire, UK

James L. Cunningham BSc PhD
Lecturer in Engineering, University of Durham, UK

Gwyn A. Evans FRCS FRCS (Ed) Orth
Director of the Children's Unit, The Robert Jones and Agnes Hunt Orthopaedic Hospital, Oswestry, Shropshire, UK

John Kenwright MA MD FRCS
Consultant Orthopaedic Surgeon, Nuffield Orthopaedic Centre, Oxford, UK

George Kirsh MB BS FRACS (Orth)
VMO, Bankstown Hospital, Sydney; Trauma Fellow, St George Hospital, Sydney, Australia

Iain W. McCall MB ChB FRCR
Consultant Radiologist, The Robert Jones and Agnes Hunt Orthopaedic Hospital, Oswestry, Shropshire, UK

W. F. G. Muirhead-Allwood BSc MB BS FRCS
Consultant Orthopaedic Surgeon, The Whittington Hospital, London, UK

John M. Rowles BM BS BMedSc FRCS (Eng)
Research Fellow to The NLDB Crash Study, University of Nottingham, UK

Alan J. Silman MSc MD MRCP FFCM
Director of the Arthritis and Rheumatism Council Epidemiology Research Unit, University of Manchester, UK

James W. Strickland MD
Clinical Professor, Department of Orthopedics, Indiana University School of Medicine; Chief, Hand Surgery Section, St Vincent Hospital, Indianapolis, USA

William F. Wagner MD
Department of Orthopedic Surgery, Indiana University Medical Center, Indianapolis, USA

Contents

1. Epidemiology in orthopaedics in the 1990s 1
A. J. Silman

2. Epidemiology of accidents in the 1990s 15
J. P. Bull

3. External skeletal fixation – which frame and why? 27
J. Kenwright, J. L. Cunningham

4. Recent advances in imaging in orthopaedics 41
I. W. McCall

5. Advances in diagnosis and treatment in closed traction lesion of the supraclavicular brachial plexus 65
R. Birch

6. Recent advances in flexor tendon surgery 77
J. W. Strickland, W. F. Wagner

7. Assessment of adolescent acetabular dysplasia 103
A. Catterall

8. Changes in the management of the child with Duchenne muscular dystrophy 119
G. A. Evans

9. The management of major disasters 133
J. M. Rowles, G. Kirsh

10. Arthroscopy and the management of shoulder problems 145
S. A. Copeland

11. The impact of prosthetic design on revision hip replacement 157
W. F. G. Muirhead-Allwood

Index 173

1

Epidemiology in orthopaedics in the 1990s

A. J. Silman

DEFINITION OF EPIDEMIOLOGY

Epidemiology can be usefully defined as the study of the distribution of diseases and their risk factors in human populations. Broadly speaking, therefore the heading 'epidemiology' in relation to the description of a disease or group of related disorders covers both its occurrence and its possible cause or causes. The former is based on *descriptive* epidemiology which describes the occurrence by age, sex, geography (both between and within countries) and by time. The latter requires *analytical* techniques such as the case control and the prospective study, where putative risk factors, suggested either by clinical observation or from descriptive studies, are formally tested for their association with the disease, normally in relation to a comparison group.

METHODS OF EPIDEMIOLOGICAL STUDY IN ORTHOPAEDICS

The occurrence of diseases can either be gleaned from routinely available and published statistics or requires special population surveys. There are numerous sources of data available and some of these are discussed below. Unlike the situation in other specialties most orthopaedic conditions have a low and variable case fatality rate and thus routine mortality data are of little value.

Cancer registration

Data on bone cancers by site are readily available from published cancer registration data (Office of Population and Census Studies a, annually) and give the number of new registrations (incidence) by age, sex and area of residence. Data by histological type are available on request. As an example, recent trends in all primary bone cancers are shown in Table 1.1. The overall population incidence was 0.9/100 000 in women and 1.1/100 000 in men from 1975 to 1984. Table 1.1 seems to suggest a small recent decline in incidence against a background of considerable variation. As it is possible in England and Wales to link cancer registration data with death notification, survival data by cancer site are available nationally and indeed by region. The completeness of cancer registration varies depending on the enthusiasm locally but it is likely to be high for relatively rare cancers such as osteogenic sarcoma in young people.

Hospital discharge statistics

Up to the last 5 years in England and Wales the

Table 1.1 Age-adjusted trends in incidence rates of primary bone cancers in England and Wales 1975–1984 for all ages to 75 years

	Standardized rate (1979 = 100*)	
Year	Males	Females
1975	93	105
1976	84	100
1977	97	86
1978	94	96
1979	100	100
1980	92	94
1981	115	119
1982	77	84
1983	85	82
1984	86	90

*All rates are relative to the 1979 rate after allowing for changes in the age distribution between individual years.

diagnosis at discharge on a one-in-ten sample of all admissions to acute hospitals was published under the Hospital In-Patient Enquiry (Office of Population and Census Studies b, annually). This system has now been superseded by the Körner system which essentially should provide the same data. The usefulness of these data for epidemiological purposes depends on the accuracy of the diagnostic coding at discharge and the likelihood that an individual with a specific diagnosis will be admitted as an inpatient. The accuracy is suspect, for example a recent report compared hip arthroplasty rates using such data (the system also records surgical procedures) with the results from operating theatre records from a few selected hospitals (Rajaratman et al 1990). The results showed that using routine data there was a considerable overestimate of arthroplasties performed, probably based on the inclusion of acute open reductions of fractured femurs.

The system is also more appropriate for some diagnoses than others. Thus it is likely that fractured femoral neck will result in admission and thus be recorded whereas only a minority of those with a prolapsed intervertebral disc will be admitted. It can be argued that if admission policy does not change over time, or between areas, then comparison of admission rates can provide a useful estimate of underlying trends in disease incidence.

Morbidity in primary care

Data are available on episodes of disease based on attendance at general practice. There have been four 12-month national morbidity surveys: in 1956, 1970–1972 (two consecutive studies; Royal College of General Practitioners 1979) and 1981–1982 (Royal College of General Practitioners 1986), with a further one planned for 1991–1992. In these surveys approximately 40–60 general practices, for the whole of a study, keep a record of the diagnosis made at every consultation and whether it represents a new episode. There is no attempt at diagnostic standardization and as a consequence incidence rates of the common disease vary considerably between practices. As a guide to morbidity rates of common diseases in the general population, however, these data are unique. Figures 1.1–1.4 show incidence rates for some common orthopaedic problems derived from this data source (Silman 1988). Figure 1.1 shows the incidence of new episodes of back pain without sciatica and demonstrates the relatively small effect of age and sex on these rates. By comparison (Fig. 1.2) the incidence of prolapsed intervertebral disc is lower, by a factor of 10, has a pronounced age peak in early and middle adult life, and is 50% higher in males. The data for all shoulder syndromes (Fig. 1.3) and

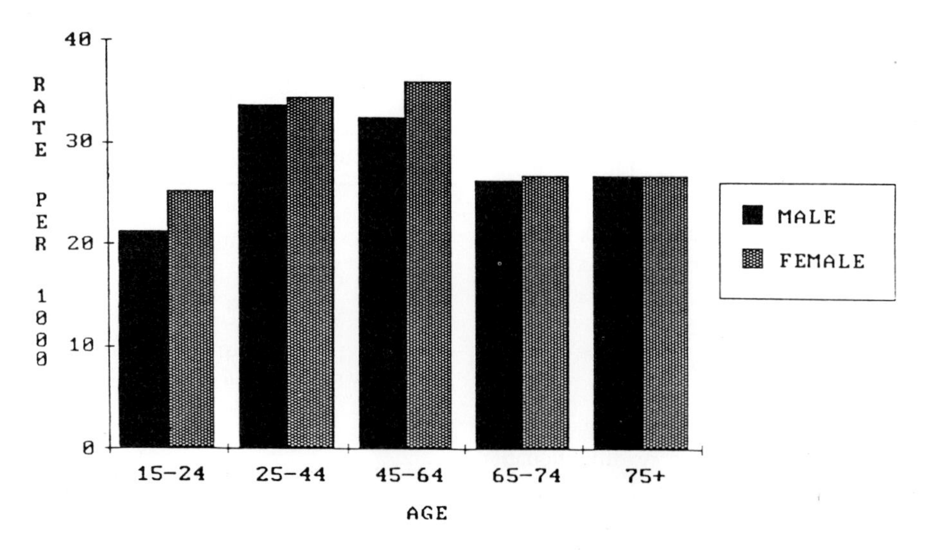

Fig. 1.1 Incidence of back pain per 1000 population according to age (no sciatica). (Reproduced with permission from Silman 1988.)

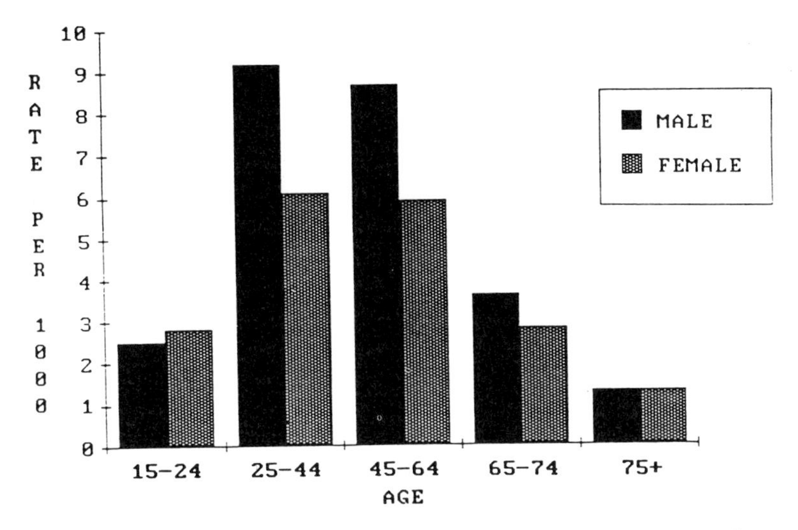

Fig. 1.2 Incidence of prolapsed intervertebral disc per 1000 population according to age. (Reproduced with permission from Silman 1988.)

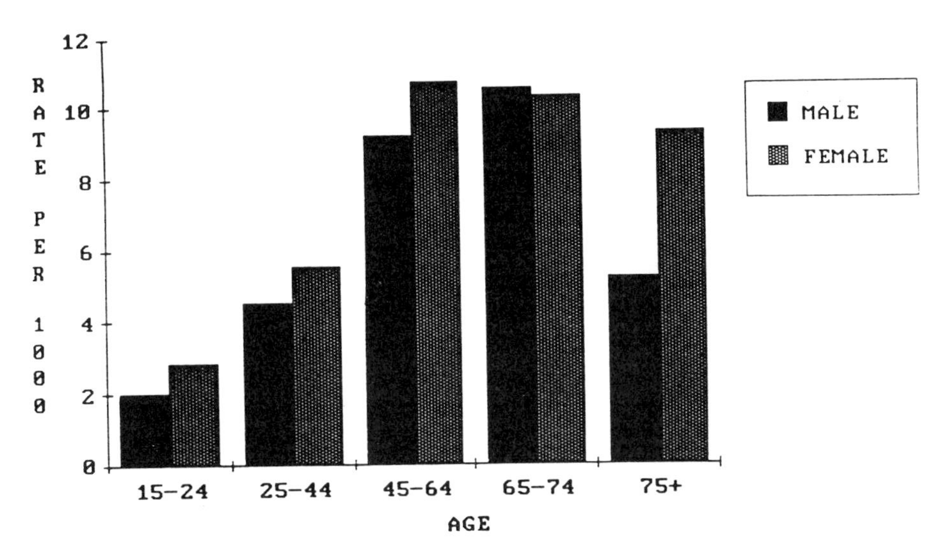

Fig. 1.3 Incidence of all shoulder syndromes per 1000 population according to age. (Reproduced with permission from Silman 1988.)

frozen shoulder (Fig. 1.4) are similar in their age and sex distribution.

Despite the diagnostic errors these are the only incidence data available in relation to shoulder problems in the UK. The major advantage of using primary care as a base for epidemiological study is the availability of a fixed denominator population of known age and sex distribution that relatively easily allows the calculation of such morbidity rates.

RECENT ADVANCES

The remainder of this review will concentrate on four disease areas where there have been recent changes in our understanding of their epidemiol-

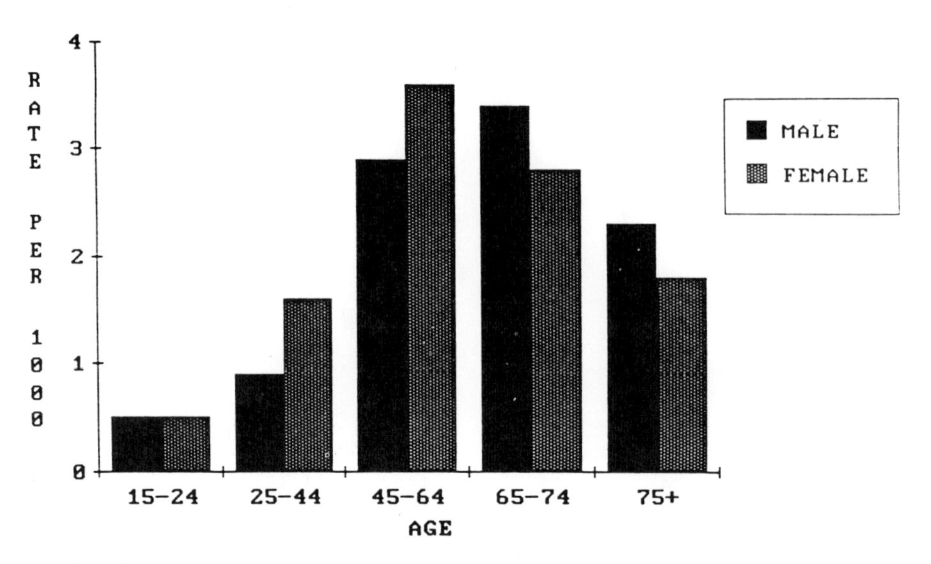

Fig. 1.4 Incidence of frozen shoulder per 1000 population according to age. (Reproduced with permission from Silman 1988.)

ogy. These are fibromyalgia, osteoporosis, osteoarthritis and rheumatoid arthritis.

FIBROMYALGIA

The term 'fibrositis', first coined at the beginning of this century, has been a convenient label for the large number of patients with ill defined musculoskeletal pain for whom a specific pathology could not be demonstrated. The past decade has witnessed a reviving interest in this syndrome with a view to better understanding its nature, aetiology and therapy. The term 'fibromyalgia' was introduced in 1976 and criteria for its diagnosis were published in 1990 (Wolfe et al 1990; Table 1.2). The hallmark clinically of the diagnosis is the presence of tender points, which are simply defined as a site in muscle, at a bony prominence or at a muscle–bone interface, that are tender to palpation (Wolfe 1990). The pathophysiological derivation of these tender areas is unclear and there remains considerable scepticism about this phenomenon. Clinically they are reproducible between observers and their co-occurrence with the chronic pain that underscores this syndrome have been taken as evidence to support them as a clinicopathological entity. It is in fact of interest that the area distal to the lateral epicondyle of the elbow is a tender point whereas the equivalent area on the medial aspect is non-tender.

Epidemiology

Despite the frequency with which patients with chronic pain are encountered there is no good descriptive epidemiology available on this disorder. Much of the data are derived from clinic populations and the frequency of any disorder is dependent on the selection and referral process that leads to such attendance. Some of the pertinent data are shown in Table 1.3. The largest series of clinic patients to be examined (Wolfe & Cathey 1983) found that only 3.7% of 1473 new attenders qualified for that diagnosis. Interestingly such a prevalence rate is not that dissimilar from that found in either general practice attenders (Hartz & Kirchdoerfer 1987) or a general medical clinic (Campbell et al 1983). It is relevant to add that the features of fibromyalgia occur in the presence of other generalized musculoskeletal disorders such as rheumatoid arthritis or osteoarthritis and it is not always possible to separate out the co-occurrence of two unrelated disorders from the isolated presence of fibromyalgia.

Table 1.2 Classification criteria for fibromyalgia (Reproduced with permission from Wolfe et al 1990)

1. History of widespread pain
Definition: Pain is considered widespread when all of the following are present: pain in the left side of the body, pain in the right side of the body, pain above the waist, and pain below the waist. In addition, axial skeletal pain (cervical spine or anterior chest or thoracic spine or low back) must be present. In this definition, shoulder and buttock pain is considered as pain for each involved side. Low back pain is considered lower segment pain

2. Pain in 11 of 18 tender point sites on digital palpation
Definition: Pain, on digital palpation, must be present in at least 11 of the following 18 tender point sites:

Occiput: bilateral, at the suboccipital muscle insertions
Low cervical: bilateral, at the anterior aspects of the intertransverse spaces at C5–C7
Trapezius: bilateral, at the midpoint of the upper border
Supraspinatus: bilateral, at origins, above the scapula spine near the medial border
Second rib: bilateral, at the second costochondral junctions, just lateral to the junctions on upper surfaces
Lateral epicondyle: bilateral 2 cm distal to the epicondyles
Gluteal: bilateral, in upper outer quadrants of buttocks in anterior fold of muscle
Greater trochanter: bilateral, posterior to the trochanteric prominence
Knee: bilateral, at the medial fat pad proximal to the joint line

Digital palpation should be performed with an approximate force of 4 kg. For a tender point to be considered positive the subject must state that the palpation was painful. Tender is not to be considered painful.

For classification purposes, patients will be said to have fibromyalgia if both criteria are satisfied. Widespread pain must have been present for at least 3 months. The presence of a second clinical disorder does not exclude the diagnosis of fibromyalgia.

Risk factors

Again there are no sound data on the age distribution of this syndrome in the population and the reported age spectrum from clinical series is subject to the same referral biases mentioned above. The syndrome has been defined at all ages with perhaps up to 25% starting in childhood. What is of interest is the approximately 7:1 female excess seen in all studies (Wolfe 1990). Whether this reflects differences in pain perception between the sexes is unclear. Some data exist to suggest that fibromyalgia patients are more likely to be from a higher socioeconomic group and be better educated than the background population rates (Cathey et al 1986). Most reports suggest that fibromyalgia patients have a range of premorbid psychological problems but in one well conducted study no such differences emerged (Clark et al 1985). A true summary of the state of the art in this field is that it is possible to recognize a subgroup, mainly female, within the population who complain of chronic pain and whose muscles at specific sites are tender to palpation. As a diagnostic label it remains convenient and the recent development of relatively tight criteria may aid understanding of response to management. It seems unlikely that any unifying pathology underlying this disorder will be identified.

Table 1.3 Prevalence of fibromyalgia syndrome in different populations

Reference	Setting	Prevalence (%) Male	Prevalence (%) Female
Campbell et al (1983)	General medical clinic	5.7	73
Wolfe & Cathey (1983)	Rheumatology clinic	2.7	75
Muller (1987)	Hospital	7.5	85
Hartz & Kirchdoerfer (1987)	General practice	2.1	88

OSTEOPOROSIS

There has been an explosion of interest in the epidemiology of osteoporosis worldwide in the past decade. In part this is related to the economic and social costs of treating the most important consequence of this disorder, fracture of the femoral neck, and in part it is related to the development of new technologies for the measurement of bone mineral content with a view to identifying those at risk of subsequent fracture and hence who need to receive prophylaxis. This review will consider the current epidemiology of osteoporosis in three parts—femoral neck fracture, vertebral crush fracture and risk factors generally for osteoporosis.

Femoral neck fracture

Femoral neck fracture is probably the most important orthopaedic disorder affecting the elderly population. The age- and sex-specific incidence rates are shown in Table 1.4 (Royal College of Physicians 1989) and demonstrate the exponential rise in incidence with increasing age, the two- to threefold

Table 1.4 Hospital discharge rates for hip fracture by age and sex in the UK in 1985

	Discharge rate (per 10 000)	
Age (years)	Males	Females
0–4	0.5	0.6
5–14	0.7	0.6
15–44	1.0	0.4
45–64	2.7	4.3
67–74	10.4	23.0
75–84	34.1	90.1
85 +	136.2	252.5

female excess and the rarity of this disorder under the age of 65. An approximate rate of 1% per annum of those over 75 is a reasonable summary measure.

The interesting question is whether there has been an increase in incidence rates in recent years. Data from the Oxford region suggest a two- to threefold increase in age- and sex-specific rates in the last three decades (Boyce & Vessey 1985; Table 1.5). Such an increase has also been observed in Sweden (Obrant et al 1989). A more recent analysis from the whole of England and Wales (Spector et al 1991) suggested that indeed there has been an increase since 1968 but that this increase began to level off around 1978–1979 and the rates have remained flat subsequently. It has been predicted that if current trends in incidence continue, given the increasing survival of the elderly, the absolute numbers of fractures will double between 1985 and 2016 (Royal College of Physicians 1989).

The data used to derive these trends are based on recorded diagnosis at discharge from hospital, collated for national statistics, which, as stated above, are known to be subject to error. It is perhaps unlikely that there has been a selective change in the error rate over the past three decades sufficient to explain the trends observed. The reasons for these trends are entirely speculative and relate to the known risk factors for osteoporosis and in addition, particularly in relation to this site of fracture, the risks of falls.

Table 1.5 Trends in incidence (per 10 000) in hip fracture in Oxford in 1954 to 1958 and 1983

	1954–1958		1983	
Age (years)	Male	Female	Male	Female
35–54	1.1	1.1	2.1	1.9
55–64	6.5	4.0	6.3	9.3
65–74	6.7	15.3	11.6	21.6
75–84	21.8	52.6	53.1	111.8
85 +	48.8	140.5	131.6	322.3

Vertebral crush fracture

The other major site of osteoporotic fracture is the dorsal and lumbar spine. Radiological interpretation is more hazardous at this site specifically as many fractures are painless and detected only on radiological screening. Further there is no clear-cut definition of what constitutes a fracture. Definitions are normally based on morphometric analyses of vertebral shape, for example the loss of anterior height relative to posterior height. In population studies these vertebral dimensions do not show a bimodal distribution and it is thus necessary to have a cut-off point between normal and fracture. The exact cut-off points to be used in epidemiological surveys are the subject of a current National Institutes of Health-sponsored international working party which should report towards the end of 1991.

Prevalence

The best data on the prevalence of vertebral crush fracture come from a radiological survey of 200 women aged over 50 (Melton et al 1989). The results are summarized in Table 1.6 and show such events to be very common in women, reaching a rate of 40% in those aged over 80. The definition used in that study was based on standard parameters of vertebral height adjusted for the dimensions seen in normal women. Other studies have been

Table 1.6 Prevalence of vertebral fractures in women aged 50 and over in Rochester, USA (Reproduced with permission from Melton et al 1989).

Age (years)	Prevalence (%)
55–59	8.3
60–64	11.7
65–69	16.2
70–74	21.9
75–79	29.0
80–84	37.4
85 +	46.5

restricted to a narrower age range: such a study of women aged 70 and over from Denmark yielded results very similar to those derived above (Jensen et al 1982). The relationship of fracture risk to bone mineral density (BMD) as measured, for example, by dual photon or dual energy absorptiometry, is not, however, clear. Again there is no sharp cutoff point in BMD below which fractures occur. Further there is no obvious linear relationship, although in general there appears to be a trend (Melton et al 1989). Interestingly, the strong effect of age is not explained by the decline in bone density with age and thus there appears to be an independent effect of age on fracture at this site.

Risk factors for osteoporosis

A number of risk factors have been proposed which are thought to increase the risk of osteoporosis. These are cigarette smoking, alcohol consumption, lack of dietary calcium, low body weight, lack of exercise and some drugs, notably corticosteroids, thiazide diuretics and thyroid hormones. In addition there is the well described female hormonal factor of ovarian failure related to early or premature menopause—perhaps the single most important factor.

Such a conclusion is strongly supported by the age and sex distribution of osteoporotic fractures and studies of bone density in pre- and post-menopausal women. The European Foundation for Osteoporosis at a recent consensus conference (Conference Report 1987) suggested that oestrogen replacement was the only established prophylaxis against fracture. The problems of compliance and the desire by women not to suffer cyclical blood loss, the risks of unopposed oestrogen on the endometrium and the possible risk of breast cancer may all mitigate against its widespread introduction.

Lifestyle

The possible role of fluoride deficiency has been ruled out recently. A trial of fluoride supplementation did not prevent fracture (Riggs et al 1990). Further the descriptive epidemiology does not support a geographical relationship between fluoride level in drinking water and risk of fracture (Cooper et al 1990).

Alcohol consumption is clearly related to osteoporosis risk (Feitelberg et al 1987) and has been shown to be inversely related to bone density as measured by dual photon absorptiometry (Stevenson et al 1989). This latter study estimated that the consumption of 5–8 units of alcohol a day (1 unit = $\frac{1}{2}$ pint of beer, 1 measure of spirit or 1 glass of wine) would take the BMD of a 50-year-old woman below the fracture threshold.

The calcium story is more controversial with an inconsistency in those studies suggesting a beneficial effect of calcium supplementation. Descriptive epidemiological studies found no relation between calcium intake and bone loss (Riggs et al 1987) or between calcium intake and risk of hip fracture (Cooper et al 1988). There may however be differential effects on men and women and on the axial and appendicular skeletons (Kelly 1990). The difficulty in defining the role for calcium has not reduced the extensive push for a greater dietary increase in calcium in the elderly, up to 1500 mg day in oestrogen-depleted women. The argument that such an input is without harm and may be of benefit is persuasive in public health terms.

OSTEOARTHRITIS

Definition

Osteoarthritis is the most frequent of all the arthritic disorders, affecting nearly 100% of the population in at least one joint site by the eighth decade of life. The epidemiology of this disorder depends on the means of diagnosis which classically has been from radiological surveys of normal populations. Historically the Kellgren & Lawrence (1963) scheme has been used to categorize both the presence and the severity of osteoarthritis (Table 1.7) but this has been subject to recent criticism on three counts. First, the system overemphasizes the presence of osteophytes which may not reflect true osteoarthritis. Secondly, it is recognized that only a proportion of individuals with radiological change would have signs and symptoms of osteoarthritis and it is this latter group on which one would wish to concentrate. Indeed the American Rheumatism Association (now the American College of Rheumatology) has formulated criteria for osteoarthritis at specific joint sites that do not rely on X-rays. An

Table 1.7 Kellgren & Lawrence grading scheme for osteoarthritis

Grade	Criteria
0	Normal
1	Doubtful narrowing of joint space, possible osteophytes
2	Definite osteophytes, absent or questionable narrowing of joint space
3	Moderate osteophytes, definite narrowing, some sclerosis, possible deformity
4	Large osteophytes, marked narrowing, severe sclerosis, definite deformity

example of such criteria for the knee joint is shown in Table 1.8 (Altman et al 1986). Thirdly, and perhaps more intriguing, is the observation from the examination of post-mortem and other skeletal remains that significant degenerative joint damage can occur, including eburnation in the presence of a normal X-ray appearance (Rogers J 1990, personal communication). Thus, taking all these considerations, the utility of the X-ray as the gold standard in the diagnosis of osteoarthritis is likely to be increasingly questioned. Further the advent of magnetic resonance imaging has highlighted widespread joint damage in a far superior way to conventional X-ray but this tool is unlikely to be used for epidemiological purposes given its expense.

Occurrence

There are virtually no data on the *incidence* of osteoarthritis, that is the rate of new cases in the population; the available data relate only to prevalence, or the rate of existing cases. The reason for this is a function of the difficulty in dating disease onset when, as explained above, the principal means of diagnosis has been radiology. The lack of incidence data makes it virtually impossible to consider trends over time, though it would be of value to know whether the disease was increasing or decreasing in occurrence.

The most recent data on prevalence come from a large population-based study in Zoetemeer in the Netherlands where 3109 males and 3476 females all underwent X-ray examination of their principal joints (Van Saase et al 1989). The main results are shown in Table 1.9 by age and sex. Grade 2 osteoarthritis (osteophytes in the absence of joint space narrowing) was virtually universal by the eighth decade and thus the data presented are confined to grade 3 or worse. There are a number of points to be made from these data. First osteoarthritis is a rare disease in those under the age of 40. Second there is not an equal sex incidence: females have a higher rate of osteoarthritis and this excess increases with increasing age. Thirdly the age and sex patterns of joint involvement are not the same, in that generalized osteoarthritis is com-

Table 1.8 Classification criteria for osteoarthritis of the knee (Reproduced with permission from Altman et al 1986.)

Clinical and laboratory	Clinical and radiographic	Clinical
Knee pain plus at least 5 of these 9:	Knee pain + at least 1 of these 3:	Knee pain + at least 3 of these 6
1. Age >50 years 2. Stiffness <30 min	1. Age >50 years 2. Stiffness <30 min	1. Age >50 years 2. Stiffness <30 min
3. Crepitus 4. Bony tenderness 5. Bony enlargement 6. No palpable warmth	3. Crepitus + osteophytes	3. Crepitus 4. Bony tenderness 5. Bony enlargement 6. No palpable warmth
7. ESR < 40 mm/h 8. RF <1:40 9. SF OA		

ESR = Erythrocyte sedimentation rate (Westergren); RF = rheumatoid factor; SF OA = synovial fluid signs of osteoarthritis (clear, viscous, or white blood cell count <2000/mm^3). An alternative for the clinical category would be 4 of 6, which is 84% sensitive and 89% specific.

Table 1.9 Prevalence (per centage) of radiographic osteoarthritis* by selected 5-year age groups and sex by selected joint site

	Males			Females		
Joint site	50–54 years	60–64 years	70–74 years	50–54 years	60–64 years	70–74 years
Right knee	2.2	5.6	7.1	2.7	4.8	16.4
Right hip	0	1.7	2.4	0	1.6	4.9
Distal interphalangeal	3.5	10.7	9.4	4.7	15.1	26.3
Cervical spine	29.1	39.0	64.6	21.7	40.7	42.0

*Grade 3 or 4 on Kellgren & Lawrence scheme.

moner in females whereas, for example, hip involvement is commoner in males. The almost universal involvement of at least one joint side is underlined by these data.

Symptomatic disease

Given the universal nature of this disorder in an ageing population it is questionable whether such radiological surveys are of value at least in defining the public health problem from osteoarthritis. One alternative approach is to consider the relation between radiographic change with symptoms (Croft 1990). The results are of interest. Thus in the knee, approximately half of those with severe radiographic change have pain compared to only around 10% of those with minimal change. By contrast 40% of those with completely normal X-rays also reported chronic knee pain, underlying the relative lack of specificity of this symptom. The results from the hip are of more encouragement. Hip pain is much more specific for osteoarthritis but nevertheless there is still a sizeable proportion of individuals with severe radiological involvement who do not report pain. It is possible that a proportion of these might have referred pain that would not be correctly identified in a survey restricted to symptoms only.

Trends in osteoarthritis

As mentioned above there is a lack of data on incidence but some information can be gathered from general practice statistics based on patient attenders (Royal College of General Practitioners 1979, 1986). Such data are not based on standardized diagnosis and are thus subject to error but the broad trends are relevant. The rate of patient attenders has increased between such general practice surveys. It is obviously difficult to argue whether this reflects a lower threshold for patient self-referral or a true change in the incidence of symptomatic osteoarthritis.

Aetiology

Osteoarthritis is a heterogeneous disorder both clinically and aetiologically and thus there are many different causal pathways. Classically, primary (i.e. cause unknown) has been distinguished from secondary (cause known) disease. This in a sense only reflects patterns of knowledge for a given patient, for example the presence of previous injury or joint disease certainly predisposes to osteoarthritis at that site. The comments in this section will concentrate solely on those cases without such an obvious precondition.

Genetics

The concept that there is a single disease entity of generalized osteoarthritis is widely accepted. It is commoner in females than in males, has a peak age of onset around the fifth and sixth decades, it is frequently associated with Heberden's nodes and has a strong genetic predisposition with an autosomal dominant pattern of inheritance (Lawrence 1977). This latter observation has not been translated into identifying the gene or genes responsible. Some preliminary data suggested an association between generalized osteoarthritis and the human leukocyte antigen (HLA) haplotype A1 B8 DR3 (Doherty et al 1990) but this seems intuitively unlikely given the functional role of the HLA region in the immune response, hardly a feature of osteoarthritis. Perhaps more promising is the investigation by the newer molecular biological techniques of mutations in the genes responsible for collagen synthesis. Recent work on two multi-case families suggested a mutation in the type II collagen gene on chromosome 12, though these families were more in keeping with an osteodysplastic syndrome than true osteoarthritis (Palotie et al 1989). This is an area of current increased interest and it is likely that other positive associations will become apparent in the next 2–3 years.

Obesity

The most studied aetiological factor has been that of obesity. There is a consistent positive association between obesity and osteoarthritis of the knee in a number of studies (Anderson & Felson 1988, Davis et al 1988). Although one explanation from cross-sectional observations that osteoarthritis can lead to obesity by reducing exercise was not borne out by a prospective study showing that obesity at a mean age of 37 years predicted the development of osteoarthritis at a mean age of 73 (Felson et al 1988), there is the more intriguing observation that obesity is also associated with osteoarthritis of the hands (Engel 1968) but not consistently with the hip (Felson 1990). Thus one explanation is that the link between obesity and osteoarthritis is not related to mechanical factors but that the obesity has a metabolic or hormonal influence. This latter is perhaps supported by the increased effect of obesity in women. Studies of possible confounders between obesity and osteoarthritis have ruled out serum cholesterol, diabetes, body fat distribution or blood pressure as explaining the influence of obesity.

RHEUMATOID ARTHRITIS

Rheumatoid arthritis (RA) is not numerically the most frequent cause of polyarthritis in the population. In terms of the burden to both the patient in terms of morbidity and disability and to health services, and in terms of cost, RA is the most important of the polyarthritic disorders.

Definition

There has been considerable discussion over the years on the diagnosis of this disorder and, in particular, its classification for study purposes. Existing criteria were thought to be too non specific and in 1987 the American Rheumatism Association published revised criteria which improved the specificity of the existing sets and provided more detailed information on the individual features (Arnett et al 1988). These are summarized in Table 1.10. Such criteria have the benefit of allowing a certain consistency in the standardization of reports but are too restrictive and possibly too inaccurate for clinical use. Their main drawback is that the criteria were derived from long-standing patients with RA attending specialist centres within the USA and their clinical appearance may not represent the experience of RA patients generally. None the less, it is probably reasonable to assume that future publications of studies of patients with rheumatoid arthritis will need to use these criteria.

Trends

One of the more intriguing suggestions recently from the study of RA has been the suggestion that it is declining both in incidence and in severity. This would be an interesting possibility both to those considering the causes of the disease and those planning health services.

The data are fairly limited on the subject but there is a remarkable consistency in the information. Data from the Mayo Clinic from the population of Olmsted County in Minnesota—that facility provides the only source of medical care for that population—would suggest that since 1960 there has been a marked decline in incidence in females, but not in males (Linos et al 1980). Data from the UK have been mainly gleaned from general practice (Silman 1989a). In two separate studies the results have been similar. First in a study continuously recording all episodes of morbidity in general practice over the 13-year period 1976–1988 there has been a decline in RA episode incidence of approximately 7.5 per 100 000 cases per year. Similarly, in the interval between two year-long studies of patient attenders at general practice between 1970–1972 and 1981–1982, there was a

Table 1.10 American Rheumatism Association 1987 revised criteria for the classification of rheumatoid arthritis

Criterion	Definition
1. Morning stiffness	Morning stiffness in and around the joints, lasting at least 1 h before maximal improvement
2. Arthritis of 3 joints or more	At least 3 joint areas simultaneously have had soft-tissue swelling or fluid (not bony overgrowth alone) observed by a physician. The 14 possible areas are right or left PIP, MCP, wrist, elbow, knee, ankle, and MTP joints
3. Arthritis of hand joints	At least 1 area swollen (as defined above) in a wrist MCP or PIP joint
4. Symmetrical arthritis	Simultaneous involvement of the same joint areas (as defined in 2 above) on both sides of the body (bilateral involvement of PIPs, MCPs, or MTPs is acceptable without absolute symmetry)
5. Rheumatoid nodules	Subcutaneous nodules, over bony prominences, or extensor surfaces, or in juxta-articular regions observed by a physician
6. Serum rheumatoid factor	Demonstration of abnormal amounts of serum rheumatoid factor by any method for which the result has been positive in <5% of normal control subjects
7. Radiographic changes	Radiographic changes typical of rheumatoid arthritis on posteroanterior hand and wrist radiographs, which must include erosions or unequivocal bony decalcification localized in or most marked adjacent to the involved joints (osteoarthritis changes alone do not qualify)

For classification purposes a patient has rheumatoid arthritis if he or she satisfies either any 4 of the above or criteria (2) and either (6) or (7). There are other possible combinations allowed but these apply to very few patients (see Arnett et al 1988).
PIP = Proximal interphalangeal; MCP = metacarpophalangeal; MTP = Metatarsophalangeal

decline in RA incidence of 20% in females but little difference in males (Hochberg 1990).

Trends in severity

Mortality rates can be used as a measure for the joint effects of both incidence and case survival and hence any trend of a decline in overall population mortality for RA would be consistent either with a fall in incidence or a reduction in severity of diagnosed cases or both. One long-term population study of trends in mortality comes from Australia and covered the period 1950–1981 (Wicks et al 1988). It is not clearly stated in that report whether it covered all mentions of RA on death certificates or only those in which RA was included as underlying cause of death. In brief, there was no significant trend apparent overall in age-adjusted death rates during this period although there was evidence of a recent decline in mortality rate in women, particularly those in the older age group. What was interesting from that data set was the observation that there was no improvement in survival of men with RA as judged by age at death, particularly against a background of falling mortality generally in the population. The inherent problem is the frequent failure to mention RA on death certificates (the source of population mortality rates) and there are a number of studies confirming the high rate of under-recording of this disease as a contributor to death.

There is a commonly accepted view among rheumatologists that RA is declining in severity and indeed a recent survey of the opinion of Australian rheumatologists confirmed this view in a large group of observers (Laurent et al 1989). Such a conclusion may, however, result from changes in the referral practice in terms of patients seen in a centre and thus may not reflect the true status of RA in the community. Changing patterns of disease severity were analysed using three indicators of disease severity: ever seropositive, ever erosive and ever having subcutaneous nodules. In that analysis the trends in severity were judged by the effect on the year of birth by comparing severity in RA patients born in different periods (birth cohorts). If there was no birth cohort effect on severity then the proportion of those with disease onset at for example, age 35–44, who were ever seropositive should be the same for all periods of birth. This was not the situation and the results from all three indicators were similar (Silman et al 1983). The data figures showed that successively more recent generations were less likely to be positive for any of the above features. Further examination showed that the trends were not linear and that there was a severity peak in patients presenting in around 1960 with the majority of the birth cohorts displaying their maximum severity around that year.

There are also data from Finland to suggest that RA is becoming less severe. At a population level there has been a marked decline in the number receiving disability pensions due to RA and further the proportion of those registered disabled with musculoskeletal conditions having RA has also fallen (Isomaki 1989).

There have obviously been a number of prospective studies of patients with RA to assess outcome but few have been repeated with more recently diagnosed cohorts from the same population to examine trends in prognosis. In one such paired survey—a 9-year follow-up study of seropositive RA in 1958—observed that 38% progressed to severe handicap (Aho et al 1989) compared to less than 3% for a similarly derived cohort follwed for 8 years up to 1982 (Aho et al 1989).

Possible explanations

A reasonable summary from the data on both incidence and severity is that there is a marked consistency with both a reduction in incidence and severity of RA in the past 20 years or so, although conclusive proof is not available. Further, if there is a pointer to a possible cause it is that these observations are more marked in females than in males. One possible explanation for this sex difference is the possible protective role of increasing use of the oral contraceptive pill (OCP). This hypothesis is based on an earlier prospective study suggesting that such use was associated with a reduction in RA risk (Wingrave 1978). There have been a large number of subsequent studies testing this hypothesis, including the same Mayo Clinic population in whom the sex difference in trend was first noted. Interestingly, in that latter population there was no evidence that OCP use could explain the trends (Linos et al 1983, Del Junco et al 1985), but other studies have suggested that the opposite is the case with most reports now finding a protective effect of OCP use. A recent consensus conference attempted to resolve the conflicting results and concluded that OCP use was likely both to postpone the development and reduce the severity of RA rather than affect the incidence per se (Silman & Vandenbroucke 1989). Such a conclusion is consistent with the epidemiological data on trends summarized above.

Data concerning other possible explanations for the decline is speculative given the lack of aetiological clues concerning the onset of RA. Whether the trends in RA reflect changing patterns of viral or other infection, as postulated by Buchanan & Murdoch (1979), remains unclear but the problems associated with this were recently summarized (Silman 1989b). Similarly the possibility that changes in therapy have influenced severity remains untested in a population setting although the evidence from clinical trials of the effectiveness of specific agents would argue against this being a major part of the story.

REFERENCES

Aho K, Tuomi T, Palosuo T, Kaarela K, Essen R Von, Isomaki H 1989 Is seropositive rheumatoid arthritis becoming less severe? Chin Exp Rheumatol 7:287–290

Altman R, Asch E, Bloch D et al 1986 Development of criteria for the classification and reporting of osteoarthritis. Arthritis Rheum 29:1039–1049

Anderson JJ, Felson DT 1988 Factors associated with osteoarthritis of the knee in the first National Health and Nutrition Examination Survey (Hanes 1). Am J Epidemiol 128:179–189

Arnett FC, Edworthy SM, Block DDA et al 1988 The American Rheumatism Association 1987 revised criteria for the classification of rheumatoid arthritis. Arthritis Rheum 31:315–323

Boyce WJ, Vessey MP 1985 Rising incidence of fracture of the proximal femur. Lancet *i*:150–151

Buchanan WW, Murdoch RM 1979 Hypothesis: that rheumatoid arthritis will disappear. J Rheumatol 6:324–329

Campbell SM, Forehand ME, Bennett RM et al 1983 Clinical characteristics of fibrositis, I. A blinded controlled study of symptoms and tender points. Arthritis Rheum 26:817–824

Cathey MA, Wolfe F, Kleinheksel SM, Hawley DJ 1986 Socioeconomic impact of fibrositis. A study of 81 patients with primary fibrositis. Am J Med 81:78–84

Clark S, Campbell SM, Forehand ME et al 1985 Clinical characteristics of fibrositis. II. A 'blinded', controlled study using standard psychological tests. Arthritis Rheum 28:132–137

Conference report 1987 Consensus development conference: prophylaxis and treatment of osteoporosis. Br Med J 295:326–327

Cooper C, Barker JDP, Wickham C 1988 Physical activity, muscle strength, and calcium intake in fracture of the proximal femur. Br Med J 297:1443–1446

Cooper C, Wickham C, Lacey RF, Barker DJP 1990 Water fluoride concentration and fracture of the proximal femur. J Epidemiol Community Health 44:17–19

Croft PC 1990 Review of UK data: osteoarthritis. Br J Rheumatol 29:391–395

Davis MA, Ettinger WH, Newhaus JM 1988 The role of

metabolic factors and blood pressure in the association of obesity with osteoarthritis of the knee. Rheumatology 15:1827–1832
Davis MA, Ettinger WH, Newhaus JM, Hauck WW 1988 Sex differences in osteoarthritis of the knee. The role of obesity. Am J Epidemiol 127:1019–1030
Del Junco DJ, Annegers JF, Luthra RS et al 1985 Do oral contraceptives prevent rheumatoid arthritis? JAMA 254: 1938–1941
Doherty M, Pattrick M, Powell R 1990 Nodal generalised osteoarthritis in an autoimmune disease. Ann Rheum Dis 49:1017–1020
Engel A 1968 Osteoarthritis and body measurements. Series 11, no 29. National Center for Health Statistics, Rockville, MD
Feitelberg S, Epstein S, Ismad F, D'Amanda C 1987 Deranged bone mineral metabolism in chronic alcoholism. Metabolism 36:322–326
Felson TD 1990 The epidemiology of osteoarthritis. Clin Rheum Dis:499–512
Felson DT, Anderson JJ, Naimark A et al 1988 Obesity and knee osteoarthritis. Ann Intern Med 109:18–24
Hartz A, Kirchdoerfer E 1987 Undetected fibrositis in primary care practice. J Fam Pract 25:365–369
Hochberg M 1990 Changes in the incidence and prevalence of rheumatoid arthritis in England and Wales, 1970–1982. Seminars Arthritis Rheum 19:294–302
Isomaki HA 1989 Rheumatoid arthritis as seen from official data registers. Experience in Finland. Scand J Rheumatol 79:21–24
Jensen GF, Christiansen C, Boesen J et al 1982 Epidemiology of postmenopausal and long bone fractures. Clin Orthop 166:75–81
Kellgren JH, Lawrence JS 1963 Atlas of standard radiographs. The epidemiology of chronic rheumatism, vol 2. Oxford, Blackwell
Kelly PJ 1990 Dietary calcium, sex hormones, and bone mineral density in men. Br Med J 300:1361–1364
Laurent R, Robinson RG, Beller EM, Buchanan WW 1989 Incidence and severity of rheumatoid arthritis—the view from Australasia. Br J Rheumatol 28(4):360–361
Lawrence JS 1977 Rheumatism populations. Heinemann, London
Linos A, Worthington JA, O'Fallon M et al 1980 The epidemiology of rheumatoid arthritis in Rochester Minnesota: a study of incidence, prevalence and mortality. Am J Epidemiol 111:87–98
Linos A, O'Fallon WM, Worthington, JW, Kurland LT 1983 Case-control study of rheumatoid arthritis and prior use of oral contraceptives. Lancet *i*:1299–1300
Melton LJ, Kan SH, Frye MA et al 1989 Epidemiology of vertebral fractures in women. Am J Epidemiol 129:1000–1011
Muller W 1987 The fibrositis syndrome: diagnosis, differential diagnosis and pathogenesis. Scand J Rheumatol (Suppl) 65:40–53
Obrant KJ, Bengner U, Johnell O et al 1989 Increasing age-adjusted risk of fragility fractures: a sign of increasing osteoporosis risk in successive generations? Calcif Tissue Int 44:157–167
Office of Population and Census Studies a Cancer registrations: England and Wales. HMSO, London (annually)
Office of Population and Census Studies b Hospital In-Patient Enquiry: England and Wales, HMSO, London (annually)
Palotie A, Vaisanen P, Ott J et al 1989 Predisposition to familial osteoarthrosis linked to type II collagen gene. Lancet *i*:924–927
Rajaratman G, Black N, Dalziel M 1990 Total hip replacements in the NHS: is need being met? J Pub Health Med 12: 56–59
Riggs BL, Wahner HW, Melton LJ et al 1987 Dietary calcium intake and rate of bone loss in women. J Clin Invest 80:979–982
Riggs BL, Hodgson SF, O'Fallon WM et al 1990 Effect of fluoride treatment on the fracture rate in postmenopausal women with osteoporosis. N Engl J Med 322:802–809
Rogers J 1990 personal communication
Royal College of General Practitioners Office of Population Censuses and Surveys Department of Health and Social Security 1979 Morbidity statistics from general practice. Second national study 1971–1972. HMSO, London
Royal College of General Practitioners Office of Population Censuses and Surveys Department of Health and Social Security 1986 Morbidity statistics from general practice. Third national study 1981–1982. HMSO, London
Royal College of Physicians of London 1989 Fractured neck of femur: prevention and management. Royal College of Physicians, London
Silman AJ 1988 Epidemiological aspects of soft tissue rheumatism. In: Hazleman B, Silman A (eds). Soft tissue rheumatism. Arthritis and Rheumatism Council, London
Silman AJ 1989a Are there secular trends in the occurrence and severity of rheumatoid arthritis? Scand J Rheumatol 79:25–30
Silman A 1989b Rheumatoid arthritis and infection: a population approach. Ann Rheum Dis 48:707–710
Silman AJ, Vandenbroucke JP (eds) 1989 Female sex hormones and rheumatoid arthritis. Br J Rheumatol (suppl 1)
Silman AJ, Davies P, Currey HLF, Evans SJW 1983 Is rheumatoid arthritis becoming less severe? J Chron Dis 36:891–897
Spector TB, Cooper C, Fenton LA 1991 Recent secular changes in hip fracture in England and Wales 1968–85. Br Med J (In press)
Stevenson JC, Lees B, Davenport M et al 1989 Determinants of bone density in normal women. Risk factors for future osteoporosis. Br Med J 298:924–927
Van Saase JLCM, Van Romunde LKJ, Cats A et al 1989 Epidemiology of osteoarthritis: Zoetermeer survey. Comparison of radiological osteoarthritis in a Dutch population with that in 10 other populations. Ann Rheum Dis 48:271–280
Wicks IP, Moore J, Fleming A 1988 Australian mortality statistics for rheumatoid arthritis 1950–81: analysis of death certificate data. Ann Rheum Dis 47:563–569
Wingrave SJ 1978 Reduction in incidence of rheumatoid arthritis associated with oral contraceptives. Lancet *i*:569–571
Wolfe F 1990 The epidemiology of fibromyalgia. Rheum Dis Clin North Am 16:681–698
Wolfe F, Cathey MA 1983 Prevalence of primary and secondary fibrositis. J Rheumatol 10:965–968
Wolfe F, Smythe HA, Yunus MB 1990 The American College of Rheumatology 1990 criteria for the classification of fibromyalgia. Arthritis Rheum 33:160–172

2

Epidemiology of accidents in the 1990s

J. P. Bull

A feature of modern life is the common use of amounts of energy far in excess of the tolerance of the human body. When the energy is accidentally misplaced injuries occur. In earlier times gravity, fire, and human and animal power were the main sources of injury. Travel by wheeled vehicles added the possibility of injury by more massive moving objects. The harnessing of fossil and, more recently, nuclear fuels and the distribution of electric power have extended the hazards. Though the earlier types of accidents still occur the combination of wide exposure and the large amounts of individually controlled energy in road traffic are now the source of the most numerous severe accidents and injuries.

In parallel with this technological development of the use of energy has been the application of scientific research to the prevention and treatment of disease. The success in controlling infectious diseases has produced a major epidemiological revolution in the last few decades; in the UK in 1950 there were still 23 752 deaths from infectious diseases and 16 362 from accidents; by 1988 infectious diseases killed 2533 and accidents 13 308. In 1950 there were 6045 fatal domestic accidents; in 1988 there were 4838. In both years road deaths just exceeded 5000 (Fig. 2.1). Compared with the success with infections, the preventive medicine of injury has, in many cases, barely kept pace with the hazards (Gloag 1988). Accidents and violence are now a leading and increasing cause of loss of life in the 15–64 age group (Blane et al 1990).

Components in the trends will be discussed later but an important general factor in the fatal—as distinct from total—accident figures is the improved prognosis of serious injuries. This followed the application of wartime clinical lessons in the management of the severely injured, particularly by the recognition of the occurrence of blood loss and the value of its adequate replacement. Consistent with these changes in care the death rate for seriously injured road casualties which was 8% before the war had fallen to 6% in 1988.

THE AVAILABLE DATA

Statistical information is fullest and most reliable for fatal accidents. Whatever notification procedures there may be, the further interest of the police and coroners ensures that the data are cross-checked more thoroughly than for non-fatal cases. Though a severely disabled survivor may present a greater social and financial burden than a fatality, information on disablement is not routinely recorded. The next level of medical information is for cases admitted to hospital as inpatients. Unfortunately since the Hospital In-Patient Enquiry was cancelled in 1985 no replacement data have appeared. Inpatient cases include the bulk of those presenting surgical problems and many valuable studies of their causes and prevention have been made by clinicians at individual hospitals. The work of Cairns on motorcyclists' head injuries, of Colebrook on burns, and Gissane on road injuries was largely instrumental in the introduction of safety helmets, safer children's nightwear and car seatbelts respectively (Bull 1988). The recently instituted Major Trauma Outcome Study should also throw new light on the causes, mortality and disabilities of serious hospital cases.

Apart from the Registrar General's listing of fatalities (Office of Population and Census Studies 1990), there are separate official statistics for each of the main sources of accidents though they differ in

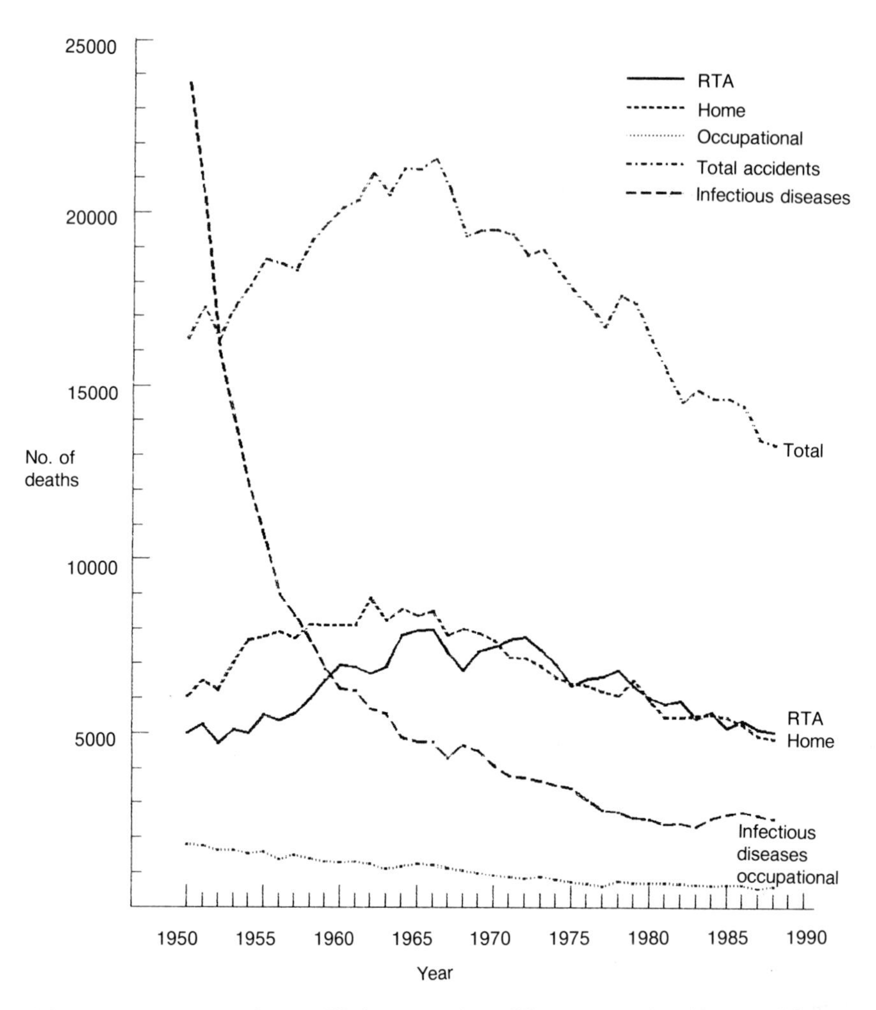

Fig. 2.1 Annual deaths in the UK since 1950 from different types of accidents and, for comparison, from infectious diseases. (Data from Annual Abstracts of Statistics, HMSO.)

definitions and scope. The most thorough data are for road traffic accidents. The information comes from standard reports from the police, who also check admission details of cases known to have gone to hospital. The casualty figures are published categorized as 'slight', 'serious' and 'fatal'. The 'fatal' are defined as those dying within 30 days of the accident. 'Serious' injuries include hospital inpatients and some outpatient fracture cases (Fig. 2.2). By definition, accidents and casualties not reported to the police are omitted, and there is serious under-reporting of several categories; for instance only about one-third of the non-fatal injuries of pedal cyclists and two-thirds of those of motorcyclists are reported (Bull & Roberts 1972). The official data are therefore deficient for these categories.

Since both the National Health Service and the Department of Transport require and go to some trouble to collect information on road traffic accidents and injuries it has long seemed desirable to be able to study the combined data. On the initiative of the Transport and Road Research Laboratory (TRRL) and the Department of Health for Scotland this has largely been achieved while still retaining the required anonymity of medical information. Further studies on the same lines are being tried in England.

Work accidents are the concern of the Health and Safety Commission (1989) who publish annual

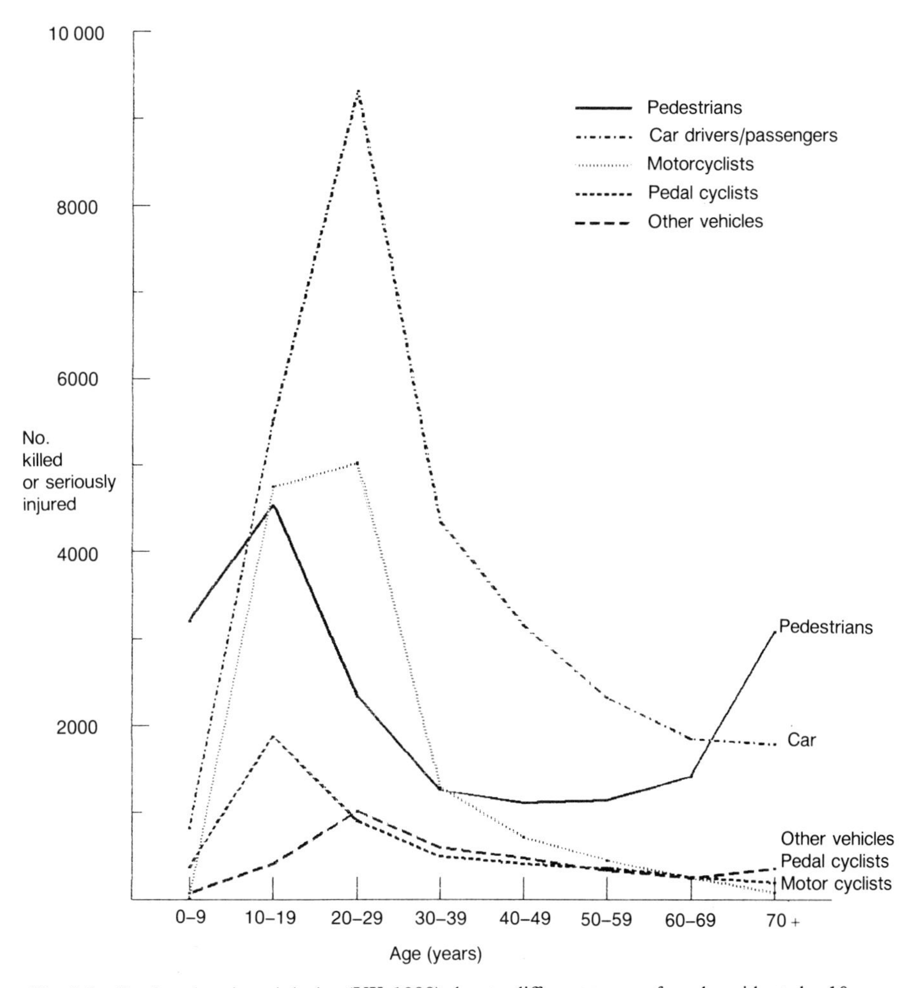

Fig. 2.2 Fatal and serious injuries (UK 1988) due to different types of road accidents by 10-year age groups. Data from Road Accidents Great Britain 1988, The Casualty Report (1989).

analyses based on statutory notification by employers. Regulations for notification of injuries changed in 1980 and again in 1985 so there is some difficulty in analysing trends.

Quite a different approach provides data on domestic accidents. The Home Accident and Safety Survey, organized by the Department of Trade and Industry, has since 1976 collected data on domestic accident cases at a moving sample of Accident & Emergency departments. The focus is on products involved in the injuries with a view to improving their safety by regulation. A parallel Leisure Accidents Safety Survey has recently been added, using the same methods (Consumer Safety Unit 1989).

TRANSPORT ACCIDENTS

As mentioned above, road traffic is now the main cause of accidental death. Of the 5052 such fatalities in the UK in 1988, 2378 (47%) were of vehicle occupants, 670 (13%) motorcyclists, 227 (4.5%) pedal cyclists and 1753 (37%) pedestrians. The corresponding 'serious injuries', approximately equivalent to hospital inpatient admissions, are reported as 68 543 but the exact numbers are uncertain because of incomplete notification.

The types of accident vary between urban and rural areas as three-quarters of pedestrian fatalities occur in built-up areas and, reflecting the higher speeds and numbers of miles driven, three-quarters of vehicle occupant fatalities are in rural areas. Motorcycle fatalities are about equally divided between built-up and non-built-up areas. There are peaks of road casualties in the morning and evening because of travel to and from work but a large number of serious injuries continue until past midnight. These include a high proportion of the alcohol-related cases.

Vehicle occupants

Much is now known about the biomechanics of injuries to vehicle occupants. When these studies first started in the late 1930s ejection from the vehicle was a common mechanism and the main value of the early lap-strap seatbelts was to prevent this. In a crash the occupant moves towards the point of impact and is injured by striking the interior of the vehicle which, itself, may be deformed and intrude inwards. A strong passenger compartment limits this deformation and controlled 'crushability' of the front of the vehicle reduces the effective velocity of the injuring contact. Seatbelts restrain forward movement and so minimize impact with the interior.

Improvements of vehicle control by steering and braking have helped in primary prevention of accidents as also have changes in road surfaces and layout (Grime 1987). On the other hand power and speed have tended to increase, offsetting some of the benefits for accident and injury prevention.

All the improvements in safety are readily defeated if the competence of the driver is impaired by alcohol. At the legal limit of blood alcohol of 80 mg% the accident risk is already about doubled. Useful reduction in accidents and injuries followed the breathalyser legislation, however more could be done; about one-quarter of fatally injured drivers (and motorcyclists) still have blood alcohol levels above the limit.

Pedestrians

In about three-quarters of pedestrian accidents the casualty is struck by a car; relatively few involve motorcycles, commercial vehicles or buses. Accidents to adults often occur in the central shopping streets of towns, while those to children are more common in residential areas. Severity of injury and mortality are related to the weight of the striking vehicle and the age of the casualty (Atkins et al 1988).

There are two peaks in the age distribution of these accidents (Fig. 2.2). The first is among children when they first start walking and using the road and, later, as they play outside and go to and from school. Such accidents are much commoner in boys than girls. The second peak is at the other extreme of life and here more casualties are female than male, corresponding to the higher proportion of elderly women. The childhood (0–14 year) peak accounts for more than a third of the seriously injured pedestrians; the peak in the elderly (70+ years) accounts for more than a third of the fatalities.

In contrast to its relatively favourable showing in other aspects of road accidents, for some years the UK has had one of the poorest records in Europe for child pedestrian accidents. Studies have been made to investigate their circumstances in order to try to devise remedies. Among preschool children three-fifths were injured while playing in the street within 100 m of home. One-third of the under-5s were on their own and another third were only accompanied by an older child. One-quarter of the school children were on their way to or from school and nearly half were on their own when injured. Prior to the accident four-fifths of the children had been running, many of them chasing each other or playing. Three-fifths did not stop at the kerb.

Elderly pedestrians often have diminished sensory and motor abilities. Sight, hearing, agility and balance may be impaired so that crossing the road becomes hazardous. Interview studies of casualties also reveal difficulties in judging the likely actions of drivers and confusion in knowing when it is safe to cross.

Alcohol is an important factor in pedestrian as in other types of accidents. Breathalyser measurements of casualties and non-accident controls suggest that at 80 mg% alcohol a pedestrian has about the same increased risk as a driver at 50 mg%. In 1988 34% of fatally injured pedestrians were found to exceed the 80 mg level and 25% had twice this level. Only rarely is excessive alcohol found in the drivers of the cars involved in these accidents.

Motorcyclists

Motorcycles offer high efficiency, high acceleration and speed and full exposure to the elements and, unfortunately, to impact with other vehicles or objects. It is therefore not surprising that they are the most dangerous vehicles on the road; their riders have some 24 times the risk of injury per mile as the driver of a car. There were 670 fatalities and at least 12 650 serious injuries in Great Britain in 1988 (Road Accidents Great Britain 1988). The riders are mostly in their teens or early 20s and they suffered characteristic leg fractures from side impacts and head and spinal injuries from being thrown forward off their machines. Injury to the brachial plexus often causes permanent paralysis. Many injuries are multiple and if not fatal carry a high possibility of later deformity or disability. Head injuries have been mitigated by helmets and some others can be prevented by heavy riding gear, but the high-impact velocities and direct exposure make further protection difficult.

Intrinsically safer designs providing retention on the machine and side-leg protectors have been produced as prototypes but have not yet found favour, either because of the weight penalty or their lack of attraction to a risk-seeking clientele.

Pedal cyclists

The age range for cycling is wide, from the preschool child to the elderly touring enthusiast. Injuries are most frequent between 5 and 25 years of age (Mills 1989). Riders share with the motorcyclist the direct exposure to the violence of impact but their own speed is usually less important than that of the striking vehicle—most often a car. Side impacts when either the car or the cycle is turning a corner are common and limb fractures are frequently the result. Since wearing of helmets has been compulsory for motorcyclists, in several series head injuries are now more frequent among pedal cyclists than motorcyclists. Helmet-wearing by cyclists would be of benefit.

Other transport

There are relatively few casualties from rail and air transport. Neither, on average, accounts for more than 1% of total accidental deaths. Those that do occur are often in spectacular disasters. Air crashes have a high proportion of fatalities.

ACCIDENTS AT WORK

The circumstances and numbers of work accidents have changed greatly in recent years in step with the changing patterns of employment and types of industry. Heavy industry with its high number and severity of accidents has declined and been replaced by lighter and service industries. In the early 1950s there were about 1800 deaths at work annually; this had fallen to about 800 in the 1970s and is currently about 600 per annum. Reduction occurred in all the main branches of industry. Over the same period fatal accidents in manufacturing fell from about 500 to 300, fatalities in construction work fell from about 200 to 130 and mining fatalities fell spectacularly from about 500 per annum in the 1950s to about 60 in the late 1980s. Fatal accident rates in mining per 100 000 employees, however, remained relatively high at about 20—corresponding rates in all industries and in manufacturing were about 2, in construction work about 10 and in agriculture 7. In 1985 13 180 major (non-fatal) industrial injuries were notified, largely from manufacturing and from construction. Some industries with a diminishing workforce appear to have rising accident rates but this may be partly due to more thorough reporting (Goddard 1988).

DOMESTIC ACCIDENTS

In the UK there were 4797 fatal accidents in homes and residential institutions in 1988 and the numbers have been fairly stable in recent years. Up to middle age most fatal casualties are male but in the elderly most are female. This is partly attributable to the preponderance of females in the elderly population (females outnumber males by 60% at ages over 65 years) and partly to their extra liability to fractures, which will be discussed later.

Fatal accident rates are also relatively high in children under 5. In infants under 1 year suffocation and choking are prominent causes of death. Between 1 and 5 years burns and house fires become more important. Non-fatal injuries due to falls on stairs and elsewhere, burns and scalds and accidental poisoning are also common at these ages.

Domestic accidents are not a frequent cause of death or injury in school children but they increase again in adult life when falls and burns become more common causes of serious and fatal injuries.

Two-thirds of fatal home accidents occur in persons over 65 years of age and two-thirds of the cases are female. Most are due to falls which cause fractures, often of the femoral neck. The injuries may not be classed as 'major' and few patients die directly from their injuries; they may survive several weeks, but respiratory or other complications then supervene. Those who do survive may well become permanently dependent following the accident; personal and social implications are thus very serious.

A number of studies have shown important medical aspects of these injuries. The falls can be due to attacks of dizziness or unsteadiness which can be secondary to medication and there is often a history of many previous falls. A second feature in postmenopausal women is the increased liability to fracture due to osteoporosis, which is a main determinant in hip, vertebral and upper limb fractures in the elderly (Cooper 1989).

Injuries from other violence

Though not strictly accidents, these cases often occur in a domestic setting; they often involve abuse of alcohol and present the same clinical problems as accidental injuries. They are not very numerous—possibly only 1–2%—but they have recently been increasing and include a relatively high number (about 6%) who require inpatient treatment (Shepherd et al 1990). The face is most commonly involved and blows from fists and feet cause bruises and sometimes fractures. Lacerations and penetrating injuries from knives and broken glass are now more frequent. Gunshot wounds are still relatively rare in the UK. Injuries from falls from a height may be very severe and multiple.

ACCIDENTS IN SPORT AND LEISURE ACTIVITIES

Many sports involve an element of risk-taking, so it is not surprising that there are accidents and injuries. Fatal accidents are not common—sport and leisure account for about 1% of the total, but they cause some 10% of Accident & Emergency attendances. A few deaths occur each year in horse-riding, motor and motorcycle racing, ball games and mountaineering. The total deaths—about 80 per year—are far exceeded by those due to drowning which number about 600 per year. These seldom occur as part of organized sport but many involve leisure swimming in unsupervised circumstances. Further cases are due to accidental falls into canals, rivers or pools. Many fatalities could be prevented if more people learned to swim and if more swimming was properly supervised.

Accidental injuries requiring hospital treatment range from the common bruises, sprains and minor fractures of the playground and sports field to serious head and spinal injuries from diving and from falls in horse riding, climbing and air sports. Proper training and equipment can greatly reduce these unneccessary injuries. Serious injuries in school rugby have been largely controlled by safer interpretation of rules and by seeing that teams are matched for weight. An epidemic of spinal and other injuries from trampolining was stopped by ensuring better supervision (Silver et al 1986).

FACTORS IN THE FREQUENCY OF ACCIDENTS AND THE SEVERITY OF INJURIES

Hazards, energies and exposure

The frequency of accidents occurring in a particular activity depends on the specific hazard of the activity and the number of persons exposed. Further, in the case of mechanical impacts the severity of the resulting injury depends on the amount of energy released, the part of the body involved and the degree of concentration of the energy on that part. The energies available in a car accident are proportional to the square of the velocity of impact. This can be modified by the 'crushability' of the vehicle and by the wearing of a seatbelt—the latter also spreads the load on to areas best able to tolerate it. A similar relation to the amount and distribution of energy occurs in burn injuries due to heat, electricity and chemicals. In poisoning the relation is more subtle; the agent typically interferes with some specific biological function such as the oxygen-carrying power of the haemoglobin and, though chemical energy is involved, the quantity of the agent rather than the amount of energy is a more practical measure of its injuring potential. The energy involved in electrocution may be quite small if an alternating current is applied so that it passes through the heart. Similarly, injury by asphyxia or drowning can be caused by a small specific application of mechanical energy—in this case to block the respiratory passages; the period and completeness of the obstruction then determine the outcome.

Demographic changes and accidents

Specific risky activities tend to be undertaken at certain ages. Cycles are popular, for example, among school children and teenagers, then motor cycles are in vogue up to young adult ages. The population at risk for different types of accident depends therefore on the age composition of the community. Within the populations at risk the specific hazard also varies with age; in general it is high in the young and inexperienced and diminishes as the activity is thoroughly learned. The risk tends to rise again as abilities begin to decline in middle age and a further factor in the elderly is that a given accident tends to cause more severe injury and a given injury is more likely to be fatal. Changes in the age distribution of the population such as are currently occurring will therefore be important in determining the numbers exposed to various hazards, their risks of accident, the severity of injuries and the resulting mortality (Fig. 2.3).

In developed countries, the average size of family has declined and, with improvements in hygiene and health care, a higher proportion of people survive into old age. The balance of these changes has caused a slowing in the growth of the UK population, like that of most western European countries, to 2–3% per annum. (In contrast, the populations of the USSR and the USA continue to increase by about 10% per annum and that of India by about 25% per annum.) Our population size tends towards stability because of lower mortality at all ages which is balanced by the lower inputs by births. In this process of stabilization the proportion of young people declines and that of the elderly increases. In 1951 16% of the population of England and Wales were under 10 and 9% were over 70; corresponding proportions in 1988 were 13 and 22%. The declines in mortality rates at various ages are relatively steady so that the main cause of any changes in the size of different age groups is variation in the birth rate. Such variations tend to

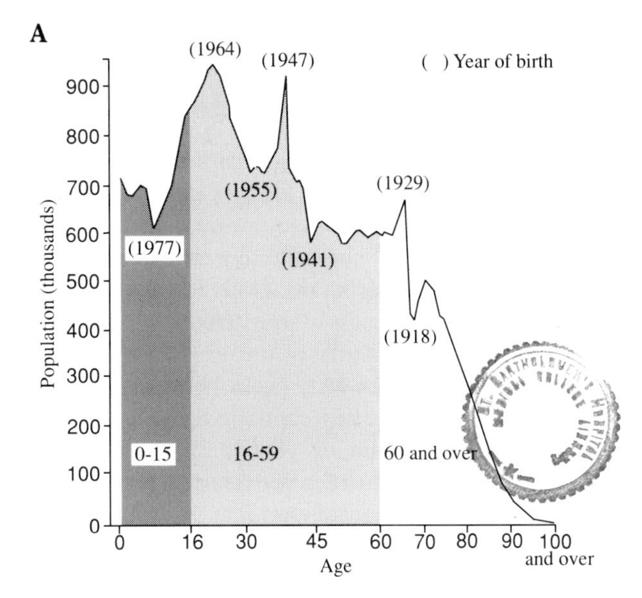

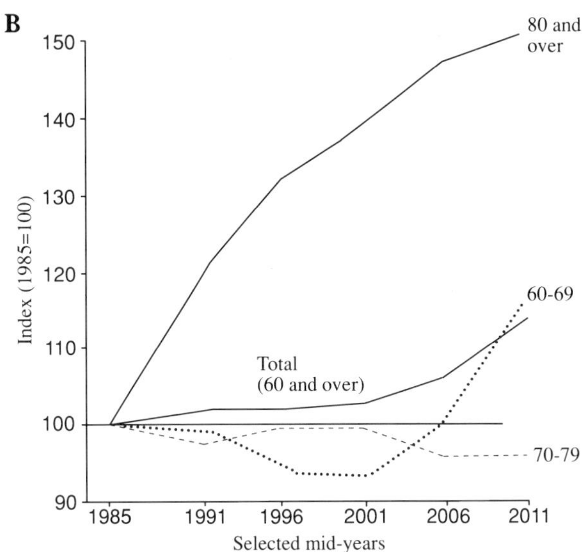

Fig. 2.3 (**A**) Distribution of the population of the UK in 1985 by single years of age, showing peaks and troughs due to variations in numbers of births. (**B**) Estimated future trends in the population in the UK of persons aged over 60. (Reproduced from Thompson 1987, Population Trends 50, HMSO.)

recur cyclically as those born in perhaps a high-birth-rate period themselves reach reproductive age. Other social and economic factors affect the extent of the peaks and troughs, but the important features in this century have been a high birth rate in the first two decades, another smaller peak in the late 1940s and a large 'bulge' in the early 1960s. Since then birth rates have been more steady though they have risen a little during the 1980s and are expected to decline slowly again in the 1990s corresponding to the secondary effects of the lower rates of the 1970s following the 1960s' peak. The repercussions of the earlier peaks will continue to work through the surviving population (Fig. 2.3). Of particular significance for injuries is the large increase in the expected proportions of the over 80s due to the high birth rates early in the century (Thompson 1987).

During the 1990s the peak of the early 1960s will appear as a 'bulge' of middle adults, but of greater significance for general economics, including those of medical care, is the prospective shortage of school-leavers and young adults due to the subsequent reduced birth rate. Since accidents are a major cause of death and disability at these ages the need for their prevention and, if they occur, their effective treatment, is further reinforced.

Changes in specific hazards

The specific hazards of many risky activities have diminished in the last few decades. For instance, fatal motorcycle accidents in the 1930s, when roads were poor and before there were driving tests, were about 1 per 400 machines per annum and they accounted for more deaths than those of car occupants. In the 1950s the rates fell to 1 death per 1000 machines and currently the rate is about 1 per 1400.

It has been shown that the early months of motorcycling are particularly hazardous. A rising trend in ownership will produce a higher proportion of novice riders, thus raising the mean specific hazard. When the number of machines later declines the proportion tends to fall and with it the average hazard. Similar considerations apply to drivers of cars so that as the driving population matures the average specific risk falls. The earlier phase is evident in newly developing countries where very high accident rates occur in the early years of motor vehicle use.

Since the 1930s, active engineering research on road safety has led to improvements in roads, road layout and traffic control. Studies of the biomechanics of injury have led to better safety design of vehicles and to specific personal protection by seatbelts in vehicles and helmets for motorcyclists. More recently regulations have required learner motorcyclists to use the smaller and safer machines and only after a staged learning sequence to be licensed for the more powerful ones. Perhaps because of this more complex procedure the use of motorcycles has declined with further benefit to the accident figures.

Mathematical models of accident occurrence

Road accidents are currently the major cause of serious injuries and attempts have been made to analyse the trends mathematically so as to understand past, and forecast future, changes. Smeed (1972) derived a formula which gave an approximate fit to the data from many countries:

$$D/P = 0.0003(N/P)^{1/3}$$

where D = number of road deaths, N = number of vehicles and P = population. This showed that though the fatal accident rate tended to rise with the number of vehicles, the rise was not proportional to its square, as might be expected from random collisions between vehicles, or even to the number itself, as might occur from striking other objects, but to its cube root. This was an empirical relationship but it implied some factor of adaptation tending to mitigate the number of fatalities in spite of an increase in traffic.

The Smeed formula fitted the accident trends quite well from the early days of recording in the 1920s through to about 1970. An unexpected change then occurred whereby road traffic accident deaths tended to decline even though numbers of vehicles and miles travelled continued to increase. An obvious factor around this time was the raising of oil prices by OPEC and the associated fuel rationing and speed limits. These doubtless played a part but the decline has continued in spite of the subsequent return to increased fuel consumption and higher speeds.

A new and more general analysis by Oppe (1989) would explain both the past and recent trends by a combination of two processes. One is the growth of traffic volume (i.e. vehicle miles driven). In the early days of motor traffic the growth was slow and then began to increase more and more rapidly. There are signs that this growth is tending to tail off and Oppe believes that it will reach a saturation maximum with no further increase in traffic volume. Increasing congestion, for instance, might be a determining factor of this maximum. Such changes can be described mathematically by a logistic sigmoid (S-shaped) curve. It is suggested that in developed countries around 1970, the sigmoid curve was at its inflection point with rate of traffic growth at a maximum and indeed the OPEC action can be interpreted as an economic reaction to this peak of demand.

The second suggested process is a social learning curve, measured in terms of fatalities per vehicle mile and made up of the various social and personal responses which tend to counteract the challenge of road traffic and the resulting accidents. This recalls the adaptive feature implied in the Smeed formula; it includes the improvements in roads, vehicles, road user behaviour and safety devices discussed above, as well as improvements in surgical care. On analogy with psychological learning studies it is suggested that this curve is a negative exponential with an early period of very rapid learning tailing off to a steady state some time in the future.

The first curve of vehicle miles is a measure of exposure and the second, deaths per vehicle mile, a measure of mean hazard; both are over time. It follows that the fatalities in a given year can be estimated by multiplying corresponding values on the two curves. Such calculations show that the model predicts the observed rise until the early 1970s and the subsequent observed decrease in road fatalities in spite of increased traffic. An interesting corollary of the model is that there is a lag of about 10 years between an extra challenge of accidents and the corresponding correcting response by the learning curve. Another implication is that there is little room for any importance to be attached to the hypothesis of risk compensation as applied to fatal road accidents.

Factors which may change the forecasts

Medical interventions

As has been mentioned, a rise is expected in the population of elderly persons and fractures in the elderly are a prominent feature of both domestic and pedestrian accidents. Effective methods for prevention and treatment of osteoporosis could make a valuable saving of personal, social and medical costs. Several methods are being investigated but it is important that they should not only be demonstrated to improve bone structure but also that fractures are prevented. Improved prophylaxis of the complications of these injuries is also required.

Another action with important medical implications is improved control of the current widespread abuse of alcohol. About one-quarter of serious accidents are estimated to be related to alcohol. Consumption is linearly related to price; though not neccessarily a vote-winner, taxing of alcohol up to its earlier equivalent price would reduce the occurrence and severity of most types of accidents and violence.

Green environmental policies

Environmental policies to limit production of greenhouse gases may well affect accident rates. Reduction in the use of fuels will tend to reduce traffic speeds which would lead to fewer and less severe accidents. (It has been estimated that reduction of mean speed by 10% will reduce road traffic accident casualties by 15%.) Other effects may be complex, depending on the change in total amount of travel, also the balance of reduced vehicle occupant exposure (moderate risk), increased pedal cycle exposure (probably higher risk), increased public transport exposure (low risk) and uncertain changes in pedestrian exposure and risk.

A transfer to nuclear power would be expected to produce less work accidents during normal operation. Should it prove impossible to exclude reactor explosions and leaks of radioactivity, overall implications for injuries remain problematical.

Segregation and 'calming' of motorized traffic

Most road injuries are attributable to the energy of motor vehicles. The benefits of separating cars from pedestrians and cyclists have been shown experimentally. Another method, 'traffic calming' whereby lower speeds are encouraged, particularly in residental areas, has proved effective in trials in the Netherlands and Germany and is proposed here.

Changes in leisure and sport activities

As has happened repeatedly in the past (e.g. with skateboards, trampolining, BMX bicycles, hang-gliding), it is likely that fashions in leisure activities will continue to introduce new hazards. Details cannot be foreseen and accident services need to be alert to the possibility of these epidemics so that appropriate damage-limitation action can be taken.

Changes in methods of violence

The high proportion of gunshot wound injuries in the Accident & Emergency departments of many city hospitals in the USA shows what might happen if numbers of weapons were allowed to increase. The media appear to encourage an impressionable audience in the use of violence and firearms. Further action may be needed to offset this influence.

CONCLUSIONS FOR CLINICAL WORK

The trends described for the main types of accident suggest that the present load of cases will remain about constant. Transport and domestic accidents may continue to decline slightly, but this may be offset by an increase in leisure and sport injuries and in those due to violence.

Current care of the present load of accident cases leaves something to be desired and recent developments of methods of audit will probably give this further emphasis. Some of the more elaborate suggestions for major injury centres may prove inpracticable. There is however still a strong case for the principles worked out and applied by Gissane (1962):

1. A 24-h specialist accident service with a large enough catchment area to justify the provision of experienced consultant staff on site, or at short call, who will care for the seriously injured through to discharge and rehabilitation.
2. Investigation and surgical facilities which, though adequate rather than elaborate, must be earmarked and always available for the injured patient so that both staff and equipment are constantly focused on his or her needs.

Experience has shown that such a service can be an excellent base for training and for research on both prevention and treatment. Since the expert management of multiple injuries becomes a matter of routine, calling in further specialist help is facilitated. When an exceptional disaster occurs the system can readily expand to cope with the extra demand (Evans 1979). This avoids requiring clinicians unaccustomed to such cases to be expected to take responsibility for patients outside their normal competence.

As in the past, there will continue to be opportunities for clinicians who care for the seriously injured to contribute to the social learning curve of prevention of accidents and improved treatment of injuries.

REFERENCES

Atkins RM, Turner WH, Duthie RB et al 1988 Injuries to pedestrians in road traffic accidents. Br Med J 297:1431–1434
Blane D, Smith GD, Bartley M 1990 Social class differences in years of potential life lost: size, trends and principal causes. Br Med J 301:429–432
Bull JP 1988 Action on the mechanism of injury. In: Strategies for accident prevention. A colloquium Department of Health and Social Security, HMSO, London, pp 17–21
Bull JP, Roberts BJ 1972 Road accident statistics; a comparison of police and hospital information. Accid Anal Prev 5:45–53
Consumer Safety Unit 1989 Home and leisure accident research, 11th annual report. Department of Trade and Industry, London
Cooper C 1989 Osteoporosis—an epidemiological perspective. JR Soc Med 82:753–757
Evans RF 1979 Disasters; the multiply injured patient. Br J Hosp Med 22:329–332
Gloag D 1988 Strategies for accident prevention. A review of the present position. Medical Commission on Accident Prevention, London
Gissane W 1962 The basic surgery of major road injuries. Ann Roy Coll Surg Engl 30:281–298
Goddard G 1988 Occupational accident statistics 1981–85. Employ Gaz 96:15–21
Grime G 1987 Handbook of road safety research. Butterworths, London

Health and Safety Commission 1989 Health and Safety Executive annual report 1987–8. HMSO, London
Mills PJ 1989 Pedal cycle accidents—a hospital based study. Research report 220. Transport and Road Research Laboratory, Crowthorne
Office of Population and Census Studies 1990 Deaths due to accidents and violence 1988. HMSO, London
Oppe S 1989 Macroscopic models for traffic and traffic safety. Accid Anal Prev 21:225–232
Road Accidents Great Britain 1988 The casualty report (1989) Department of Transport HMSO, London
Shepherd JP, Shapland M, Pearce NX et al 1990 Pattern, severity and aetiology of injuries in victims of assault. JR Soc Med 83:75–78
Silver JR, Silver DD, Godfrey JJ 1986 Injuries of the spine sustained during gymnastic activities. Br Med J 293:861–863
Smeed R 1972 The usefulness of formulae in traffic engineering and road safety. Accid Anal Prev 4:303–312
Thompson J 1987 Ageing of the population: contemporary trends and issues. Pop Trends 50. HMSO, London pp 18–22

3

External skeletal fixation—which frame and why?

J. Kenwright J. L. Cunningham

External skeletal fixation has been in use for about 150 years: Malgaigne in 1840 described a metallic band to be applied externally for the treatment of fractures (Malgaigne 1853–1854) and the system devised by Lambotte in 1902 used half-pins attached to a bar, the overall appearance being very similar to that of some modern frames. There have been many developments over ensuing decades, and these have led to more reliable devices with the ability to stabilize fractures of increasing complexity at different anatomical sites.

External skeletal fixation can be and has been used to stabilize nearly every type and pattern of fracture, osteotomy, arthrodesis, or leg-lengthening procedure; there is a multiplicity of indications, some of which may appear bizarre.

Much has been written about these various treatment methods and about the design and use of new frames, but there are still major controversies surrounding two areas. The first concerns the indications for external skeletal fixation; when is this treatment method prescribed for an individual fracture type, if there are the alternatives of modern functional casts or effective new implants? The second controversial area relates to the choice of device or system to be made available within a hospital and which particular frame is to be used for an individual patient's problem. There are an increasing number of fixation systems available, all constructed according to sound engineering principles utilizing modern and sophisticated materials. The most appropriate frame for a given indication should be chosen after consideration of the mechanical conditions needed for stability and the biological demands of the fracture.

In this review, indications for external skeletal fixation will be discussed as well as the factors to be considered when choosing a frame. Discussion about the use of external fixation for the treatment of spinal pathology, for skull traction, or for the fixation of facial fractures has been excluded.

CONTROVERSIES ABOUT INDICATIONS

Under certain conditions, external skeletal fixation offers overwhelming advantages over other methods of treatment. These advantages will be reviewed here, followed by a discussion of inherent drawbacks of the method, and examples will be quoted where controversy exists.

The main advantages offered by external skeletal fixation as a method of treatment are as follows:

1. External fixation can achieve effective stabilization of the fracture and surrounding soft tissues where there is a combination of serious fracture and severe soft-tissue injury. Under these conditions, fractures can be stabilized to a greater degree than when using casts and the level of immobilization attained seems to be close to the critical level for the healing of soft tissues. Many wounds which do not heal when using casts or traction heal rapidly after the application of external skeletal fixation without any other treatment. This critical level of immobilization which will enhance wound healing is not known, but external skeletal fixation appears to be as effective as internal fixation for acute injuries and yet does not increase the need for local dissection of bone ends and damaged soft tissues, as does internal fixation. Infected non-union is still one of the most disabling conditions in orthopaedics and any fracture treatment which will enhance early wound healing without the drawback of infection should be utilized. This indication must apply to the use

of external skeletal fixation for open diaphyseal fractures if there is any concern about delay in healing of the skin or of other soft tissues. It has been shown convincingly in a study with random selection to treatment group that the use of external fixation, as opposed to plate fixation, for grade II and III tibial fractures leads to lower wound and fracture infection rates (Bach & Hansen 1989).

2. The frame configuration employed for stabilization can be designed to allow access for further wound or fracture treatment without obstruction by external casts or splints.

3. Fracture stability can be achieved rapidly, simply and effectively. These qualities may be particularly important in the treatment of polytrauma where a protracted programme of operative treatment may be needed within the first 12 hours of injury. External skeletal fixation may be particularly indicated for the treatment of severe pelvic fractures, where early temporary stabilization can decrease morbidity and mortality. The application of an anterior frame, even for fracture dislocations of the pelvis with major posterior instability, can lead to rapid improvement in the patient's general condition in circumstances where haemorrhage appears to be uncontrollable; more definitive treatment of the fracture dislocation can be effected later (Slatis & Karaharju 1975; Fig. 3.1). Open-book and vertical shear injuries are commonly associated with severe bleeding and are suitable for urgent use of an external fixator. Similarly, stabilization of the adjacent skeleton is an important accompaniment to repair of major vessels and external fixation enables stability to be achieved in a rapid and effective manner.

4. Stability may be obtained where other methods fail due to severe comminution. Shattered fractures of the lower radius or pilon fractures of the tibia may be beyond the capacity of internal fixation and will be poorly controlled if casts are applied; stabilization in near anatomical position can be achieved by the use of external skeletal frames, although the frame configuration will need to embrace the adjacent joint and traction (ligamentotaxis) may need to be incorporated between the pins on each side of the injury.

5. Joint and muscle rehabilitation can be started immediately after frame application provided external fixation pins or screws have been inserted so as to allow effective function.

6. Arthrodesis performed for damaged or infected joints requires stabilization and external fixation has many advantages under these conditions, enabling sufficient immobilization to achieve

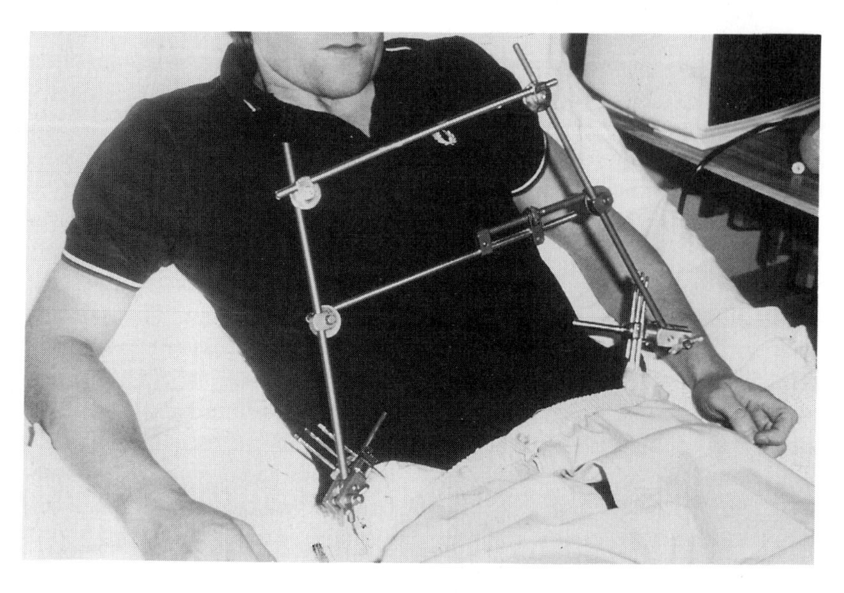

Fig. 3.1 The use of the Slatis quadrilateral frame is appropriate for many pelvic fractures with predominantly anterior instability. Though it looks cumbersome, the frame can be applied rapidly and safely but should allow for abdominal distension.

a sound arthrodesis, and avoiding the use of implants. Special demands are made of the method of fixation when attempting arthrodesis after total knee replacement, especially if infected (Fidler 1983, Cunningham et al 1989).

7. Most external skeletal frames allow adjustment of stability of fixation to be made during treatment according to the biological needs of the fracture. It is well recognized that fracture healing is very sensitive to its mechanical environment and this can be controlled by altering the fixation system. Frames may be dismantled progressively or devices used which have in-built units which can be adjusted to allow either progressive loading (dynamization) of the fracture or the passive application of micromovement.

8. Accurate control of fracture or osteotomy position can be achieved with the use of external frames, and corrections can be made to fracture or osteotomy position during treatment. Such adjustment can be made in one stage or gradual change can be effected. Use is made of this advantage in bone transport, leg lengthening, epiphyseal distraction and in the progressive correction of bone or soft-tissue deformity.

It seems therefore, that external skeletal fixation might be the panacea for many orthopaedic problems and that any fracture which requires immobilization and control of position might best be treated using this method, as there are so many advantages over both cast treatment and internal fixation.

There are, however, a considerable number of disadvantages associated directly with the method.

1. *Screw or pin tract loosening and infection.* These complications have always been recognized as a great nuisance, and the initial enthusiasm for external skeletal fixation waned rapidly because of the high incidence of such problems. With the development of modern frames and screws, and meticulous care of screw tracts at the time of insertion and in the ensuing weeks, the incidence of problems has reduced. It might be predicted that further improvements in frame and screw technology would lead to a disappearance of this problem, but this is unlikely. Screws will always have to pass from the external environment through mobile soft tissue, and if the screws are loaded through the action of bearing weight on the leg, there will always be a predisposition to loosening due to loading leading to fatigue failure and micromovement of the screws as well as infection. Usually screw tract infection is a benign problem but this is not always the case. There is a definite incidence of cavity or sequestrum formation (Fig. 3.2), and of infection spreading from the screw tract to the primary operation (Green 1981). Secondary surgery may then be needed and unattractive scars result. Despite a low incidence of major or troublesome late complications, the risk of their development is ever-present.

2. *Damage to neurovascular structures.* Surgical damage to neurovascular structures at the time of insertion of screws should not occur but can do so because of the close proximity of major structures to essential sites of screw or pin insertion. Safe

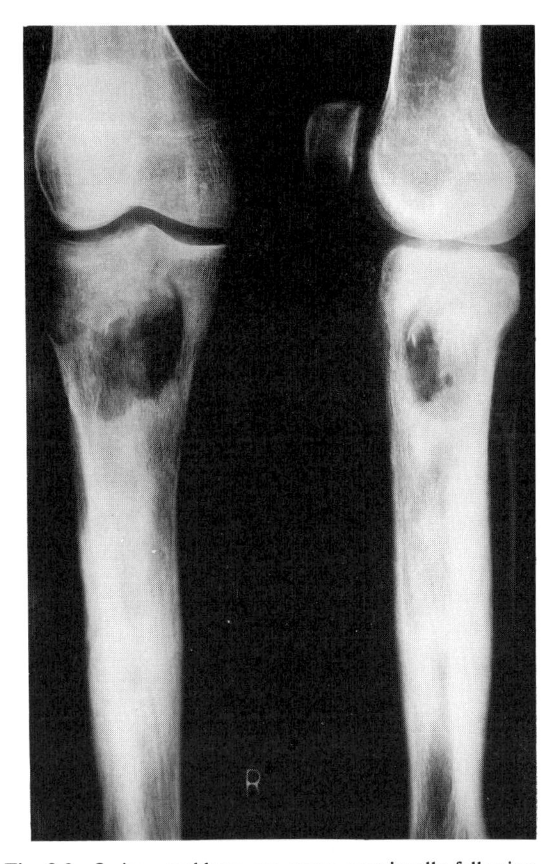

Fig. 3.2 Serious problems can occur occasionally following screw tract infection and there may be cavity formation, as seen here. Infection which persists in screw tracts after screw removal needs early surgical treatment.

corridors have been described for insertion, but for complicated fractures some modification of the angles of insertion may be needed, and damage to nerves and vessels can occur, particularly when transfixation pins or wires are used. Corridors have been defined as safe, unsafe and hazardous (Behrens & Searls 1986) but when using circular frames for the complex problems for which these frames are needed, it is usually impossible to employ only safe corridors. A careful review of a series of patients treated will nearly always show an incidence of disability from such complications. Whichever type of device is used, the insertion of screws in the arm needs to be made under direct vision since both above and below the elbow there is a special risk of neurological damage.

3. *The problem of joint stiffness.* Inhibited mobilization of joints and muscles can be reduced by careful planning of pin sites, so as to minimize penetration of muscles or tendons; the screws inserted into the first metacarpal for the treatment of distal radial fractures must not be inserted through the extensor mechanism with the fingers in the extended position or finger flexion will be prevented. In certain other sites, however, there is inevitable inhibition of function, due to the passage of pins or screws; this applies particularly to the region of the lower femur where penetration of the fascia lata will lead to inhibited knee joint movement. Many patients are also too apprehensive to overcome the inhibition of uncomfortable screw tract sites.

4. *Intra-articular fractures.* In the treatment of intra-articular fractures, the maintenance of an accurate reduction is crucial and internal fixation is usually the more precise technique for the achievement of this aim. External fixation systems cannot control accurately the position of several bony components. An added disadvantage of external skeletal fixation under these circumstances is the necessity to bridge the joint for fixation and thereby prevent early joint rehabilitation. External fixation may have to be used for severely comminuted intra-articular fractures or where there is gross contamination or infection but in general, the main objectives in the treatment of intra-articular fractures are best met by internal fixation. In juxta-articular fractures similar disadvantages prevail in that immobilization through an external frame means the fixation must bridge the joint. Some joint stiffness usually follows such treatment but the method is usually only applied to the most serious injuries, where some disability from stiffness can be anticipated whatever treatment method is chosen. Where the method has been employed for lower radial fractures, however, the permanent stiffness seems to be much less of a problem than anticipated, and the functional results are consistently better than when using casts for such injuries (Kongsholm & Olerud 1989). Embracing the knee joint with external fixation is nearly always associated with serious permanent joint stiffness (Fig. 3.3).

5. *Metaphyseal and osteoporotic bone.* Under these conditions the bone–screw connection may fail at an early stage during treatment, particularly when using unilateral frames; transfixing pins or wires will cause less of a problem as fixation will not rely so heavily on an intact bone–screw interface.

6. *Delayed union.* When treating diaphyseal fractures using external skeletal fixation, delayed union is seen frequently. To a large degree, this is

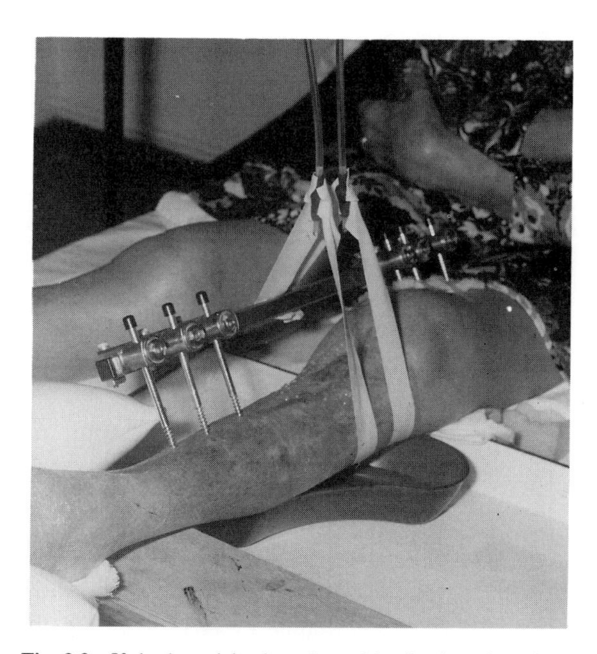

Fig. 3.3 If the knee joint is embraced by fixation, there is nearly always permanent joint stiffness. This frame has been applied for treatment of chronic osteomyelitis, and wound irrigation of a cancellous bone graft of an upper tibial fracture non-union is in progress.

associated with the severity of the initial injury, but there is a general consensus of opinion that the fixation frame itself frequently inhibits healing because it enforces inappropriate mechanical conditions upon the healing fracture; this problem is seen commonly with tibial diaphyseal fractures. It is claimed that the problem can be overcome by using frames which allow progressive dynamization. Even if the mechanical environment is adjusted to the different phases of fracture healing, there may still be delayed union when treating diaphyseal fractures and this is especially troublesome if there are also associated serious screw tract problems. Such infections may declare themselves at any stage during the treatment programme and necessitate frequent hospital visits with repeated courses of antibiotics.

There is always a race between the time to healing and the development of screw tract problems when treating tibial diaphyseal fractures with external skeletal fixation. If problems develop forcing early removal of the frames, the fractures often do not heal in casts. Such problems lead to unpredictable management and it is probably more appropriate to use intramedullary nail fixation for unstable closed tibial fractures and casts for stable ones. The fracture healing times may not be different from those seen when using external fixation with dynamization for injuries of equal severity, but rehabilitation will be less troublesome with no fear of pin tract infection.

It can be seen, therefore, that there are disadvantages as well as advantages of external skeletal fixation as a method of treatment and these have to be balanced for each patient's problem before the treatment method is selected. External skeletal fixation has not replaced and will not replace other methods of treatment.

THE IDEAL FIXATION SYSTEM

Engineering scientists ask for design requirements and constraints before embarking on any design project. These are easy to define for external skeletal fixation systems but are difficult to achieve and some demands are mutually exclusive. This, together with the vast increase in the use of external skeletal fixation, has led to the development of many different types of fixator.

The perfect fixation system would include the following features:

1. Stability: the frame would give very considerable stability using a small number of fixation screws. There would be a very stable screw–clamp junction, this being the weakest point on most fixators. Fixation would be sufficient to stabilize complex leg fractures and yet allow significant weight-bearing.
2. Simplicity: the fixation system would be user-friendly so that it can be applied rapidly by infrequent users with little assistance.
3. Adjustable geometry: with the ideal fixation system it should be possible to attach the device according to local mechanical and anatomical needs; adjustment of the fracture or osteotomy should be possible in all axes, including rotation.
4. Adjustable elasticity: the ideal frame would allow adjustment of the overall elasticity of fixation so that loading of the fracture can be changed during the healing phase according to the biological needs.
5. Comprehensive: an ideal system should be elaborate enough to deal with complex problems including pelvic fractures, fixation across joints, arthrodesis, leg lengthening and bone transport and should include the small components necessary for treatment of wrist, hand and foot injuries.
6. A comprehensive range of screws, pins or wires is needed so that configurations can be constructed with a minimal number of screws, with minimal stress levels at the bone–screw interface, and yet with sufficient stability to prevent deformity.
7. Light-weight and not bulky: the frame should be of light-weight construction for convenience and for use on children, although patients hardly ever complain of the weight of any fixator. Similarly the frame should not be bulky so as to allow easy mobilization of the limb; there should not be a risk of inadvertent injury of the opposite limb due to protruding parts.
8. Inexpensive: this will be of varying importance for different communities. Cost should not, however, prevent availability of fixators.
9. Ease of service and replacement: frames should be robust so as not to fail during use and service for re-use should be easy.

In certain developing countries in the world points 8 and 9 take on special importance, and in such communities there is often a very high incidence of problems which require external skeletal fixation. No one frame system embraces all these ideal features but the features should be considered when selecting fixation systems for a given hospital, so that a range of frames is available which will meet the demands of the practice encountered. It is also important to select for an individual patient the frame which will best suit his or her needs and to preplan frame and screw placement before operation. The surgeons on the team need to train in the correct use of the frames, such as they might do for the use of internal fixation, so as to prevent problems associated with learning and to reduce the time of operation.

ENGINEERING CHARACTERISTICS OF FIXATORS

When planning an external fixation for an individual clinical problem, it is important to consider the engineering characteristics of the fixation system to be used, so that a frame with the appropriate geometrical configuration can be chosen to match the biomechanical and biological demands. A considerable amount of knowledge is available about the mechanical behaviour of many commonly used fixation systems. These data have been obtained from several sources including measurement of fixator stiffness and fracture gap motion for different fixators under a variety of loadings on simulated fractures in both synthetic materials and on cadaveric bone. Finite element and analytical models have also been used to enable the stiffness of a given geometry of external fixator to be predicted accurately. Experimental studies have demonstrated the effect of different stiffnesses of the same fixator and hence different mechanical conditions at the fracture site on fracture healing (Lewallen et al 1984, Williams et al 1987). Retrospective reviews of patients' progress in practice has added further to knowledge of performance of frames (Burny 1979, de Bastiani et al 1984, Kenwright et al 1986, 1991).

The information from these studies can be applied in a clinical environment, but it is important to recognize the limitations of such studies. In vitro laboratory studies are always performed under idealized conditions with secure placement of bone screws, and the loading of the fixator is carefully controlled. These conditions do not always exist in a clinical situation when fractures may be comminuted, bone may be osteoporotic and screws may be inserted in a suboptimal manner; for patients of considerable weight, loading of the fixator may be unpredictable and overloading can also occur in people with unreliable behaviour. In vivo studies on experimental models can demonstrate biological processes, but again extrapolation to the clinical situation may be inadvisable; in addition to any species-related differences, other clinical factors may intervene in patients, particularly with relation to the high-energy types of fracture which are so common in people. There are, however, certain engineering characteristics of external fixator frames which should be considered during frame selection and application.

Frame mechanics

Fixator devices have been classified into two groups—pin fixators and ring fixators (Behrens 1989). Pin fixators consist of stiff pins which require firm anchorage in the bone and form part of the frame configuration; in ring fixators there is an exoskeleton of bars and the transfixion wires merely suspend the bone. Pin fixators may be classified as simple pin clamp-type in which each pin or screw is attached to the bar by its own clamp, clamp-type in which several pins are attached to each multi-pin clamp which in turn has an articulation with the bar. Pin fixators can be applied in a unilateral manner to one surface of the limb.

Such devices have been tested in the laboratory, and their stiffness or rigidity is determined from the linear portion of the load deflection curve (Fig. 3.4). Loads can be applied axially, in bending in the anteroposterior and lateral planes and in torsion. Each loading mode will generate a different value of frame stiffness, which can then be compared between the different fixators which are available (Kempson & Campbell 1981, Chao et al 1982, Chao & Hein 1988). Changing the configuration within a given frame-type will change the overall stiffness or rigidity of the frame (Moroz et al 1988). However, it should be noted that a given change in fixator configuration will not have a proportionate

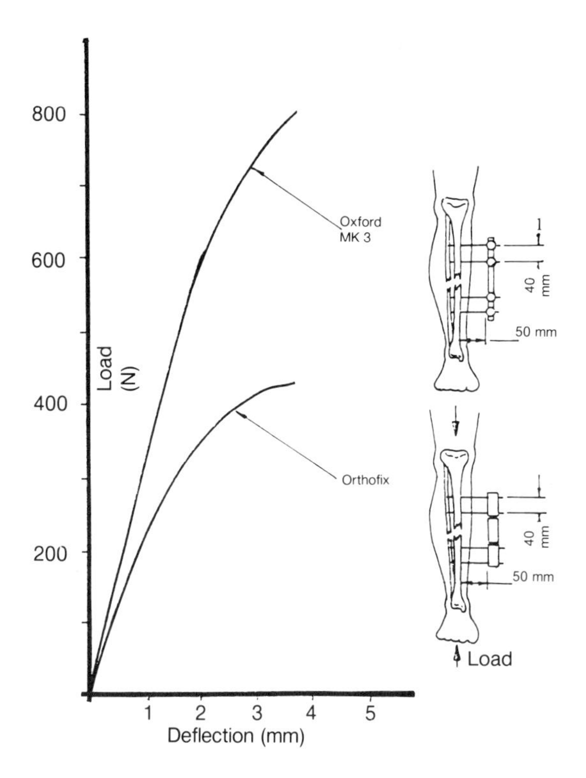

Fig. 3.4 The load deflection curve for a fixation system of defined configuration can be tested on simulated fractures for different loading directions in the laboratory: the stiffness or rigidity of the system is determined from the linear portion of the curve, and is expressed in N/mm. This figure compares the axial stiffness of two unilateral fixation systems and demonstrates the axial flexibility of the Orthofix system.

effect upon the different modes of stiffness (Finlay et al 1987). The most important factors influencing rigidity within any pin fixation system have been found to be the number of pins or screws used, the screw diameter and the distance from the bone to the support column of the fixator (Briggs & Chao 1982). Pin separation distance and the stiffness of the support column will also influence overall fixator stiffness. Bilateral frames are generally stiffer than unilateral frames, although unilateral frames which use a large-diameter bone screw can give comparable values of stiffness to some bilateral frames.

Many of the developments in the area of fixator design have been aimed at increasing stability with as few components as possible so as to maintain a non-obtrusive external skeleton. In the intact tibia, for example, the moments which act during weight-bearing are much higher in the sagittal plane than those in the coronal plane; torsion and compression of the frame are also important in walking. Most pin external fixators also tend to be least rigid in anteroposterior bending (sagittal plane) and torsion (assuming the fixator to be applied medially to a bone such as the tibia) and this applies to both unilateral and bilateral frames. Studies have shown that bilateral configurations with pins passing through the limbs are weak in resisting sagittal moments and that a half-frame applied anteriorly (AO half-frame) has a very high resistance to this sagittal moment and hence will minimize deformation of the frame on weight-bearing (Behrens & Johnson 1989, Gasser et al 1990). Fixation stiffness can also be improved by the use of two unilateral frames placed at right angles or by the use of triangulation. Ring fixators' stiffness is increased by these same factors as well as by an increase in wire tension, the placement of wires at 90° to one another, and by changing the rigidity of the external frame by increasing the number of rings and decreasing their diameter (Fleming et al 1989).

The failure point of a fixator is usually defined as the load beyond which an irreversible displacement of the frame occurs, this usually results from slippage in one or more of the joints of the device. It is important to know this failure point for any fixation system, particularly if high levels of loading occur in clinical use, for example, in early weight-bearing in a fracture in which there is no bone contact. In leg lengthening there is an axial tension associated with the distraction in addition to the axial force of weight-bearing; these forces summate and may lead to high axial force levels which can exceed the failure load of the frame and result in deformity at the osteotomy. When unilateral frames are used for leg lengthening the failure load can easily be exceeded if free weight-bearing is permitted.

Laboratory loading tests on frames which use crossed tensioned transfixion wires held by a circular or semi-circular frame, several of which are connected together with rods to construct a frame, can demonstrate considerable levels of stiffness in all modes of loading, other than axial loading, where there can be considerable elasticity (Gasser et al 1990, Paley et al 1990). Such frames theoretically allow weight-bearing to be applied with minimal risk of frame distortion and hence angulation of the fracture or osteotomy. The relatively low axial stiffness of such frames will allow considerable axial micromovement across the fracture or osteotomy to be achieved on weight-bearing, which may lead to enhanced bone healing while maintaining stability.

Bone–screw mechanics

The bone–screw connection is the Achilles heel of external fixation, and as such presents a major clinical problem. The decision to remove the fixator is often governed by screw loosening or screw tract infection, rather than fracture healing.

The geometry of an external fixator results in large bending loads being carried by the screws which give rise to high local stresses in the bone at the sites of screw insertion (Pope and Evans 1982, Huiskes et al 1985). Unilateral fixators give rise to significantly higher stress in the cortex adjacent to the frame than in the distal cortex while bilateral fixators give similar values of stresses in both cortices. The maximum stress which occurs in the bone around the screw can be of a sufficiently high value to cause local failure of the bone, particularly when the fracture is so unstable that none of the applied load is taken through the fracture itself. As fracture healing progresses, and the tissue formed between the bone ends becomes sufficiently stiff to take appreciable load, there will be a marked decrease in the loading of the bone–screw interface for a given loading of the fracture. Cyclical loading of screws has been shown in cadaveric studies to result in a decrease in the strength of the bone–screw interface (Harris et al 1981). In vivo micromotion of the screw relative to the surrounding bone may cause local bone resorption and lead to screw loosening (Pettine et al 1986). Stresses in the bone at the bone–screw interface can be reduced by the use of a large-diameter screw and by reducing the distance from the bone to the external support column; pretensioning of screws, as employed in internal fixation, may reduce the amount of micromotion of the screw relative to the bone and prevent resorption. Poor placement of pins during insertion and drilling, which causes thermal necrosis of the surrounding bone, will also predispose to screw loosening. Stresses at the bone–screw interface can be reduced easily by the prevention or reduction of weight-bearing, but this may not best meet the biological needs of the fracture. A compromise has to be made between the provision of the necessary mechanical stimulus for the healing fracture tissue and the need to minimize the stresses at the bone–screw interface—achieving this balance is a constant challenge.

Characteristics which permit dynamization

Many experimental and clinical studies have shown that some degree of micromovement and loading of fracture callus is needed for healing to progress effectively (Sarmiento et al 1977, 1989, McKibbin 1978, Wu et al 1984, Goodship & Kenwright 1985). The exact mechanical characteristics of the optimal loading regime are not known but it is probably important for some degree of strain to be applied from the early days after fracture. It is known that fractures can heal with different histological patterns according to the degree of gap present at the fracture site and the mechanical conditions which apply (Chao & Aro 1989); in most fractures treated by external skeletal fixation, healing progresses by secondary (indirect) methods with external and endosteal callus formation. Accurate reduction that will allow osteonal healing either of the primary or gap type must be infrequent except under rigorously controlled experimental conditions. It is, therefore, probably important when planning treatment to utilize a fixator which will allow some degree of micromovement to act across the fracture, even in the early stages after injury. When considering the micromovement requirements of the fracture site it is important to note that the stiffness of a particular configuration of fixator as tested in the laboratory will not directly reflect the actual movement which occurs throughout the fracture site (Seligson et al 1981, Kristiansen et al 1987). For example, in a fracture treated with a unilateral frame, axial loading of the fracture will give mainly axial motion, but will also give considerable bending and shear motions at the fracture site, and movement patterns will vary throughout the fracture callus. Also considerable torsional forces act during stance phase in walking.

The term 'dynamization' embraces both the application of micromovement and of loading to the fracture and can be effected by increasing the load placed upon the fracture, by encouraging patient activity or by one of the following methods:

1. The use of an elastic frame with overall low rigidity (Burny 1979).
2. Progressive dismantling of the frame (Behrens and Johnson 1989).
3. Increased weight-bearing with a frame with low stiffness in the axial mode (de Bastiani et al 1984).
4. Biocompression: Lazo-Zbikowski et al (1986) have proposed the use of a unilateral frame which allows free sliding. The patient's weight-bearing controls the axial strain applied to the fracture and it is hypothesized that a feedback mechanism will then ensure the most appropriate strain at the fracture for each stage of healing.

Similar dynamization techniques which permit progressive self-loading of the fracture are built into certain other fixation systems. It would seem appropriate in the present state of knowledge to use one or other of these systems for treatment of diaphyseal fractures of the tibia at an early stage after injury. Some degree of loss of dynamization can, however, occur with all sliding and rolling fixators due to friction between the sliding or rolling components and also these frames depend critically upon the functional loading of the leg by the patient if fracture movement is to occur. Devices have been constructed which allow passive micromovement to be imposed across the healing fracture via an external pump. Such devices do not therefore depend on functional loading (Kenwright & Goodship 1989).

CHOICE OF FIXATION SYSTEM

The most appropriate external fixation devices need to be selected for a particular hospital according to local needs and careful preplanning is needed for each patient's problem. Considerable improvisation can be made with many modern devices and the scope of possibilities is described in the manuals for each system. In the following section, the place of different fixation systems will be reviewed, and particular emphasis will be placed upon situations where real difficulties may be encountered if the wrong type of frame is used. The devices will be divided into pin frames and ring frames.

Pin frames of unilateral type (e.g. Orthofix, AO, half-frame Hoffmann, Shearer, Dynabrace)

These frames are perfectly adequate for 90% of problems encountered in most hospitals and improvisation will enable the treatment of an even greater proportion. The advantages of such frames are that they can be applied rapidly and will control most diaphyseal fractures. Dynamization is possible with the majority of these frames, either because low-rigidity configurations can be constructed or because special features are built in which allow axial micromovement to be achieved. Such frames are very suitable for physeal distraction and hemichondrodiatasis (Aldegheri et al 1989); at the time of growth plate rupture a slow steady rupture occurs; with tensioned wire frames there is a sudden painful disruption due to the spring-action of the wires.

The achievement of adequate stability may be difficult when treating serious open femoral fractures with these frames but many are suitable for short-term stabilization for patients whose general condition is critical. Considerable difficulty may also be experienced when attempting to control position in complex leg lengthenings, particularly of the femur, and angulatory deformities occur frequently when lengthening congenitally short limbs (Fig. 3.5). Some protection from weight-bearing is needed in all these circumstances. There is also a distinct limitation in the ability of these frames to allow adjustment of position of an osteotomy or fracture unless there is a joint in the fixator lying between each cluster of pins. The presence of a fixed bar, remote from the axis of the bone, means that the ability to adjust for angulatory—and particularly rotatory—deformity is limited.

These frames are also not generally suitable for progressive correction of deformities, though in several bone transport can be effected.

The versatility of unilateral fixators is also limited. If it is necessary to cross a joint for fixation, such as at the ankle joint, or to fix a pelvic fracture or fractures both above and below the knee with interconnection, unilateral fixators are less than

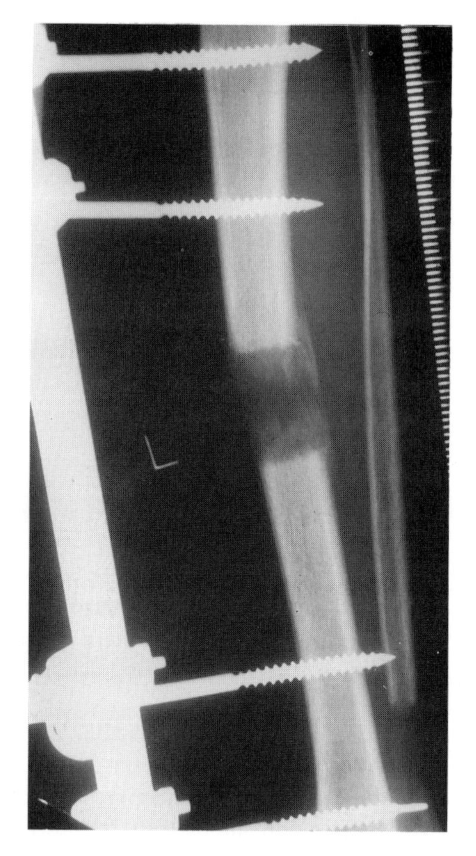

Fig. 3.5 In leg lengthening performed for congenital shortening large axial forces may develop following lengthening increments; if weight-bearing is also allowed the axial forces add together and if a unilateral frame is used, deformity may develop. Under these conditions the torques which act on the clamps can easily exceed their slippage torque.

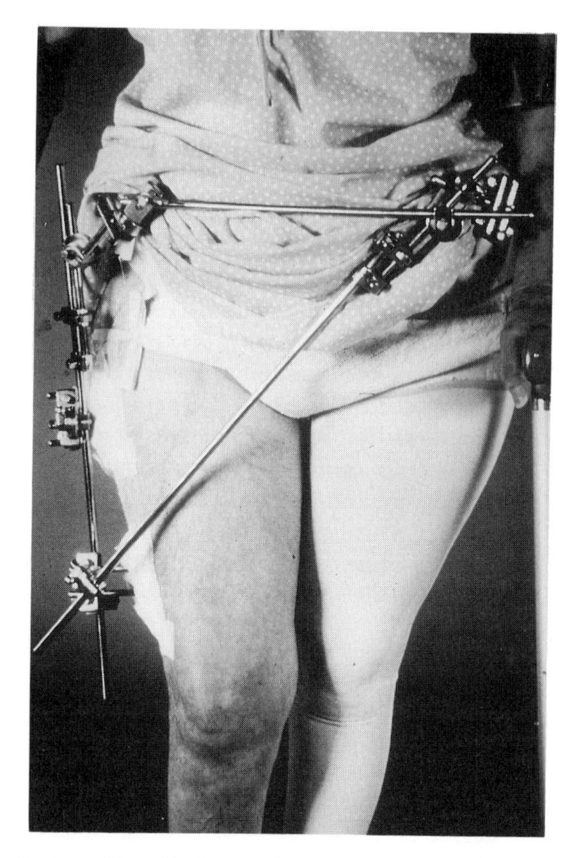

Fig. 3.6 Hip arthrodesis performed for treatment of previous septic arthritis needs a frame which offers considerable adaptability as well as stability.

ideal. Improvisation can be effected using several linked frames, but it is important to preplan for these complex types of operation to ensure the appropriate frame configurations can be constructed.

Pin frames of comprehensive type
(e.g. Hoffmann)

These frames enable a progressive build-up of components and allow the treatment of complex fractures. Such frames are ideal for treatment of pelvic fractures (Fig. 3.1) and serious juxta-articular or intra-articular injuries around the elbow, wrist, knee or ankle. They are also suitable for major arthrodesis including that of the hip joint (Fig. 3.6). All situations can be dealt with but complex, bulky configurations develop which may obstruct plastic surgery and make rehabilitation more difficult.

Circular frames

The indications for the use of these frames have become clear following the pioneering work of Ilizarov, and this type of frame undoubtedly has a major place to play in the treatment of problems requiring complex reconstruction. Circular frames offer specific advantages. The frames give sufficient stability for even the most complicated diaphyseal fracture complex, and at the same time, enable weight-bearing to be effected. The frames resist rotatory and angulatory deformation and yet allow considerable axial elasticity. This enables weight-bearing to produce axial micromovement and may thus predispose to favourable healing for osteotomies and fractures. Ilizarov (1990) and also Cattaneo from Lecco (Paley et al 1989) have shown proliferative healing of osteotomies and fractures when using these frames, which appear to offer an optimal balance between stability for control of position and elasticity in the axial direction. A further major advantage of circular frames is that they enable manipulation of bone fragments to be effected progressively during treatment and yet give sufficient stability for bone healing to proceed, and for the patient to mobilize. From a practical point of view, the thin tensioned wires appear to be associated with low levels of pin tract infection. There would, therefore, appear to be special indications for the use of this type of frame and these include:

1. The stabilization of complicated segmented diaphyseal fractures where it is extremely difficult to maintain positional control; the use of the cross wires transfixing the different segments and of olive wires allows control of fragments (Fig. 3.7).
2. Bone transport in patients where there are defects in the skeleton. Segments of bone can be moved axially or even transversely, in a progressive and controlled manner. Bone transport must rank as one of the major recent advances in orthopaedics; its most common application is for reconstruction of long bony defects in diaphyseal fractures. When circular frames are used, segments of bone can be carefully controlled and manipulated and monofocal, bifocal and trifocal transport has been described (Paley et al 1989). Bone fragments can easily move out of line and circular frames enable adjustment of fragment position either by the use of extra rings or by the application of controlling forces through olive wires. These frames, whilst allowing significant axial micromovement, resist translational shear which might inhibit new bone formation in the regenerating, lengthened limb segment. Bone transport can now be considered as a reliable alternative to massive staged onlay graft, to free vascularized grafts, or amputation, for treatment of major bone defects.
3. Infected non-union may necessitate very prolonged use of external skeletal fixation throughout the programme of reconstructive surgery. Under these circumstances, unilaterally applied external skeletal fixation often leads eventually to major problems with screw tracts, so that the fixation system has to be removed. If tensioned wires are used there may be a longer life span of effective fixation even if some loosening develops with lysis around wires. These frames, unlike unilateral fixation, are not totally dependent upon a firm bone–screw connection and can probably be maintained for very long periods. Similarly wires will be more effective in osteoporotic or metaphyseal bone.
4. Major leg lengthening. In certain pathologies there is a high risk that deformity will develop during lengthening, and circular frames enable prevention or correction of such deformities. Circular frames are particularly suitable for control of double-level lengthenings in any one bone. Simultaneous correction of deformity within the limb can

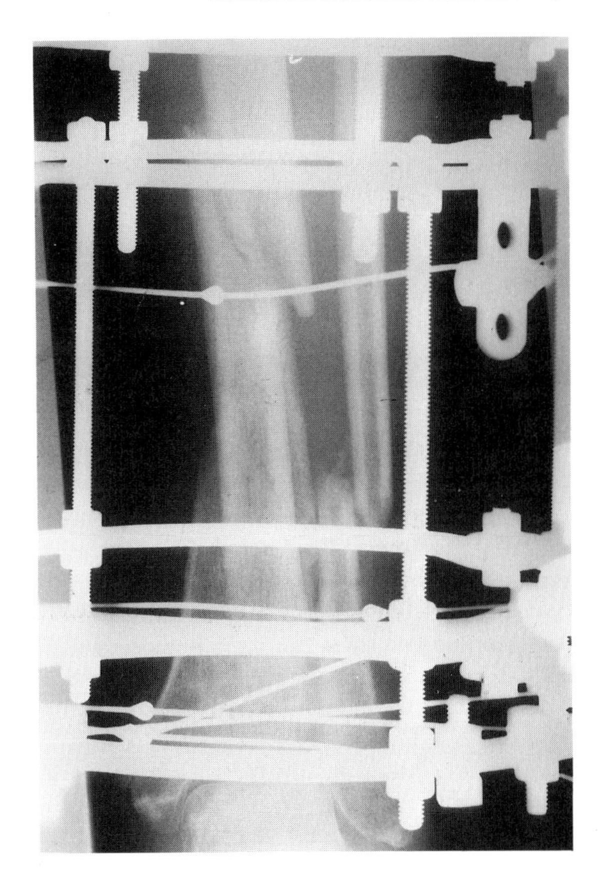

Fig. 3.7 Complex fractures with considerable comminution may need the use of circular frames which employ multiple transfixing and olive wires; nearly all fractures can be stabilized in this way, even if juxta-articular.

be made progressively with the use of a circular frame. The circular frame is particularly useful for lengthening the congenitally short limb associated with congenital dysplasia of the fibula. In these conditions varus deformity of the femur or valgus deformity of the tibia occurs frequently when unilateral frames are applied; correction of such deformity is difficult when using unilateral frames even if the clamps allow some adjustment; circular frames circumvent these problems and deformity can be corrected progressively at the time of each lengthening increment.

Circular frames also enable progressive correction of deformity in both bone and soft tissue, and are particularly useful for two- or three-plane deformity correction. The deformities should be corrected one at a time and accurate preplanning is needed so that hinging is at the correct levels and that inappropriate translations do not occur. Soft-tissue corrections without osteotomy can also be performed for the deformity of severe talipes equino varus (Grill & Franke 1987).

There are, however, distinct disadvantages associated with the use of circular frames. The application time for these frames is prolonged and even after adequate training and familiarization with the multiple components an average simple application takes approximately 3 h. There is a significant risk of damage to neurovascular structures when using the crossed tension wires. The incidence of this is not described in the literature, but must be more frequent when using multiple crossed pins as safe corridors are difficult to define for so many pins, and the margin for error in many safe corridors is small. It is not possible in many situations to insert all the wires through safe corridors and hazardous corridors have to be used. The damage thus created probably explains the greater discomfort often experienced when using circular frames. It is claimed that major structures may tolerate perforation by thin wires but permanent disability must follow such injury, and the risk of compartment syndrome must also rise. Oedema of the whole limb segment is seen much more frequently with circular frames than with unilateral frames. Inhibited muscle function also follows the use of multiple transfixing wires. The advocates of this method describe this as only a minor problem in view of the thin nature of the pins, but in practice, many pins crossing a muscle compartment must inhibit function, particularly in a nervous or depressed patient. A special problem surrounds use of the frame for control of the femur, in that multiple pins have to be inserted in the proximal segment and problems with tracts in this region are commonplace (Fig 3.8). Injury to assistants through the spiking of gloves during pin insertion is also a common occurrence with these frames. It would seem, therefore, that circular frames should not be used if the clinical problem can be treated with a simple device.

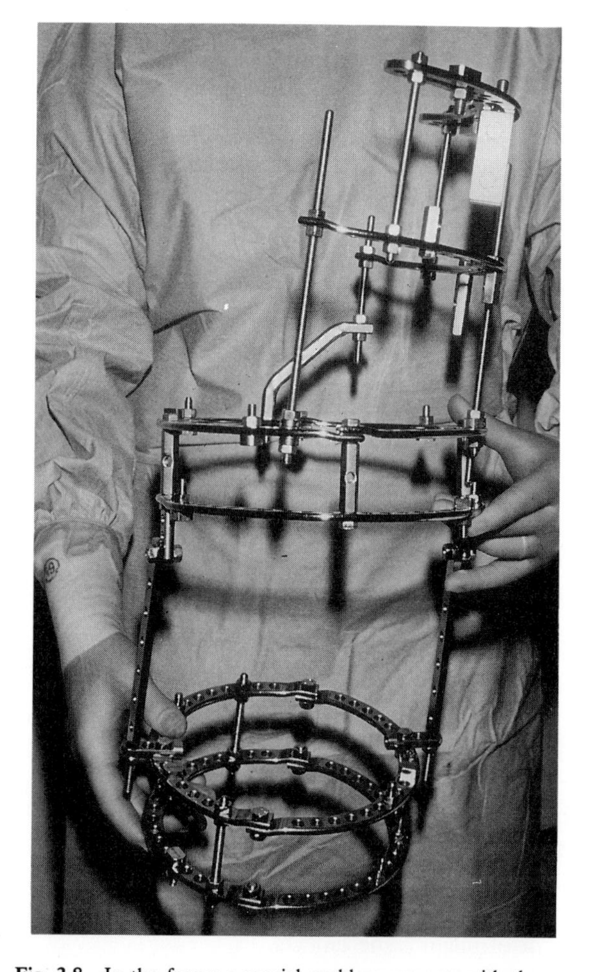

Fig. 3.8 In the femur a special problem presents with the use of circular frames: troublesome proximal transfixing wires should be avoided. Preconstruction of frames performed with the patient and the radiographs before operation can save considerable time at operation.

CONCLUSIONS

External skeletal fixator design is at an advanced stage and many comprehensive and effective systems are available. It is important to preplan the treatment carefully for an individual patient, taking into account the demands that will be placed upon the frame in order to achieve sufficient stability for fracture or osteotomy control and to enable rehabilitation to proceed. It is also important for the frame to allow the mechanical environment at the fracture or osteotomy site to give appropriate mechanical conditions during healing which will not inhibit bone healing.

It is suggested that a limited number of devices should be available within a given hospital and for these to be chosen according to the types of problem which present. Unilateral frames with appropriate characteristics for changing the rigidity of fixation will deal with 90% of problems encountered in general orthopaedic practice (Fig. 3.9). However, in units where polytrauma is managed regularly, it is important to have systems available which are comprehensive, so as to be able to stabilize serious juxta-articular and pelvic fractures. If surgical problems are encountered which require complex correction of deformity and control of bone segments, then a circular frame will be needed.

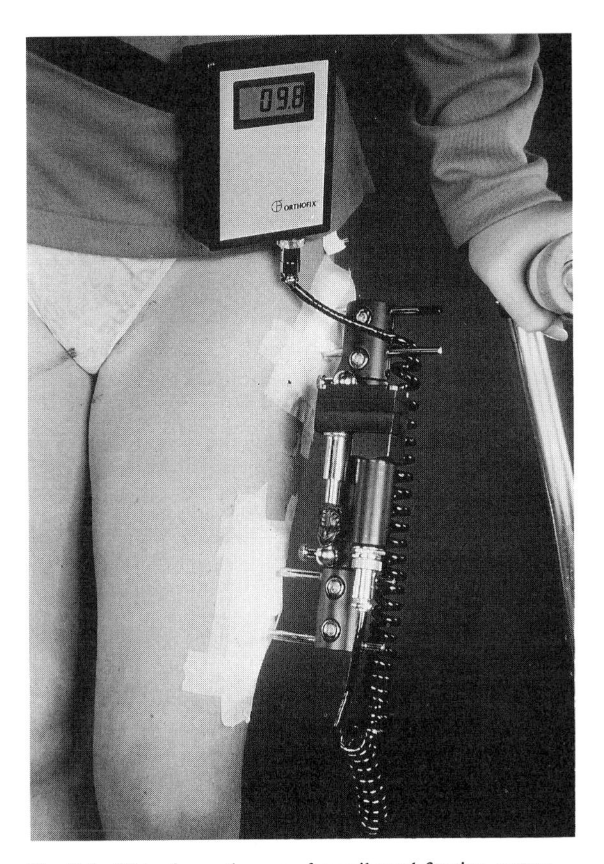

Fig. 3.9 This shows the use of a unilateral fixation system for femoral lengthening with an attached module, which allows lengthening to be accomplished automatically in very small increments. Such unilateral frames are suitable for most problems in general orthopaedic practice.

REFERENCES

Aldegheri R, Trivella G, Lavini F 1989 Epiphyseal distraction: hemichondrodiatasis. Clin Orthop 241:128–136

Bach AW, Hansen ST 1989 Plate versus external fixation in severe open tibial shaft fractures. Clin Orthop 241:89–94

Behrens F 1989 A primer of fixator devices and configurations. Clin Orthop 241:5–14

Behrens F, Johnson W 1989 Unilateral external fixation. Methods to increase and reduce frame stiffness. Clin Orthop 241:48–56

Behrens F, Searls K 1986 External fixation of the tibia. Basic concepts and prospective evaluation. J Bone Joint Surg 68B:246–254

Briggs BT, Chao EYS 1982 The mechanical performance of the standard Hoffmann-Vidal external fixation apparatus. J Bone Joint Surg 64A: 566–573

Burny F 1979 Elastic external fixation of tibial fractures; study of 1421 cases. In Brooker AF, Edwards C (eds) External fixation: the current state of the art. Williams & Wilkins, Baltimore, p 55

Chao EYS, Aro HT 1989 Biomechanics and biology of external fixation. In: Coombs R, Green S, Sarmiento A (eds) External fixation and functional bracing. Orthotext, London

Chao EYS, Hein TJ 1988 Mechanical performance of standard Orthofix external fixator. Orthopaedics 11:1057–1069

Chao EY, Kasman RA, An KN 1982 Rigidity and stress analyses of external fracture fixation devices–a theoretical approach. J Biomech 15:971–983

Cunningham JL, Richardson JB, Soriano RMG, Kenwright J 1989 A mechanical assessment of applied compression and healing in knee arthrodesis. Clin Orthop 242:256–264

de Bastiani G, Aldegheri R, Renzi Brivo L 1984 The treatment of fractures with a dynamic axial fixator. J Bone Joint Surg 66B:538–545

Fidler MW 1983 Knee arthrodesis following prosthesis removal. J Bone Joint Surg 65B:29–33

Finlay JB, Moroz TK, Rorabeck CH et al 1987 Stability of 10 configurations of the Hoffmann external fixation frame. J Bone Joint Surg 69A:734–744

Fleming B, Paley D, Kristiansen T, Pope M 1989 A biomechanical analysis of the Ilizarov external fixator. Clin Orthop 241:95–105

Gasser B, Boman B, Wyder D, Schneider E 1990 Stiffness

characteristics of the circular Ilizarov device as opposed to conventional external fixators. J Biomed Eng 112:15–21
Goodship AE, Kenwright J 1985 The influence of induced micromovement upon the healing of experimental tibial fractures. J Bone Joint Surg 67B:650–656
Green SA 1981 Complications of external skeletal fixation; causes, prevention, treatment. C Thomas, Springfield, Illinois
Grill F, Franke J 1987 The Ilizarov distractor for the correction of relapsed or neglected club feet. J Bone Joint Surg 69B:593–597
Harris JD, Evans M, Kenwright J 1981 Safe stress levels at the screw interface of an external fixator for long bone fractures. In: Stokes IAF (ed) Mechanical factors and the skeleton. John Libbey, London
Huiskes R, Chao EYS, Crippen TE 1985 Parametric analysis of pin-bone stresses in external fixation devices. J Orthop Res 3: 341–349
Ilizarov GA 1990 Clinical application of the tension-stress effect for limb lengthening. Clin Orthop 250:8–26
Kempson GE, Campbell D 1981 The comparative stiffness of external fixation frames. Injury 12:297–304
Kenwright J, Goodship AE 1989 Controlled mechanical stimulation in the treatment of tibial fractures. Clin Orthop 241:36–47
Kenwright J, Goodship AE, Kelly DJ et al 1986 Effect of controlled axial micromovement on healing of tibial fractures. Lancet ii:1185
Kenwright J, Goodship AE, Adams M et al 1991 Axial movement and tibial fractures—a controlled randomised trial of treatment. J Bone Joint Surg 73B (in press)
Kristiansen T, Fleming B, Neale G et al 1987 Comparative study of fracture gap motion in external fixation. Clin Biomech 2:191–195
Kongsholm J, Olerud C 1989 Plaster cast versus external fixation for unstable intra-articular Colles' fractures. Clin Orthop 241:57–65
Lambotte A 1913 Surgical treatment of the fractures. Masson, Paris
Lazo-Zbikowski J, Aguilar F, Mozo F et al 1986 Biocompression external fixation; sliding external osteosynthesis. Clin Orthop 206:169–184
Lewallen DG, Chao EYS, Kasman RA, Kelly PJ 1984 Comparison of the effects of compression plates and external fixators on early bone healing. J Bone Joint Surg 66A:1084–1091
McKibbin B 1978 The biology of fracture healing in long bones. J Bone Joint Surg 60B:150–162
Malgaigne JG 1853–1854 Considérations cliniques sur les fractures de la rotule et leur traitement par les griffes. J Conn Med Prat 16:9
Moroz TK, Finlay JB, Rorabeck CH, Bourne RB 1988 Stability of the original Hoffmann and AO tubular external fixation devices. Med Biol Eng Comput 26:271–276
Paley D, Catagni MA, Argnani F et al 1989 Ilizarov treatment of tibial non-unions with bone loss. Clin Orthop 241:146–165
Paley D, Fleming B, Catagni M et al 1990 Mechanical evaluation of external fixors used in limb lengthening. Clin Orthop 250:50–57
Pettine KA, Kelly PJ, Chao EYS, Huiskes R 1986 Histologic and biochemical analysis of external fixator pin–bone interface. Orthop Trans 10:337
Pope MH, Evans M 1982 Design considerations in external fixation In: Seligson D, Pope M (eds) Concepts in external fixation. Grune, New York
Sarmiento A, Schaeffer JF, Beckerman L et al 1977 Fracture healing in rat femora as affected by functional weight-bearing. J Bone Joint Surg 59A:369–375
Sarmiento A, Gersten LM, Sobol PA et al 1989 Tibial shaft fractures treated with functional braces. J Bone Joint Surg 71B:602–609
Seligson D, Powers G, O'Connell P, Pope MH 1981 Measurement of fracture gap motion in external fixation. J Trauma 21:798–801
Slatis P, Karaharju EO 1975 External fixator of the pelvic girdle with a trapezoid compression frame. Injury 7:53
Williams EA, Rand JA, An KN et al 1987 The early healing of tibial osteotomies stabilized by one or two-plane external fixation. J Bone Joint Surg 69A:355–365
Wu J-J, Shyr HS, Chao EYS, Kelly PJ 1984 Comparison of osteotomy healing under external fixation devices with different stiffness characteristics. J Bone Joint Surg 66A:1258–1264

4

Recent advances in imaging in orthopaedics

I. W. McCall

The massive strides that have been made in computer development have had a profound effect on diagnostic imaging over the last 10 years. The speed with which digitally based data can be acquired and manipulated has increased dramatically, producing some significant advances in both time of acquisition and image resolution in computerized tomography (CT) which have been obvious to all clinicians. Technical developments in the type and array of detectors have also increased the resolution and quality of the image. Software developments have provided many helpful devices such as three-dimensional reconstruction of bone or soft-tissue images (Fig. 4.1), metal artefact removal and quantitative bone mineral estimation. Similar developments have also taken place in nuclear medicine where emission CT systems have become more widely available. More recently, the development of an imaging system based on the magnetic qualities of the hydrogen proton have been made possible by the enormous power of modern computers. These developments have improved the demonstration of soft tissues very significantly, especially within joints and in the spine. The aim of this article is to describe some of the areas where these developments have improved imaging in orthopaedics and, although stressing the role of magnetic resonance imaging (MRI) in this regard, to discuss it in conjunction with CT and sonography.

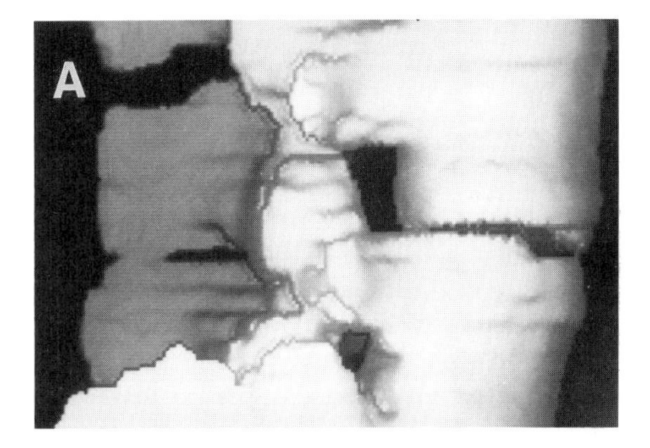

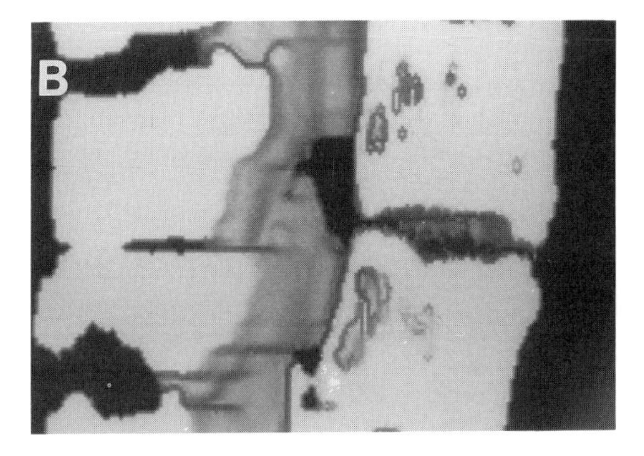

Fig. 4.1 Three-dimensional reconstruction of the spine. The bone can be viewed from (**A**) outside or (**B**) as a section viewing the foramen from within the spinal canal.

MAGNETIC RESONANCE IMAGING

This technique exploits the magnetic properties of the hydrogen proton, which is extensively distributed throughout the body. Each hydrogen nucleus behaves as a small magnet and, under carefully defined conditions, the proton can draw energy from an applied magnetic field. On removal of this applied field, these magnetic effects die away but persist long enough for measurements to be made. The amount of energy taken from the field is a measure of the number of nuclei present and the rate at which the nuclei lose that energy gives information about their environment.

Under normal circumstances, the hydrogen protons in the human body have a random orientation and their small magnetic fields cancel, leaving no net magnetization. In the presence of a magnetic field, some of the spin will align in the direction of the field, yielding a net magnetization.

Transverse magnetization is then induced by adding energy in the form of a radiofrequency pulse applied perpendicular to the static magnetic field. Following the radiofrequency pulse, if there is no further perturbation the displaced magnetization will gradually return to the longitudinal axis. This phenomenon of return to equilibrium is termed relaxation and is characterized by two time constants, designated T1 and T2. T1 relaxation is also termed spin-lattice relaxation as the nuclei lose the extra energy they gained from the radiofrequency pulse to their local environment. At a time T1, 63% of the longitudinal magnetization will have recovered and most tissues have T1 values in the range of 200–2000 ms. T2 relaxation (also termed transverse or spin-spin relaxation) is a measure of the time required for the spins, which have been induced to rotate in phase by the radiofrequency pulse, to lose that coherent rotation. T2 reflects a loss of transverse magnetization owing to the interactions of adjacent nuclei. By definition, in the time T2 63% of the maximum transverse magnetization will be lost. Most tissues have a T2 value between 20 and 300 ms.

Both longitudinal and transverse relaxation occur simultaneously but independently and are properties of all normal and pathological tissues and fluids. The relative contribution of each of these properties can be influenced by the choice of pulse sequences.

Image contrast results from a complex relationship between signal intensity, tissue type, specific proton magnetic parameters and the timing characteristics of the pulse sequences. It is also affected by blood flow. The absence of protons in air results in very low signal and if the protons are tightly bound, they have very short T2 relaxation times and no appreciable signal as in tendons or bone. On T1 weighted images subcutaneous fat and bone marrow have the brightest signal while hyaline cartilage is less bright and muscle even less so. Cystic fluid, urine, ligaments, tendons and bone have little or no signal intensity. On T2 weighted images, however, cystic fluid and urine have the brightest signal followed in decreasing order by subcutaneous fat, bone marrow and muscle. Tumours, thus, have characteristics which depend on the relative proportion of fat, hydrated tumour cells and fibrosis.

Blood has special imaging characteristics. Signal intensity varies with the rate and character (whether lamina or turbulent) of flow, the direction of flow in relation to the slice sequence and the pulse sequence selected. In most spin echo sequences, major vessels show no signal because the excited protons exit the section before detection takes place. However, short TR-TE sequences, as found in gradient echo sequences, may produce a bright signal from blood. The state of the haemoglobin will affect the imaging appearances in a case of haemorrhage.

Because adjacent normal and pathological tissue can have identical intensities at a given pulse sequence, and thus be obscured, at least two pulse sequences are obtained in most diagnostic examinations.

The choice of pulse sequence is also influenced by the likely localization of a lesion. If it is situated in fat then a T1 weighted examination will produce optimal contrast between the low-intensity tissue and the surrounding high-intensity fat, whereas if a lesion is located in muscle, which has a relatively short T2 relaxation time, then nearly all pathological processes will be of higher intensity.

The presence of metal artefacts can seriously detract from MR images by producing focal loss of signal, often with regional distortion.

The quality of the image is dependent on many parameters, including the overall magnet strength but the design of the receiver coil is very important and specific coils are produced for different anatomical areas.

KNEE

Double-contrast arthrography has been used successfully for many years to define the nature and complexity of meniscal tears by the interposition of the contrast medium and air between the surfaces of the tear with the knee stressed in either valgus or varus. Using surgery as the gold standard, accuracy rates of 95% have been recorded for the medial meniscus and, in particular, the posterior horn, while results for the lateral meniscus were lower at

81% for tears, but 95% for the demonstration of a normal lateral meniscus (Levinsohn & Baker 1980, Thiju 1982). Arthroscopy has reduced the use of arthrography but horizontal tears of the inferior surface of the posterior horn may be difficult to evaluate by arthroscopy (Levinsohn & Baker 1980). Arthrography has previously been unsatisfactory in examining the patella but the addition of CT will allow demonstration of early ulceration of the articular cartilage and even local softening can be seen as it absorbs the contrast into the cartilage (Fig. 4.2).

Lateral subluxation of the patella is usually at its maximum at 20% of flexion of the knee, which is difficult to image with plain X-rays but the transaxial mode of CT shows any angulation or lateralization very accurately (Stanford et al 1988). CT with direct sagittal imaging can also demonstrate the cruciates clearly but should be reserved for those cases where the standard lateral arthrographic view is equivocal or to distinguish between an absent or torn anterior cruciate ligament (Pavlov et al 1979). The collateral ligaments cannot, however, be imaged directly by these techniques.

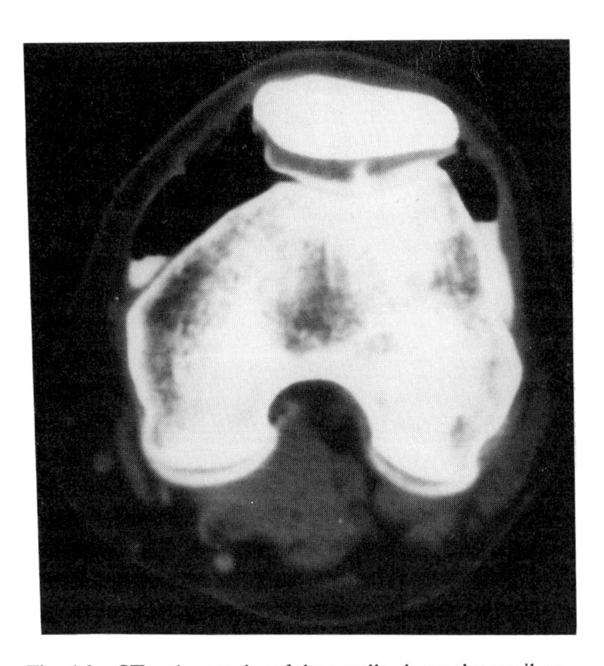

Fig. 4.2 CT arthrography of the patella shows the cartilage thickness clearly and also demonstrates an area of chondromalacia in the cartilage surface, which has absorbed the contrast medium. The detail of the cartilage surface is not so well demonstrated with magnetic resonance.

Despite these good results MRI has become the major method of imaging the internal structure of the knee. Imaging protocols include T1 weighted spin echo or gradient echo, 4–5 mm slices in the sagittal and coronal planes, and gradient echo T2 weighted images for an arthrographic effect. Three-dimensional gradient echo acquisition, however, is particularly valuable as this allows multiple thin slices with high signal-to-noise ratios and the potential for reformatting in any plane, which assists in the assessment of the cruciate ligaments (Adam et al 1989). On MRI the meniscus appears as a triangular structure, which is black (low signal) on both T1 and T2 weighted images. This is in contrast to the intermediate signal of the adjacent articular cartilage and white (high signal) on the T2 image of synovial fluid and articular cartilage. A tear in the meniscus allows synovial fluid to enter between the torn surfaces (of the tear), thus creating a small increase in the signal intensity in these zones on the T1 weighted image and a bright signal on T2 (Fig. 4.3).

Comparison of the MRI features with the findings at arthroscopy has indicated a 97% sensitivity for medial meniscus tears and 92% sensitivity for the lateral meniscus with a slightly lower specificity of 89% for the medial and 91% for the lateral, giving an overall accuracy of 94 and 92% respectively (Mink et al 1988). Polly et al (1988) quote similar figures of 98% accuracy for tears in the medial meniscus and 90% for the lateral meniscus. Some authors have suggested a 100% negative predictive value (Reicher et al 1987, Mink et al 1988) but occasional errors may involve the evaluation of the free edge of the meniscus where small radial tears may not be visible. However, false-positive examinations are more common than false-negative studies and occur mostly in the posterior horn of the medial meniscus, where increased signal intensity may be seen within the meniscus on T1 but not on T2 weighted images (Glashow et al 1989) (Fig. 4.4). These appearances probably reflect early myxoid degeneration in the centre of the ageing meniscus (Reicher et al 1985) but may also be due to partial volume effect between the curving meniscal surface and the fatty tissue of the capsule (Herman & Beltran 1988). The arthroscopist

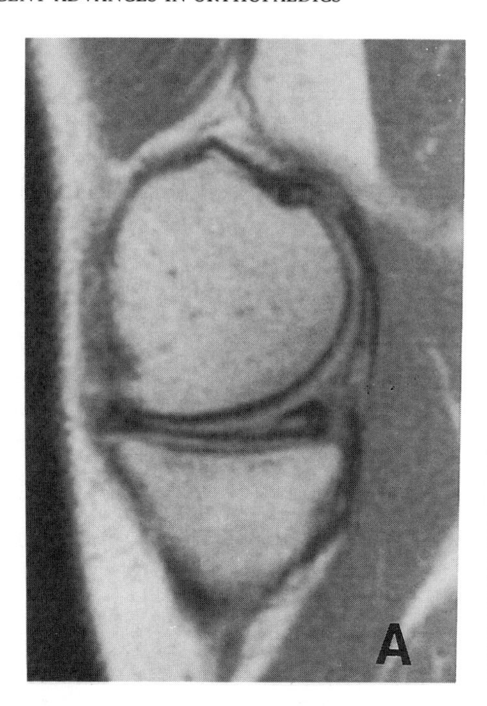

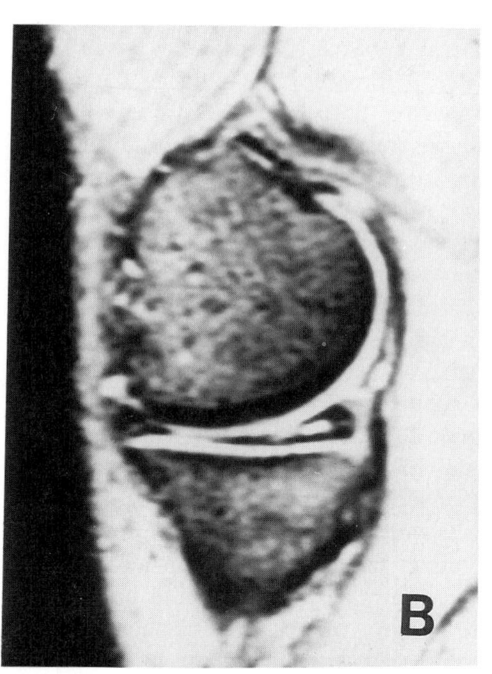

Fig. 4.3 (**A**) The T1 weighted image shows an intermediate signal within the substance of the posterior horn of the medial meniscus extending to the surface of the meniscus, indicating a horizontal tear. (**B**) On T2 there is increased intensity reflecting the synovial fluid within the tear. The cartilage and synovial fluid cannot be differentiated on this T2 weighted sequence.

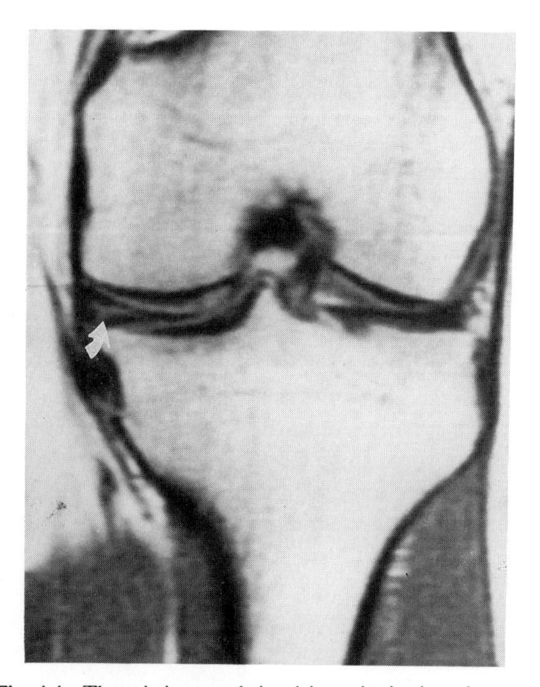

Fig. 4.4 There is increased signal intensity in the substance of the medial meniscus which does not extend to the margin (arrow). The articular cartilage is thinned on the lateral condyles and the lateral meniscus is degenerate.

should, however, examine these areas closely to exclude a tear completely. A significant number of patients with clinical evidence of meniscal tears are found to be normal arthroscopy (Reicher et al 1987), and therefore the use of MRI with its high negative predictive value for meniscal tears should result in a significant reduction in morbidity, invasive examinations, and cost.

The ligaments in and around the knee joint are seen as low-density linear structures on MRI. The anterior cruciate is best demonstrated in the sagittal plane with 15° of external rotation in the joint and the posterior cruciate may be demonstrated on the same sagittal slice. Complete rupture of the cruciates is seen as a loss of continuity and some displacement of the ligament with areas of increased signal intensity on both T1 and T2 weighted images (Fig. 4.5). Tears of the collateral ligaments are demonstrated by the loss of continuity with the cortical bone of the tibia or femur, but minor strains or partial tears may be overlooked as continuity of the ligament is maintained, although ill defined areas of high signal intensity are seen

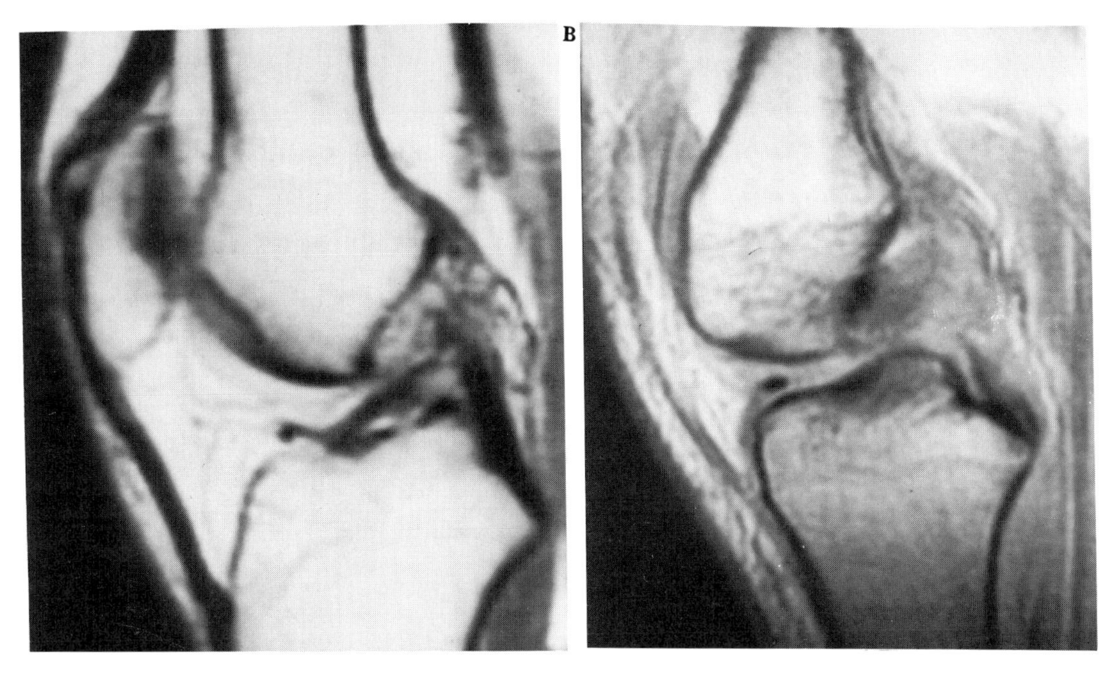

Fig. 4.5 (**A**) The anterior cruciate has lost its continuity and is posteriorly displaced, indicating a tear. (**B**) The anterior and posterior attachments of the posterior cruciate ligament are all that are seen following a tear of the posterior cruciate.

within the ligament on both T1 and T2 weighted images.

Accuracy rates of 95% have been reported for complete tears of the anterior cruciate ligament (Mink et al 1988). The clinical tests of anterior cruciate instability, such as the anterior drawer sign, produce accuracy rate of only 78% when compared with MRI (Lee et al 1988b). The data with regard to partial tears are less clear and careful technique is required to assess partial disruption of the anterior cruciate ligament. Posterior cruciate tears are rare, but in a large series of over 600 consecutive patients, 11 had tears demonstrated on MRI and confirmed by arthroscopy, of which 4 were clinically unsuspected. No false-negative MRI studies were found (Grover et al 1990).

Articular cartilage is seen as an intermediate signal on T1 weighted spin echo sequence and a differentiation of articular cartilage thinning from fibrocartilage degeneration—both of which may be a cause of joint space narrowing—can be made (Fig. 4.4). Optimum visualization, however, is achieved using gradient echo acquisition, with varying flip angles which have enabled the differentiation of articular cartilage from the synovial fluid. Early patella cartilage damage may be difficult to identify and CT with contrast may be required to show these lesions. Cartilaginous defects, such as osteochondritis and avascular necrosis of the subchondral bone, are well demonstrated by MRI. The extent of the bone lesion is shown to be greater than suspected on the plain radiographs and the overlying cartilage is well visualized and loss of continuity can be accurately predicted (Hartzmann et al 1987). Loose bodies within the joint are readily visible, but occasionally osteochondromatosis may be overlooked despite being definitely present on plain films (Hartzman et al 1987).

Sonography of the knee is of limited value but is useful in the diagnosis of popliteal cysts (Gompels & Darlington 1982) and their differentiation from popliteal artery aneurysm, although this is also accurately achieved with MRI. Evaluation of menisci, and cruciate ligaments have been reported (Selby et al 1986, Laine et al 1987) but the reliability is not established and the advent of MRI obviates the clinical value. The demonstration of patellar tendonitis or haematoma, which is hypoechoic with a low level of internal echos, may, however, be of clinical value and real-time sonography will demonstrate motion abnormalities of torn tendons (Fornage & Rifkin 1988).

SHOULDER

Double-contrast arthrography with CT has also been the prime investigation for recurrent subluxation or impingement syndromes of the shoulder. Standard radiographic anteroposterior views with tube angulation allow an accurate assessment of the rotator cuff. Complete tears are identified by an absence of the tendon and contrast entering the subacromial and often the subdeltoid bursae (Fig. 4.6a), while with partial tears of the inferior surface the contrast only enters the substance of the rotator cuff. Accuracy levels of 90% have been found when correlated with surgical findings for rotator cuff tears (Mink et al 1985). Calcification within the supraspinatous tendon is best demonstrated on plain films prior to arthrography. The glenoid and anterior capsule is best evaluated in the CT scans where the normal labrum is seen as a smooth outline, whereas tears may produce distortion, lines of contrast within the substance of the cartilage, or a complete absence, leaving only the bone outline (Fig. 4.7a). The anterior capsule may be stripped from the surface of the glenoid and a Hill-Sachs deformity in the posterior margin of the humerus is easily identified on CT when present (Fig. 4.7b). Correlation between CT arthrographic evaluation and surgical findings has shown an accuracy of 97% for anterior labral tears (Wilson et al 1989) and a slightly lower rate for posterior labrum (Rafii et al 1987). The size of the anterior capsule varies considerably, although the frequency of anterior labral lesions increased to 86% when the attachment was in the medial third of the neck of scapula (Wilson et al 1989).

Sonography of the shoulder joint, with high-resolution real-time sector scanners, has also been used to demonstrate the rotator cuff, which appears normally as a homogeneous, moderately echogenic arc of tissue, situated between the deltoid muscle superiorly and the humeral head inferiorly, and which tapers towards its insertion (Middleton et al 1986, Crass & Craig 1988). A tear is seen as a well defined discontinuity or hypoechoic focus within the substance of the cuff, while severe degeneration and rupture may produce a complete absence of

A

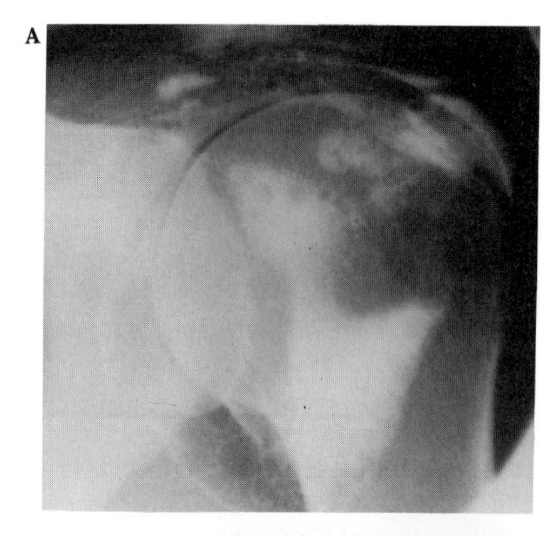

B

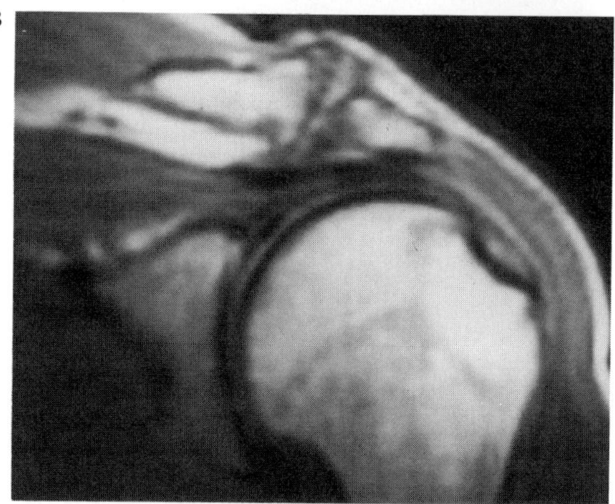

Fig. 4.6 (**A**) Complete rotator cuff tear. The contrast is seen in the subacromion and subdeltoid bursae. (**B**) The rotator cuff is completely ruptured with only a thin residual line. The supraspinatous muscle is impinged by a hypertrophied acromioclavicular joint.

an ultrasound signal. In some cases, however, an echogenic focus may be seen within the cuff; this has been reported to be due to granulation tissue in partial-thickness tears (Crass & Craig 1988) and has been found to be the least predictive sign of a tear (Brandt et al 1989). Soble et al (1989) report an accuracy of 87% but with a positive predictive value of 75% and specificity of 84%, while Brandt et al (1989) found a lower accuracy level of 79% and a negative predictive value of 75%. Inaccuracies may be due to the acromion obscuring the rotator cuff or misinterpretation of the biceps tendon for the rotator cuff. False-positive echogenic foci are due to

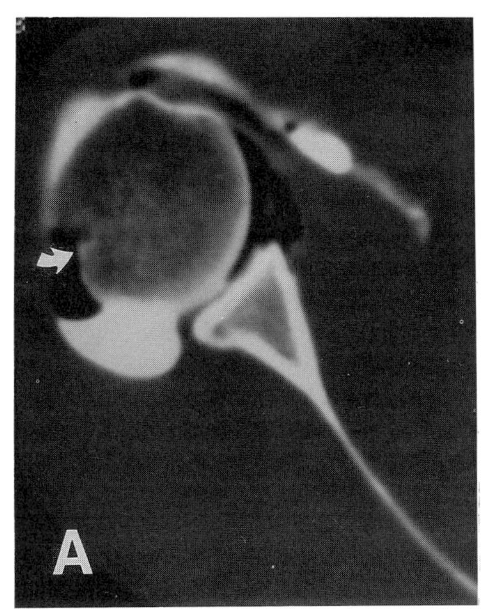

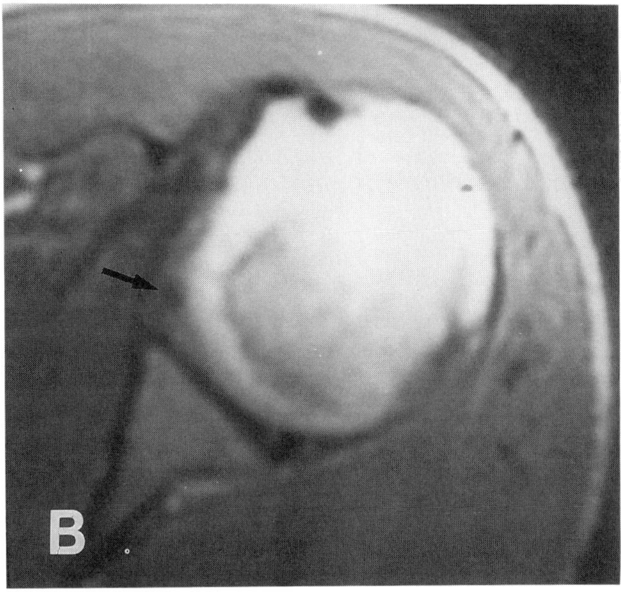

Fig. 4.7 (**A**) The anterior labrum has been completely torn and is separated from the bony margin of the glenoid, which is outlined by air. The posterior rim of the glenoid is clearly outlined by contrast. The Hill–Sachs defect of the posterior humeral head (arrow) is also clearly delineated. (**B**) The low-intensity signal of the anterior labrum is shown (arrow) separated from the bony margin of the glenoid on the T1 spin echo (SE) image. The Hill–Sachs defect is seen on the posterior surface of the humeral head.

granulation tissue, fibrous tissue or soft-tissue calcification within the substance of the cuff. These factors make sonography very operator-dependent and careful technique is essential. It may, however, be used for screening patients as the high negative predictive value reported by some authors will avoid those with a normal scan undergoing arthrography.

Recent studies, however, suggest considerable promise for MRI in the examination of patients with shoulder disorders (Seeger et al 1988b, Zlatkin et al 1988). The glenoid labrum is of low-intensity signal on T1 in relation to the bone and the appearance of injury due to dislocation includes severe attenuation, indistinct borders, and increased signal intensity either diffusely or as a discrete band (Fig. 4.7); this is confirmed by surgery (Seeger et al 1988a). The rotator cuff and its associated muscles can also be easily assessed by MRI in any plane, the former appearing as a well defined arc of low signal intensity on T1 over the humeral head merging with the intermediate signal of the muscle mass of the supraspinatous (Fig. 4.8). Patients with chronic shoulder pain and dysfunction may have degeneration of the rotator cuff and impingement of the muscle by the hypertrophied acromioclavicular joint (Fig. 4.6). Rotator cuff degeneration has been classified in three grades with early tendinitis (grade I) showing a localized increase in signal below the tendon at its insertion, associated with an intact outline of the tendon itself. Progressive signal increase within the thinned tendon heralds the grade II (Fig. 4.8) which is difficult to differentiate from a partial rotator cuff tear and may indeed represent this. Finally, complete rupture of the tendon (grade III) is demonstrated as interruption of the tendon continuity by increased signal intensity, which is particularly obvious on the T2 weighted images due to the interposition of the synovial fluid extending from the joint, traversing the tear and communicating with the subacromial bursa above it. Retraction of the muscular tendinous junction may occur (Fig. 4.6) with eventual replacement of the atrophic cuff by fat and fibrous tissue (Holt et al 1990). The MRI sensitivity of all rotator cuff tears is 91% with a specificity of 88% (Zlatkin et al 1989b). Similar findings of 92 and 100% respectively have also been reported by Burk et al (1989). The presence of calcification within the tendon and its

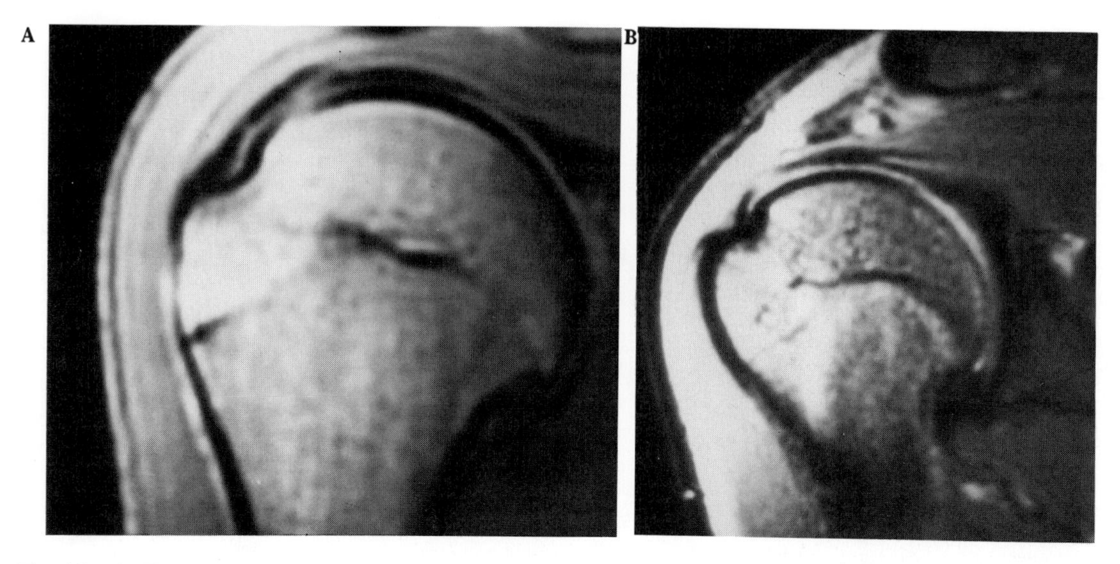

Fig. 4.8 (**A**) The rotator cuff is intact and continuous with a normal supraspinatous muscle. (**B**) There is high signal within the rotator cuff due to oedema. There is no retraction of the musculotendinous junction.

sheath cannot be diagnosed adequately on MRI and plain films are essential prior to the investigation. MRI is likely to become the principal method of examination of the shoulder but the quality of images is variable at the present time due to difference in surface coil systems. Further work on this aspect will lead to improvements.

WRIST

Trauma is a frequent indication for imaging the wrist and a careful clinical examination with high-quality plain X-rays is often all that is necessary to diagnose or exclude a fracture. Advanced imaging methods may be required if the injury is complex or involves only the soft tissues. Scintigraphy with technetium 99 methlyene diphosphonate (Tc99 MDP) provides a very accurate demonstration of occult bone damage and, if positive, CT may identify the locality of a subtle fracture, particularly those involving the hook of hamate (Norman et al 1985) and injury to the distal radioulnar articulation (Mino et al 1985). The role of CT in soft-tissue injury is limited. Abnormal movement patterns or alignment of the carpal bones such as rotational subluxation of the scaphoid or dorsal and volar intercalated segmental instability may be seen on dynamic plain films or video but arthrography is the gold standard for diagnosis of intercarpal ligament disruption (Fig. 4.9). Recent technical improvements include fluoroscopic video recording of the injection (Gilula et al 1987) and digital subtraction imaging (Resnick et al 1984) to show the passage of contrast through the ligamentous disruption. Some tears, however, have only been demonstrated by injecting the intercarpal or radioulnar joints and three compartment injection techniques have recently advocated (Zinberg et al 1988).

The examination of the wrist by MRI has received less attention than the spine or the knee, as the detail required is greater. However, development of a specific dual-surface coil array with off-axis imaging has improved resolution significantly (Zlatkin et al 1989a). The ligamentous structures consist of low-signal bands and the plane of imaging that identifies them best will depend on their alignment, but both coronal and sagittal views are often required. When normal, they appear as a continuous band on at least two contiguous images, whereas a tear appears as a distinct area of discontinuity within the ligament with increased signal intensity on T2 weighted images or a complete absence of the ligament. Using these criteria to diagnose scapholunate tears, Zlatkin et al (1989a)

A

B

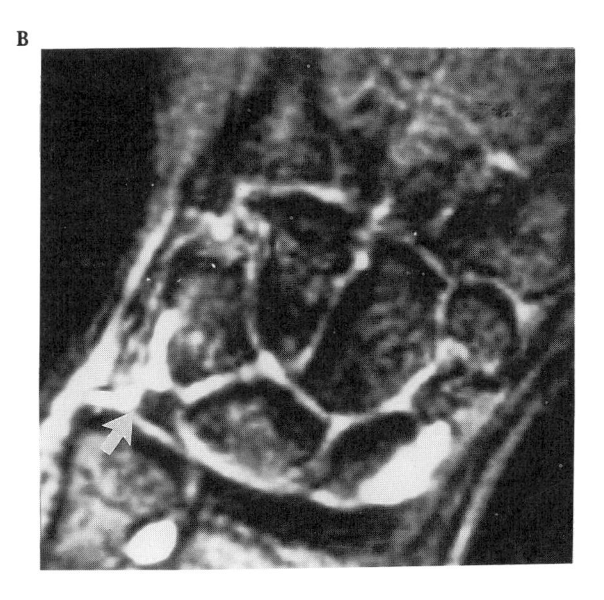

Fig. 4.9 (**A**) Wrist arthrogram showing contrast outlining the articular surfaces of all three wrist compartments, indicating a rupture in the proximal ring of intercarpal ligaments. (**B**) T2 weighted gradient echo image of wrist showing the triangular cartilage (low signal) separated from the ulna (arrow) and an effusion (high signal) in the joint and in the radioulnar joint.

have reported a sensitivity of 0.93, specificity 0.89 and an accuracy of 0.95 in comparison with arthrography on 41 patients, and an accuracy of 0.95 for a retrospective evaluation in a smaller group of 20 cases who underwent arthrotomy or arthroscopy. Lunatotriquetral tears have proven more difficult to diagnose but high accuracy levels are still reported and in a small series, tears of the volar radiocarpal ligaments have also clearly demonstrated.

Disruption of the triangular fibrocartilage, which has a low signal intensity, appears as a linear band of increased signal intensity of T1 near the radial insertion site of the disc and high signal intensity on T2 weighted images. Partial tears have also been described as irregularity and thinning of the inferior surface on T1 weighted images. Accuracy levels of 95% for complete ruptures are reported but partial tears were not confirmed by surgery or arthroscopy.

MRI has also been found to be valuable for diagnosis of other tendon abnormalities such as tenosynovitis and ganglion of formation, especially using gadolinium diethylenetriamine pentacetic acid (DTPA) to enhance the inflammatory tissue (Fig. 4.10). Evaluation of the tendons and median nerve in carpal tunnel syndrome, which is commonly due to a volumetric increase within the carpal canal secondary to synovitis of the flexor tendons, may prove to be a valuable use of this technique (Middleton et al 1987).

HIP

The hip is adequately assessed on the plain films, in most cases due to the close apposition of the articular surfaces in this ball-and-socket joint. However, the acetabulum is a complex bone and this is well demonstrated on CT, particularly with multiplanar reconstruction. In the neonate, however, the poorly ossified femoral head can only be assessed by the overall relationship of the femur to the pelvis, or by arthrography. Sonography, however, shows the cartilaginous femoral head effectively, and is the most accurate non-invasive imaging modality for identifying congenital dislocation of the hip in the period up to 6 months of age (Harke et al 1984, Novick 1988) and the real-time

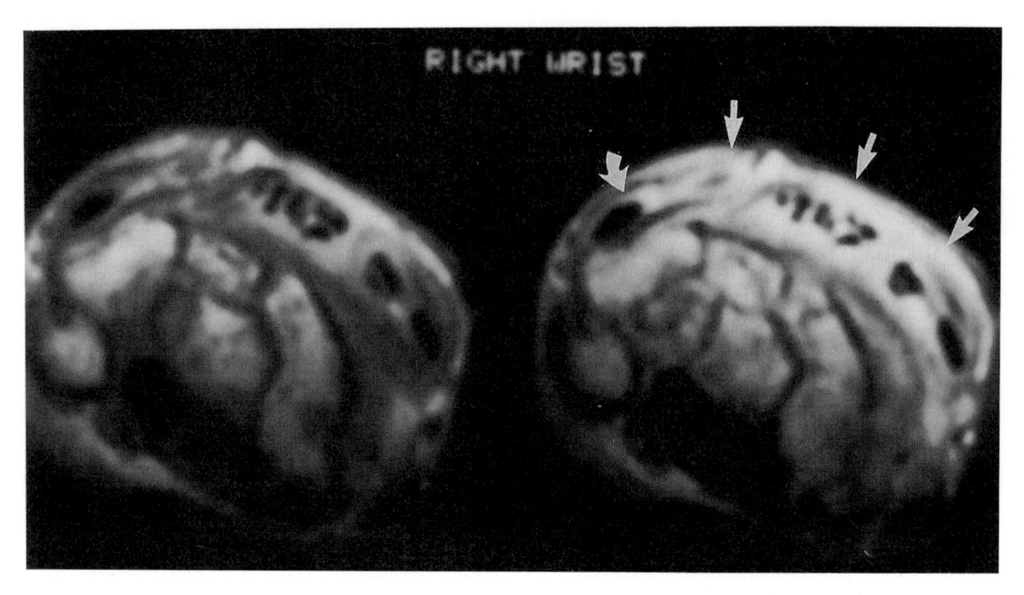

Fig. 4.10 Axial T1 weighted image of the wrist before and after gadolinium DTPA. The intermediate signal intensity of the tendon sheath of the extensor tendons is seen to become a high-intensity signal after enhancement (arrows) due to the extensive inflammation. The flexor tendons are clearly seen in the carpal tunnel.

assessment of joint movement is very valuable. CT has, however, proved to be of value in demonstrating the anteroposterior relationship of the head to the acetabulum, particularly after reduction and in plaster (Hernandez 1984) and three-dimensional imaging with CT and MRI may prove to be useful in the more complex cases (Lang et al 1989). Sonography is also of value to demonstrate enlarged bursae around joints and in particular the popliteal cysts and psoas bursa (Fig. 4.11). Effusions within the hip are difficult to assess on plain films and sonography has been accurate in their demonstra-

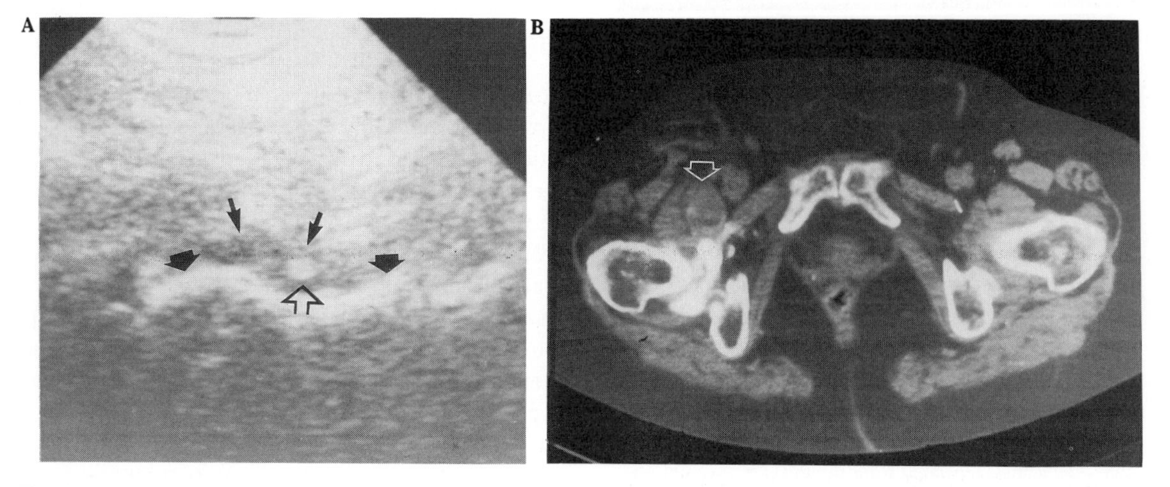

Fig. 4.11 (**A**) Sonography of the hip shows the echogenic femoral cortex (➧) and above this an oval echo-poor zone which is the enlarged psoas bursa (→). Within the bursa lies a small round echogenic lesion (⇨) which is hypertrophied synovium. (**B**) The CT scan shows the enlarged bursa with some thickening of the wall (arrow).

tion, particularly in cases of irritable hip syndrome in childhood (Wilson et al 1984).

Scintigraphy using a pinhole collimator is of value in identifying avascular necrosis of the femoral head in both children and adults and MRI has also been identified as a valuable diagnostic tool in the early demonstration of avascular necrosis. The normal femoral head has a high-to-intermediate signal on T1 due to the presence of marrow surrounded by the low signal of the cortical and subarticular bone. In early avascular necrosis there is a loss of signal from the marrow which becomes dark. Studies suggest that these findings are more sensitive than isotopes (Thickman et al 1986) and may be seen in patients at risk, such as those on steroids, even when the joints are asymptomatic (Mitchell et al 1988). CT with multiplanar reconstruction is of value to demonstrate the areas of fragmentation, sclerosis and subchondral collapse and to assess the overall shape of the head in relation to the acetabulum.

SPINE

CT has had a profound effect on the imaging of the spine. The wide tissue differentiation has enabled the dural sac, disc and ligaments to be visualized without the use of contrast medium. The ability to image the spine transaxially provides a true assessment of the canal dimensions and their relationship of canal shape to its contents. The presence of epidural fat enhances the differentiation of the canal's soft-tissue contents; this is good in the lumbar spine but less effective in the thoracic and cervical spine, where the nerve roots are difficult to visualize individually. Furthermore, the cord and intradural nerve roots cannot be defined within the dural sac and therefore an intradural tumour or compression can only be inferred by its effect on dural sac dimensions or if intrathecal contrast is used. CT is, however, excellent at depicting the vertebral bodies; bony foramina, intradiscal gas and calcification are easily visualized and differentiated.

MRI resolves many of these problems. In particular, the delineation of the cord and nerve roots within the dural sac is achieved without the use of contrast and the substance of the cord can also be fully analysed. Although the nerve roots are best demonstrated if surrounded by fat on T1 weighted images, the absence of fat is less of a problem as the cerebrospinal fluid in the nerve root sleeves can be utilized as a contrast medium due to its high signal on the T2 weighted images (Fig. 4.12). MRI has one further main advantage in that unlike CT, it can differentiate the nucleus pulposus from the annulus due to the higher water content of the former, which has a bright signal on the T2 weighted images. Thus early degeneration of the disc which results from a reduction on proteoglycans, and therefore in water content, can be demonstrated by T2 weighted images (see Fig. 4.15). Intradiscal calcification cannot, however, be differentiated from air as both have a low signal intensity.

A

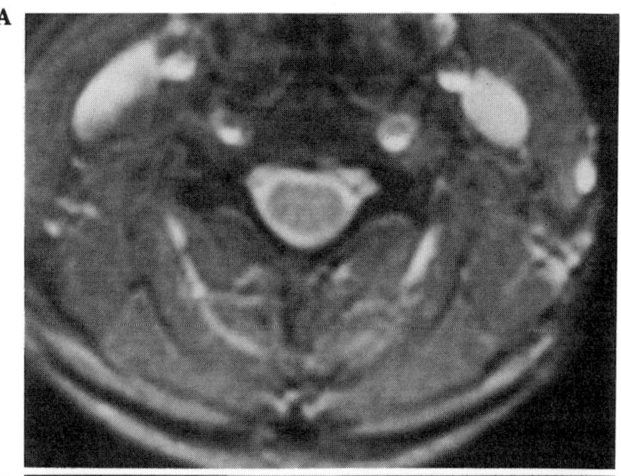

B

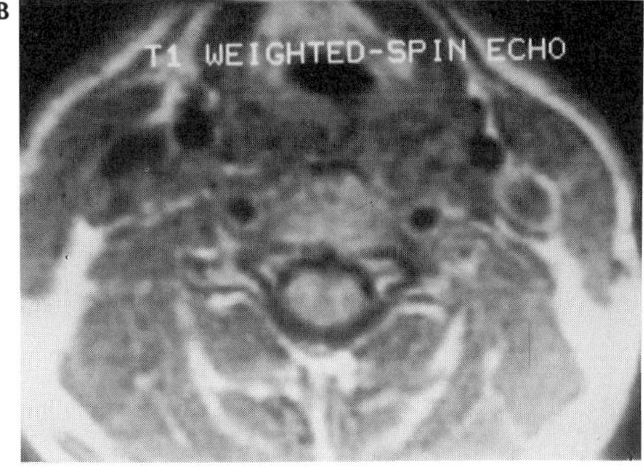

Fig. 4.12 Transaxial MR images of the cervical spine. The white and grey matter of the cord can be differentiated by the higher-intensity signal of the grey matter. The cord is surrounded by cerebrospinal fluid which is high-signal on the (**A**) T2 weighted image and (**B**) low-signal on T1. The nerve roots are seen surrounded by high signal on both T2 and T1 due to cerebrospinal fluid in the former and epidural fat in the latter.

MRI can directly image the spine in any plane, although the sagittal and transaxial planes are the most commonly used. Spinal CT images can only be acquired in the transaxial plane but by reconstructing parallel slices over a block of tissue, images can be produced in any plane. However, the anatomical detail is not as good as MRI. The highlight mode on CT can be used to provide a myelographic effect, although the cord still cannot be identified separately (Fig. 4.13).

A

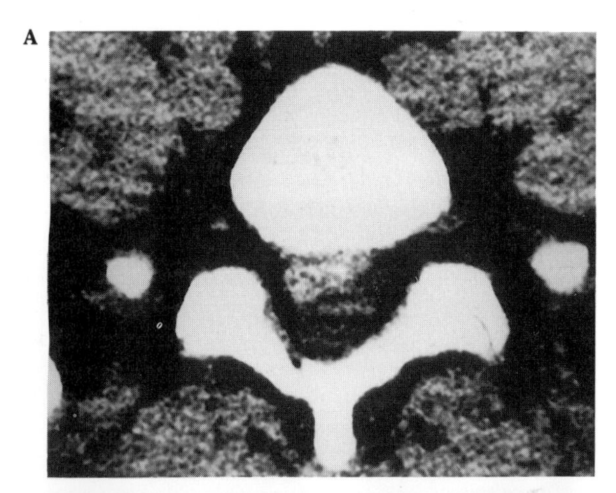

B

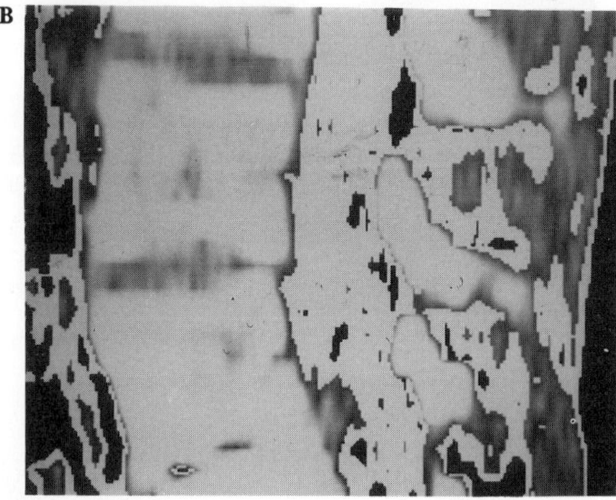

Fig. 4.13 (**A**) Axial CT: the higher attenuation of the herniated disc fragment is seen compressing the dural sac. The increased attenuation is in part due to some calcification within the prolapsed nuclear tissue. The loss of continuity with the disc and the sharp angled outline suggest sequestration and migration. (**B**) This is confirmed on the sagittal reconstruction, which shows the highlighted cerebrospinal fluid and the indentation of the dura behind the body of L5 and L5/S1 disc space.

Herniation of nucleus pulposus

Diagnosis of nucleus pulposus herniation with nerve root compression has been achieved using myelography for many years with a satisfactory level of accuracy, although reports have varied from 70 to 97% (Holmes & Rothman 1979, Herkowitz et al 1982, Jackson et al 1989). Disc herniation at the L5/S1 level may prove difficult if the epidural space is wide or the dural sac is short. Myelography also involves a lumbar puncture and postmyelographic headaches are not uncommon: the extent of the diagnostic zone is that of the dural sac and nerve root sleeves. Thus the diagnostic accuracy of nerve root compression due to nerve root canal and foraminal stenosis is low (Stockley et al 1988). Myelography does, however, have some value in the assessment of cerebrospinal flow in cases of severe spinal stenosis.

CT has now substantially replaced myelography in most centres as nuclear herniation and nerve root compression can be clearly demonstrated and migration of disc fragments lying away from the disc behind the vertebral body can be defined, particularly using the reconstruction mode with highlighting (Fig. 4.12). Accuracy rates of 92% have been reported (Freis et al 1982, Teplick & Haskin 1983), although Bell et al (1984) and Jackson et al (1989) found lower levels of 79 and 74% accuracy respectively of unenhanced CT.

The main area of diagnostic inaccuracy with CT lies in differentiating a bulging annulus from a true disc protrusion. A smooth convex curve, which also extends around the lateral margins, indicates an annular bulge but assessment of the degree of nerve root compression may sometimes be difficult, although sagittal reconstructions may be helpful. CT cannot easily differentiate between disc protrusion and extrusion or between the latter and sequestration without migration. The main disadvantage, however, lies in the fact that the lower cord is not visualized and tumours of the conus medullaris or intrathecal nerve roots, which can mimic herniated disc prolapses, may be missed. The routine use of low doses of intrathecal contrast with CT has been advocated to obviate these problems but this reintroduces the need for a lumbar puncture with its associated side-effects.

MRI resolves some of these problems. The disc

prolapse can be clearly demonstrated in both the sagittal and transaxial plane on both T1 and T2 weighted scans and nerve root compression can be diagnosed (Fig. 4.14) The posterior fibres of the annulus and the posterior longitudinal ligament are visualized as a low signal on T1 and T2 and thus a break in this line will differentiate a protruded from an extruded nucleus (Fig. 4.15). Accuracy of MRI in relation to radiculography has been reported as 88% against 75% (Szypryt et al 1988) and in relation to CT myelography as 90.3% against 77.4% (Forristall et al 1988).

A high accuracy for diagnosis of herniated nucleus pulposus is, however, dependent on the close correlation of clinical and radiological findings as radiologically demonstrable herniations have been demonstrated in 20% of asymptomatic subjects (Hiltselberger & Witten 1968, Wiesel et al 1984). Finally, the spinal cord can be imaged routinely and tumours of the conus are easily diagnosed (Fig. 4.16), although even with this technique they may occasionally not be visualized (Epstein et al 1989). Intradiscal nerve roots can also be seen and arachnoiditis may be demonstrated as clumping of the nerve roots without the need for myelography (Fig. 4.17).

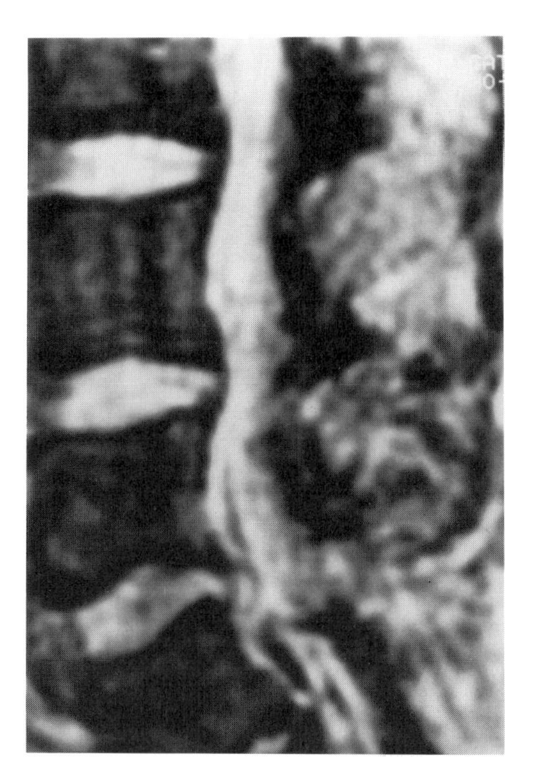

Fig. 4.14 The sagittal T2 weighted image shows an acute nuclear protrusion at L5/S1, which has the high signal of hydrated nuclear material outlined by the low signal of the intact outer rim of annulus.

Spinal stenosis

A major advantage of the transaxial nature of CT is that the true area of the canal can be demonstrated and central stenosis diagnosed by measuring the area of the dural sac. This is normally 1.45 cm^2 but is considered clinically stenotic below 0.75 cm^2 (Schonstrom et al 1984). The entry and midzone of the nerve root canal (Lee et al 1988a) can be followed carefully and stenosis compressing the nerve root due to hypertrophy of the lamina or superior articular process can be measured — 3 mm is taken as the lower level of normal (Mikhael et al 1981). Nerve root compression by bone or soft tissue in the foramina is best demonstrated with sagittal reconstruction and both front/back and cranio/caudal stenosis may be seen (Fig. 4.18). The accuracy of CT has been extensively assessed, although again with a varying range from 79 to 89% (Bell et al 1984, Modic et al 1986a). The assessment of lateral recess stenosis was less accurate—75% (Stockley et al 1988)—but this study did not use sagittal reconstructions. MRI also demonstrates central spinal stenosis and narrowing of the nerve root canals on the transaxial scans and the more peripheral sagittal slices will demonstrate foraminal narrowing. Alghouth the bony definition is less clear on MRI, comparison studies with CT have shown very high correlation between the two techniques (Schnebel et al 1989).

Failed back surgery

Despite high preoperative diagnostic accuracy for disc prolapse, some patients still fail to benefit from operation. Careful evaluation prior to further treatment is essential. In the past important control studies on asymptomatic postoperative patients have not been available but CT in the immediate postoperative period in this group shows a clearly delineated uniform shadow of 60–85 HU protruding into the canal in nearly 50% of patients,

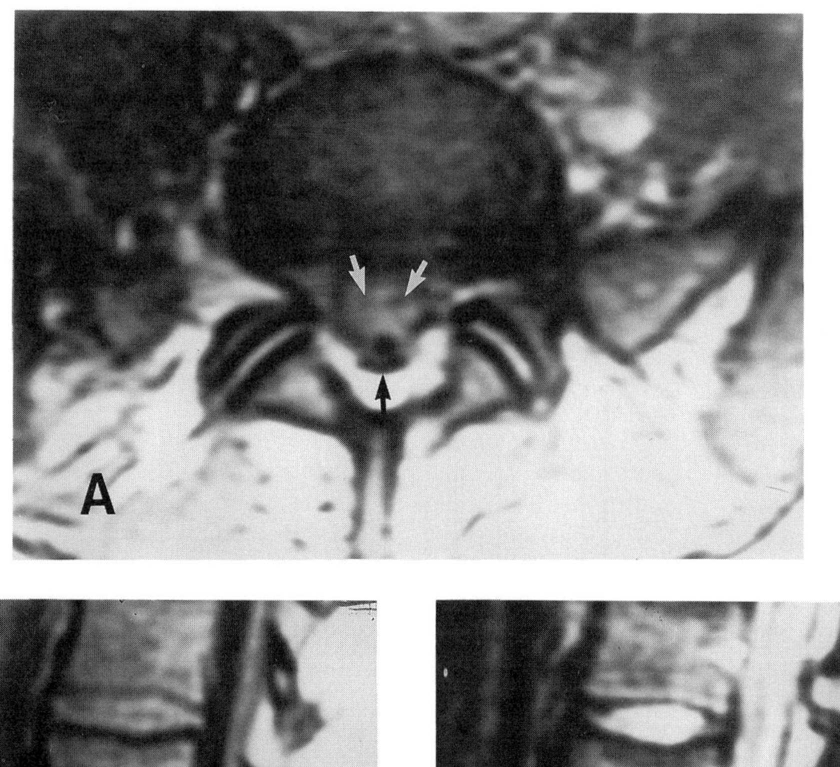

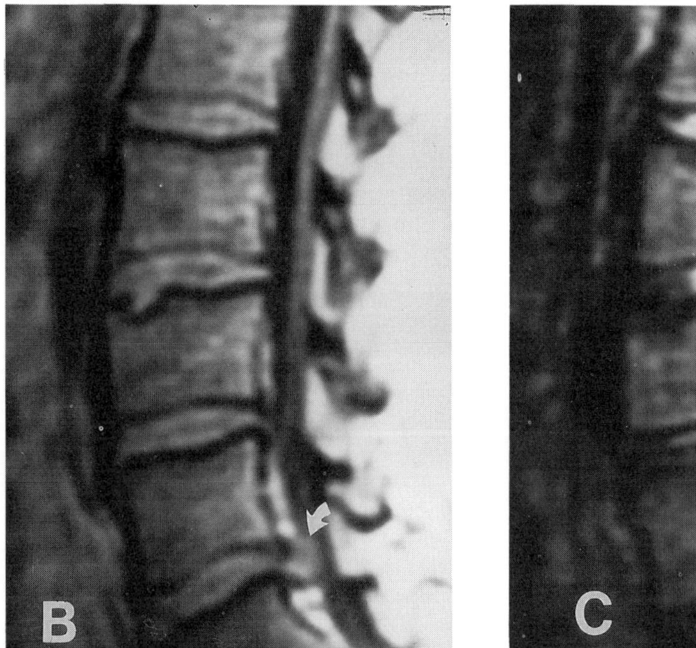

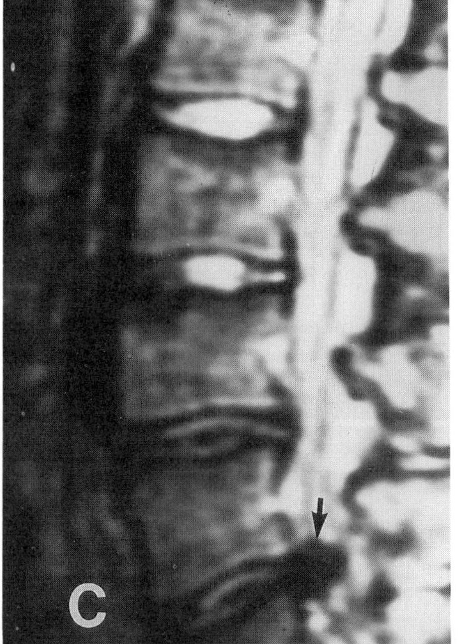

Fig. 4.15 A large nuclear herniation of long standing (white arrows) shows considerable narrowing of the dural sac (black arrow) on (**A**) the axial and (**B**) sagittal images at L5/S1. The prolapse has broken through the low-signal outer annular fibres (white curved arrow) and is also of low signal on (**C**) the T2 weighted image (black arrow), indicating a long-standing degenerate fragment. The signal from the lower two discs is markedly reduced on T2 due to degeneration and loss of hydration. A small anterior interosseous disc herniation is seen at L3/4.

suggesting persistent disc herniation. In 84% new heterogeneous material was present due to haematoma, which evolves gradually into scar tissue without significant alteration of shape (Montaldi et al 1988). Care must therefore be taken when diagnosing persistent disc herniation in patients

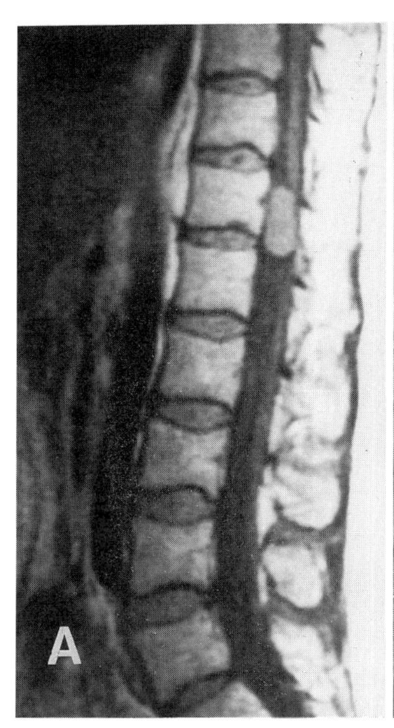

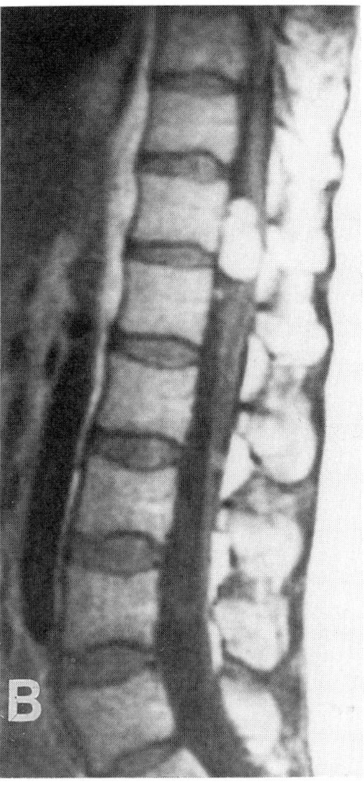

Fig. 4.16 (**A**) The conus is compressed at T12 by a large ependymoma which enhances after injection of gadolinium DTPA (**B**).

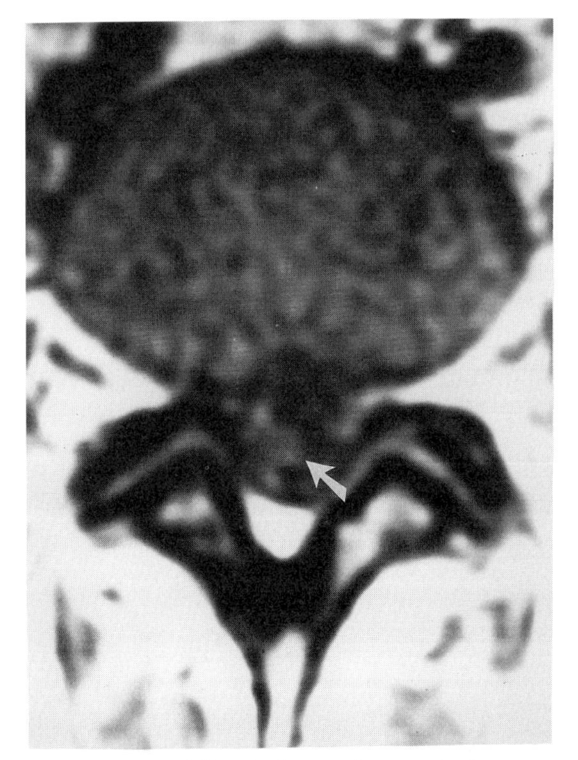

Fig. 4.17 Arachnoiditis—the intermediate signal of a group of nerve roots matted together and situated laterally in the dural sac is surrounded by the low signal of the cerebrospinal fluid on the T1 weighted axial scans.

with poor surgical results in the early postoperative period. Recurrence of symptoms may be due to a further disc herniation, but epidural fibrosis may also be a cause of persistent symptoms.

CT and MRI are both able to demonstrate epidural fibrosis. In the former there are diffuse areas of tissue of lower attenuation than the disc which obliterate the epidural fat and distort the dural sac. Enhancement often occurs with intravenous contrast media (Fig. 4.19; Dixon & Bannon 1987). In MRI the scar is hypo-or isointense on T1 weighted spin echo and hyperintense on T2 relative to the annulus intensity (Bundschuh et al 1988b). Scar formation has also been shown to enhance on T1 weighted images after the injection of gadolinium DTPA (Heuftle et al 1988) (Fig. 4.20), although images should be undertaken soon after the injection as disc tissue will gradually enhance after a period of time. Recurrent disc prolapse on MRI will appear as either hypo- or isointense with annulus on T1 and T2 sequences, but may have a rim of enhancement. MRI correlation with surgery showed accuracy levels of 96% (Ross et al 1990). Frocrain et al (1990) found a much lower concordance with surgery using CT than MRI: 44 of 45

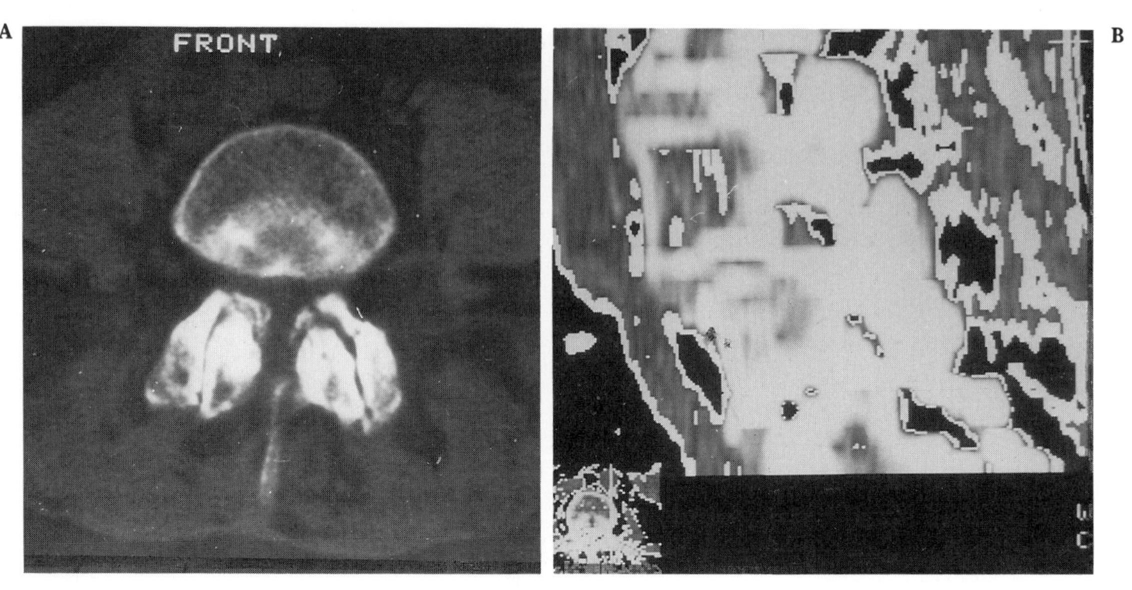

Fig. 4.18 (**A**) Osteoarthritis of the facets, with bony hypertrophy of the articular processes, has resulted in central spinal stenosis. (**B**) A sagittal reconstruction of lower lumbar CT scan shows front–back narrowing of the L5/S1 foramen.

patients correlated with surgical findings with MRI.

It is important to differentiate recurrent disc herniation from epidural fibrosis as the quantity and severity of fibrosis was similar in a comparative group of symptomatic and asymptomatic postoperative subjects, indicating that epidural fibrosis per se is not a major cause of the failure after back surgery (Cervellini et al 1988).

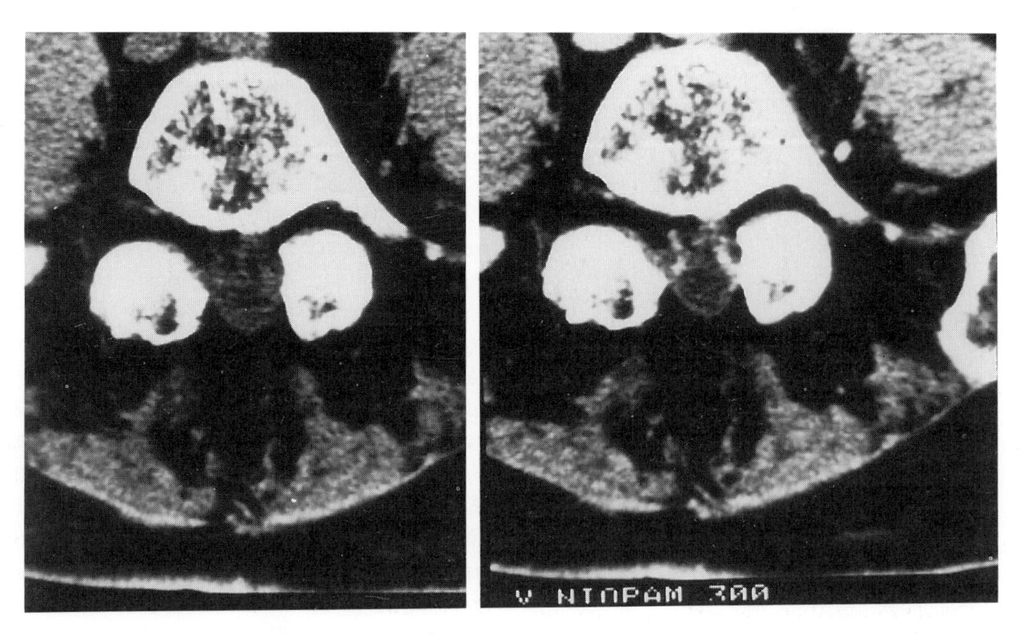

Fig. 4.19 The areas of fibrosis around the dural sac are clearly demonstrated after enhancement with intravenous iodinated contrast medium.

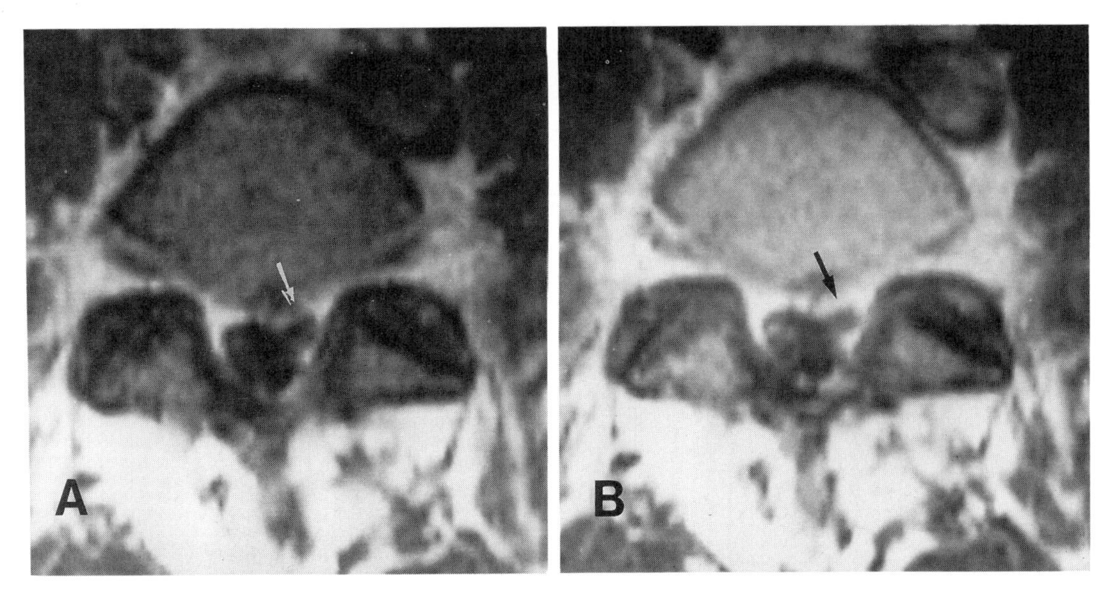

Fig. 4.20 (**A**) There is a low-density mass in the left lateral recess on T1 weighted image (arrow). (**B**) After gadolinium DTPA there is marked enhancement in this region with a high-intensity signal due to fibrosis surrounding the low-intensity signal of this nerve root (arrow).

Cervical spine

Cervical radiculography with water-soluble contrast medium accurately demonstrates the cervical nerve roots and cord and compression can be visualized very clearly. It does not differentiate between a plain disc herniation and degenerative osteophyte formation but this may be surmised from the plain films or more accurately by undertaking CT as an integral part of the examination. The combined examination has a reported accuracy of 92% (Modic et al 1986b). CT alone does not define the nerve roots clearly due to the absence of epidural fat, but narrowing of the foramina by osteophyte formation is clearly defined and reconstruction of the axial images in the oblique plane may improve visualization further. The diagnosis of cord or nerve root compression can, however, be achieved by MRI without the use of intrathecal contrast medium. The initial results suggested that MRI was less accurate than CT/myelography with only 74% (29/39) agreement between the findings and surgery (Modic et al 1986), although the main inaccuracy lay in defining the type of compression (bone versus soft tissue) rather than the level. The use of gradient echo T2 weighted scans which provide an excellent myelographic effect, demonstrating the cord and dural sac, will clearly differentiate disc material from osteophyte as the compressive force (Fig. 4.21); Kulkarni et al 1988). Three-dimensional imaging may also improve the demonstration and differentiation of low-intensity osteophyte and high-intensity disc and of foraminal stenosis by enabling contiguous slices with an improved signal-to-noise ratio to be produced (Tsuruda et al 1990).

An uncomplicated disc prolapse will also be clearly demonstrated on the T1 weighted sagittal scan but its precise relationship with the dural sac is more difficult to evaluate as posterior vertebral cortex, longitudinal ligament and cerebrospinal fluid in the dural sac all have a very low signal intensity on this imaging sequence (Fig. 4.21). MRI will also demonstrate the compression of the dural sac and cord by the posterior elements such as hypertrophy of the ligamentum flavum or degenerative changes in the facet joints. In these circumstances, the cord is pinched between the anterior disc and osteophyte and the posterior elements (Fig. 4.21). This is demonstrable on myelography and on axial CT without intrathecal contrast with the assistance of sagittal reconstruction of the CT images.

While highlighting can demonstrate the narrow-

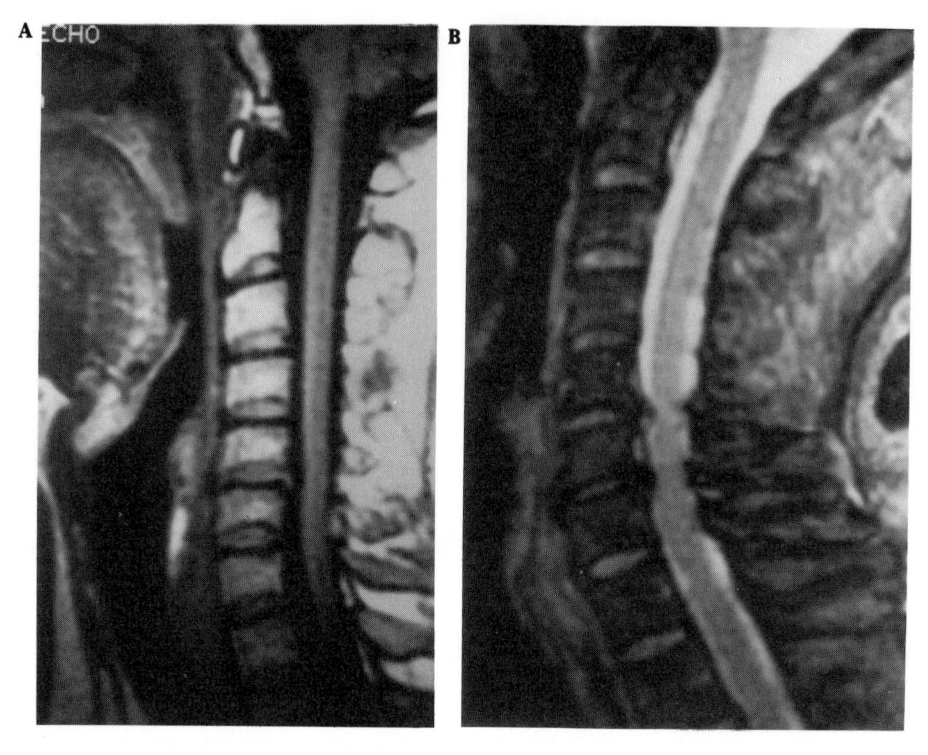

Fig. 4.21 (**A**) Sagittal MRI of cervical spine. The T1 weighted image shows intermediate signal of the disc prolapse at C5/6. The relationship with the cord is difficult to assess. (**B**) A T2 gradient echo scan on a different patient shows a disc prolapse at C5/6, with an intermediate signal differentiated from an osteophyte at C6/7 with a low signal. The ligamentum flavum hypertrophy and bony indentation of the canal posteriorly are well shown and the degree of compression of the cerebrospinal fluid and cord is clearly demonstrated.

ing effect on the dural sac it cannot demonstrate the cord directly. Although MRI is sensitive for the demonstration of disc lesions and neural compression, such abnormalities can be present in asymptomatic subjects: severe or moderate-sized lesions are present in 14% of subjects younger than 40 and 28% of those over 40. Of all asymptomatic subjects, 8% had a herniated disc and 9% had foraminal stenosis. Significant cord compression was present at 9% of disc levels in the over-40 age group (Boden et al 1990). Careful clinical correlation with MRI findings is therefore essential.

The value of MRI is particularly pronounced in patients with rheumatoid arthritis where the evaluation of cord compression has always been difficult as the patients are often unable to tolerate myelography. In these cases the cord may be compressed by granulation tissue and/or instability at either or both the atlantoaxial and subaxial levels. MRI can demonstrate the granulation tissue around the odontoid process as an intermediate signal on T1 weighted images and an increased signal on T2 spin echo images (Pettersson et al 1988) which may also enhance with gadolinium. A clinical myelopathy and/or significant delay in central motor latency has been shown to relate on MRI to a cord width of 6 mm or a canal diameter of 9.5 mm in flexion (Dvorak et al 1989). The relationship of the odontoid to the cord is also clearly defined and distortion of the cervicomedullary region with the angulation reduced to less than 135° may correlate with neurological symptoms (Fig. 4.22, Bundschuh et al 1988a).

Spinal trauma

Conventional radiography has been employed successfully for many years to evaluate spinal fractures and remains the initial investigation, although CT has now become an invaluable adjunct for detailed

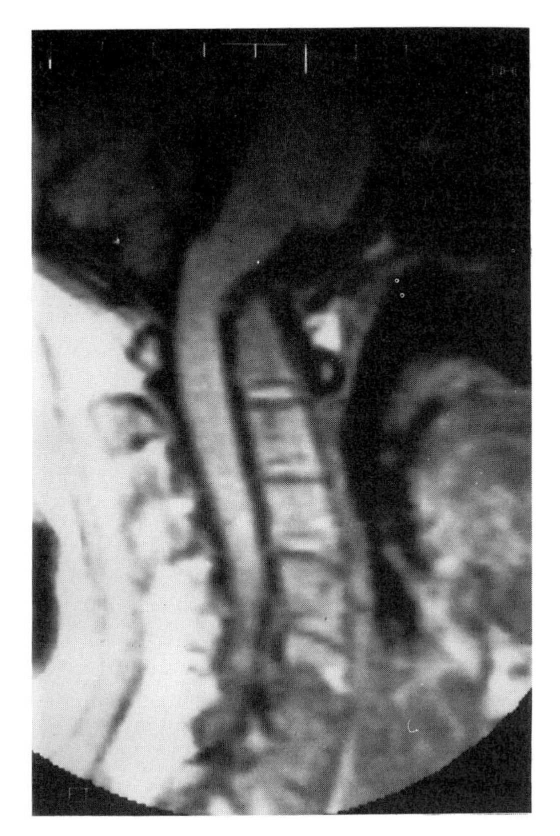

Fig. 4.22 Rheumatoid arthritis. There is upward subluxation of C2 with erosion of the odontoid. The cervicomedullary junction is compressed and the angle is 112°.

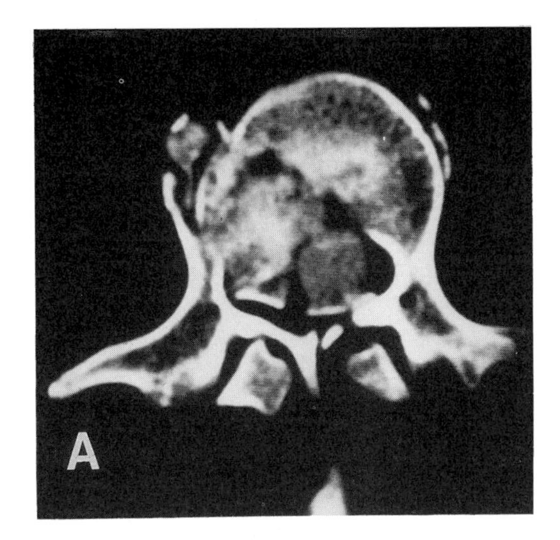

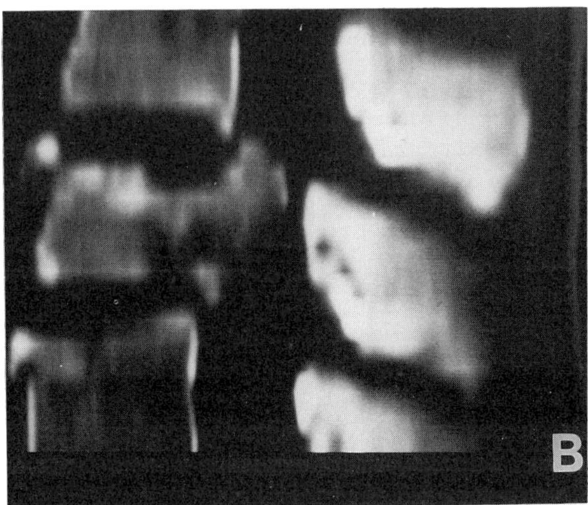

Fig. 4.23 The extent of fragmentation of the vertebral body is well shown on CT. (**A**) The lamina and pedicle base are fractured. (**B**) The extent of encroachment on the canal is seen on the transaxial scans and sagittal reconstruction.

assessment and classification of the fractures (Denis 1984, Ferguson & Allen 1984). Compression or wedge fractures represent a failure of the anterior column and are due to hyperflexion injuries. They are well demonstrated on plain films and usually do not require CT, except at the cervicothoracic junction where sagittal reconstructions may assist visualization. Axial compression or 'burst' fractures represent a failure of both anterior and middle columns and CT is particularly valuable to identify displaced fragments in the neural canal and associated lamina fractures with separation of the pedicles, which may affect subsequent stability and increase the risks of further neurological damage (McAffee et al 1983, Shuman et al 1985; Fig. 4.23). Sagittal and three-dimensional reconstruction will give an excellent overall view of the relationship of the fragments to the remainder of the canal. Dislocation with or without fractures is usually seen on plain films in the cervical and thoracolumbar spine but posterior column fractures of the lamina and lateral mass may be difficult to appreciate and CT is often invaluable to identify small loose fragments which may hinder reduction. CT does not, however, visualize the cord but this is now possible with MRI. Acute intraspinal haemorrhage appears as a reduced signal on T1 weighted images within 24 h of injury due to the presence of deoxyhaemoglobin which is also hypointense on T2 (Beers et al 1988). Cord contusion and oedema have a high signal intensity on T2 weighted images

(Fig. 4.24; Beers et al 1988). In the later stages of acute intraspinal haemorrhage, a central area of hypointensity is surrounded by an area of hyperintensity, due to the formation of methaemoglobin. The T1 images are often unremarkable but may show cord enlargement due to swelling.

Kulkarni et al (1987) have suggested that a significant degree of neurological recovery occurred with cord contusion or oedema but not with the haemorrhage pattern. Soft-tissue injuries outside the spinal cord will also be seen in the acute phase as high-intensity areas on T2 weighted images, due to oedema or haemorrhage (Fig. 4.24). MRI may be particularly valuable in patients with hyperextension injuries, where often little is seen on the radiograph or CT scan. Goldberg et al (1989) found prevertebral haematomas in all cases; these were hyperintense on T2 weighted images and also demonstrated features of cord compression, due to cervical spondylosis and central cord contusion.

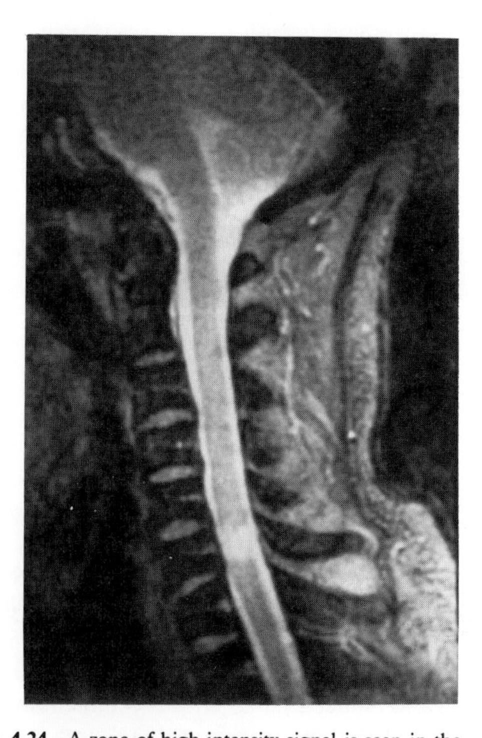

Fig. 4.24 A zone of high-intensity signal is seen in the cervical cord on this T2 weighted image, indicative of oedema due to cord injury. There is also high-intensity signal from the interspinous ligament at the same level, consistent with a hyperflexion rupture.

MUSCULOSKELETAL TUMOURS

With the advent of endoprosthetic replacement and sophisticated oncological treatment, the detailed imaging of all musculoskeletal tumours has become a matter of major importance.

Both CT and MRI have proven to be of great value in the detection, staging and characterization of bone tumours and they also play a significant role in the follow-up period. Soft-tissue masses can be diagnosed extending from bone lesions by both techniques but the better soft-tissue contrast resolution of MRI makes it more appropriate (Fig. 4.25). The rationale for treatment regimes depends on the extent and spread of the disease and needs to be accurately delineated. MRI provides a more reliable assessment of marrow involvement in primary bone tumours (Fig. 4.23), such as osteosarcoma and Ewing's sarcoma, when compared to scintigraphy or CT (Berquist 1987, Pettersson et al 1987). Fat suppression techniques may be of particular value. Involvement of neurovascular tissue can be established by both techniques, although intravenous contrast enhancement may be required with CT. Tumour matrix calcification and ossification, while clearly seen on CT, may be undetectable on MR. Cortical destruction is best assessed with CT.

Soft-tissue masses may be surprisingly difficult to define on clinical examination, particularly from body lesions such as exostosis or diffuse lesions such as muscle oedema. Sonography, CT and MRI can all demonstrate soft-tissue lesions clearly and are particularly valuable in verifying the normal. In this regard, sonography is clearly the cheapest and most easily accessible technique, which makes it an ideal initial screening tool (Golding & Wilson 1988).

Some conditions have specific diagnostic characteristics. Lipomas are highly echogenic on sonography, have a well defined low attenuation on CT and have characteristic high-intensity signal on T1 and T2 (Dooms et al 1985). Haemangiomas show serpiginous fluid-filled cavities with clear-cut walls on sonography while established haematomas are echo-free. On MRI haemangiomas have a high signal on T2 weighted pulses and signal intensity equivalent to muscle on T1 with areas of fat interspersed (Cohen et al 1988; Fig. 4.26).

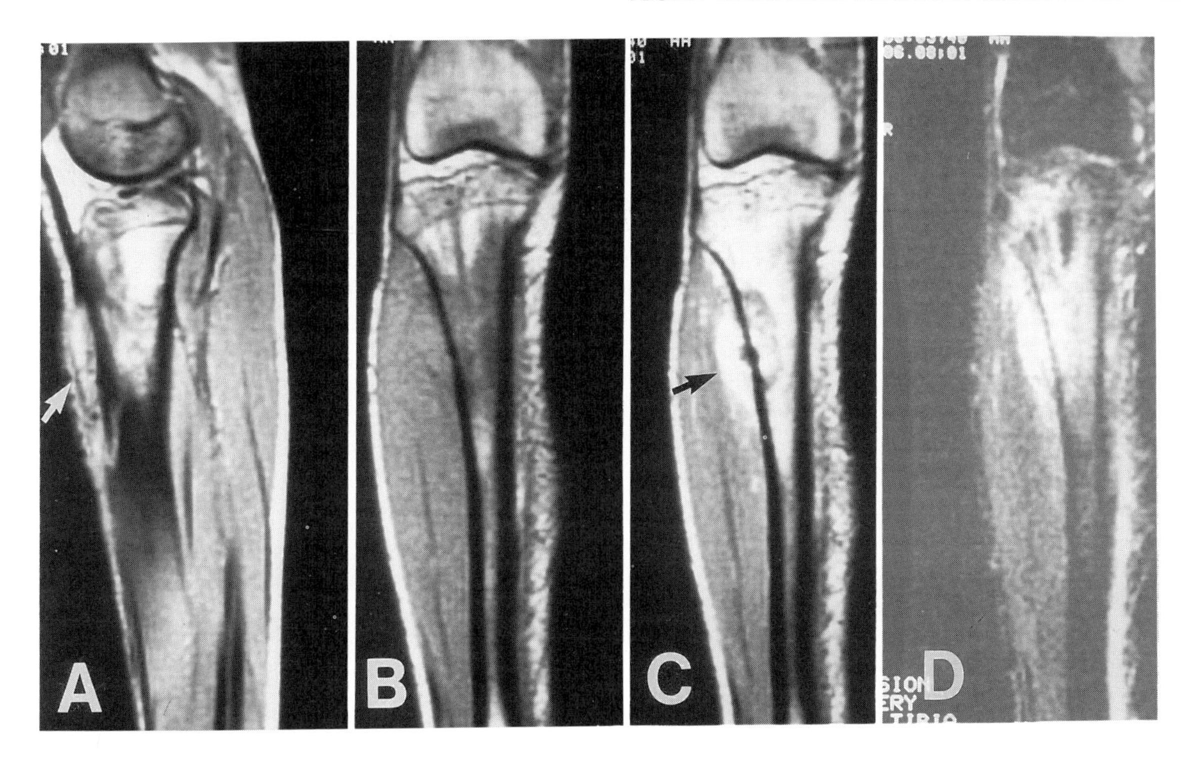

Fig. 4.25 An adamantinoma of the tibia is demonstrated. (**A**) The precontrast lateral shows a high-signal soft-tissue mass anterior to the tibia. The full extent of the marrow and soft-tissue involvement on the anteroposterior view (**B**) is only seen by the extensive increase in signal throughout the epiphysis and diaphysis (arrow) with (**C**) gadolinium enhancement or (**D**) on the fat-suppression sequence.

Haemorrhage in muscle can be clearly demonstrated on sonography as an echogenic mass or as a diffuse interdigitating material separating the normal herring-bone pattern of muscle (Wilson et al 1987). On MRI there is a characteristic increase in signal on both T1 and T2 (De Smet et al 1990). Myositis ossificans may be diagnosed very early by sonography before plain film changes appear and has a characteristic three-layer pattern with an echogenic ring in the mid layer on sonography (Fig. 4.27; Thomas et al 1991) The calcified ring may be seen early on CT but is difficult to image on MRI (Kransdof et al 1989). Soft-tissue masses, however, do not usually have features sufficiently characteristic to suggest a histological diagnosis and the images are more likely to reflect the underlying morphology of the lesion (fat content, cyst formation, haemorrhage etc.). There are also no clear features on MRI to differentiate benign from malignant lesions (Kransdorf et al 1989); a correct diagnosis of malignancy has been made in only 41%, although CT has been reported to be a better discriminator—88% of cases (Weekes et al 1985). Because of the absence of an MRI signal from calcification all scans should be interpreted with corresponding plain radiographs or CT scans.

CONCLUSIONS

This short review has highlighted the success of the newer diagnostic techniques and the dramatic recent developments in MRI. The absence of known biological hazards, the high level of tissue differentiation and spatial resolution and the ability to image in multiple planes have enabled MRI to become the dominant force in the imaging of the spine. For many peripheral joints, particularly the knee, it has substantially replaced the invasive contrast procedures, and its general use is only restricted by the availability of machines. CT remains an important investigation, in particular where bone lesions are present or when calcifica-

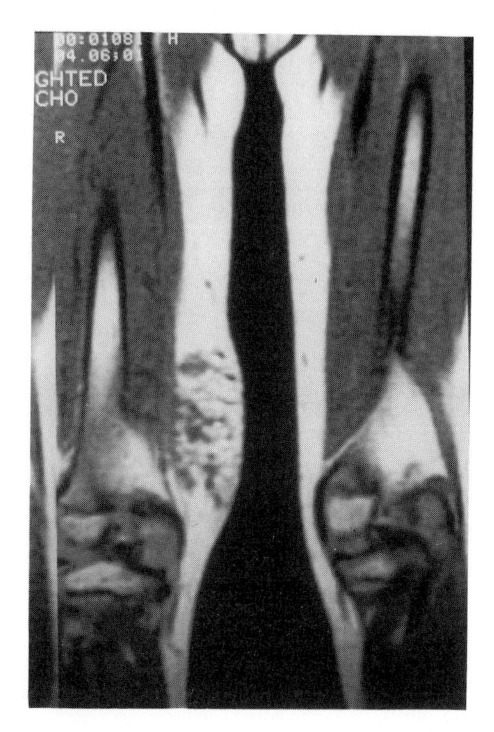

Fig. 4.26 The serpiginous pattern of the haemangioma has an intermediate signal on the T1 weighted images and is interposed by high-intensity signal of fat.

tion is suspected. Arthrography of the smaller joints is at the present time still occasionally required. The role of sonography is still disputed but it is of value in soft-tissue lesions and in the demonstration of joint effusions and ligamentous injury. In joints the anatomical detail is variable and it is very operator-dependent. It is, however, available in every imaging department, is inexpensive and may therefore be a useful initial investigation in these categories of disorders.

A

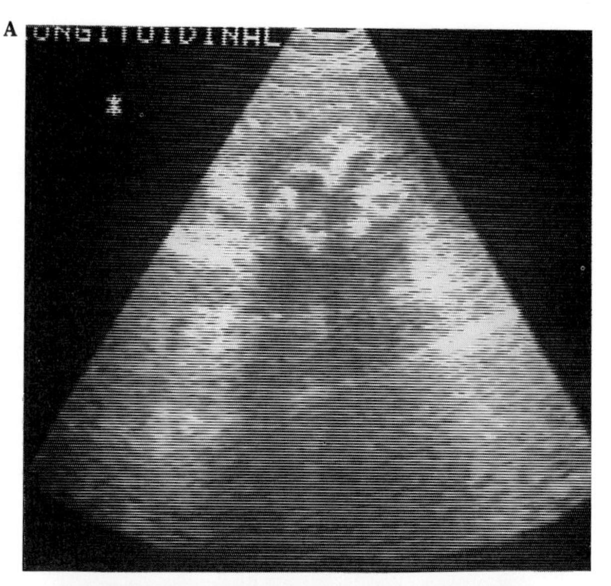

B

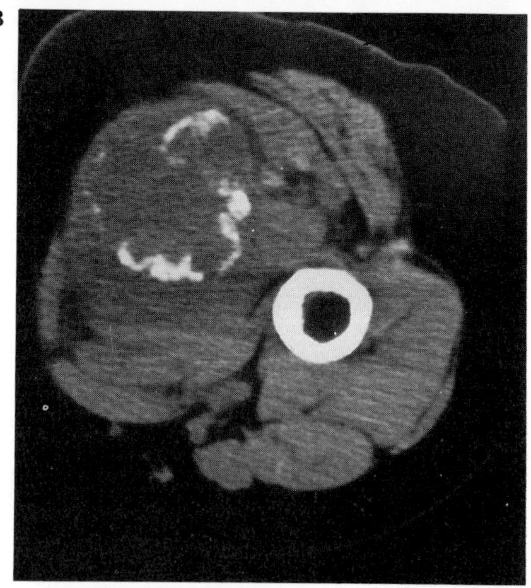

Fig. 4.27 (**A**) The sonographic zone of demarcation of heterotopic bone formation is clearly identified (3.5 MHz). The inner echo-poor core is surrounded by an undulating ring of reflective mineralized tissue, with an outer lucent zone adjacent to normal muscle. (**B**) The CT demonstrates an undulating zone of mature bone encompassing an area of uniformly reduced attenuation.

REFERENCES

Adam G, Bohndorf K, Drobnitzky K, Guenther RW 1989 MR imaging of the knee: three dimensional volume imaging combined with fast processing. J Computer Assist Tomogr 13:984–988

Beers GJ, Raque GH, Wagner GG et al 1988 MR imaging in acute cervical spine trauma. J Computer Assist Tomogr 12:755–761

Bell GR, Rothman RH, Booth RE 1984 A study of computer assisted tomography. A comparison of metrizamide myelography and computed tomography in the diagnosis of herniated lumbar disc and spinal stenosis. Spine 9:552–556

Berquist TH 1987 Bone and soft tissue tumours. In: Berquist TH, Ehman RL, Richardson ML (eds) Magnetic resonance of the musculo-skeletal system. Raven, New York, pp 85–108

Boden SC, McCowin PR, Davis DO et al 1990 Abnormal magnetic resonance scans of the cervical spine in asymptomatic subjects. J Bone Joint Surg 72A:1178–1184

Brandt TD, Cardone BW, Grant TH et al 1989 Rotator cuff sonography: a reassessment. Radiology 173:323–327

Bundschuh C, Modic MT, Kearney F et al 1988a.

Rheumatoid arthritis of the cervical spine: surface-coil MR imaging. AJR 151:181–188
Bundschuh CV, Modic MT, Ross JS et al 1988b Epidural fibrosis and recurrent disc herniation in the lumbar spine: MR imaging. Am J Neuroradiol 150:923–932
Burk DL, Karasick D, Kurtz AV et al 1989 Rotator cuff tears: prospective comparison of MR imaging with arthrography, sonography and surgery. AJR 153:87–92
Cervellini P, Curri D, Volpin L et al 1988 Computed tomography of epidural fibrosis after discectomy; a comparison between symptomatic and asymptomatic patients. Neurosurgery 23:710–713
Cohen EK, Cressel HY, Perosco T et al 1988 MR imaging of soft tissue haemangiomas correlation with pathological findings. AJR 150:1079–1081
Crass JR, Craig EV 1988 Non invasive imaging of the rotator cuff. Orthopaedics: 11:57–64
De Smet AA, Fisher DR, Heiner JR, Keene JS, 1990 Magnetic resonance imaging of muscle tears. Skeletal Radiol 19:283–286
Denis F 1984 Spinal instability as defined by the three column spine concept in acute spinal trauma. Clin Orthop 189:65–76
Dixon AK, Bannon RP 1987 Computer tomography of the postoperative lumbar spine: the need for optimal dose of intravenous contrast medium. Br J Radiol 60:215–222
Dooms GC, Hricak H, Sollitto RA, Higgins CB 1985 Lipomatous tumours and tumours with fatty component, MR imaging potential and comparison of MR and CT results. Radiology 157:479–483
Dvorak J, Grob D, Baumgartrer H et al 1989 Functional evaluation of the spinal cord by magnetic resonance imaging in patients with rheumatoid arthritis and instability of upper cervical spine. Spine 14:1057–1064
Epstein NE, Bhuchar S, Gavin R et al 1989 Failure to diagnose conus ependymomas by magnetic resonance imaging. Spine 14:134–137
Ferguson RL, Allen BL 1984 A mechanistic classification of thoracolumbar spine fractures. Clin Orthop 189:77–88
Fornage BD, Rifkin MD 1988 Ultrasound examination of tendons. Radiol Clin North Am 26:87–107
Forristall RM, Marsh HD, Pay NT 1988 Magnetic resonance imaging and contrast CT of the lumbar spine: comparison of diagnostic methods and correlation with surgical findings. Spine 13:1049–1054
Freis JW, Abodeely DA, Vijungco JG, Yeager VL, Gaftey W R 1982 Computed tomography of herniated extruded Nucleus pulposus. J Comput Assist Tomogr 6:874–887
Frocrain L, Duvauferrier R, Husson JL et al 1989 Recurrent post operative sciatica: evaluation with MR imaging and enhanced CT. Radiology 170:531–533
Gilula LA, Hardy DC, Tolty WG, Reinus WR 1987 Fluoroscopic identification of torn intercarpal ligaments after injection of contrast material. AJR 149:761–764
Glashow JL, Katz R, Schneider M, Scott WN 1989 Double blind assessment of the value of magnetic resonance imaging in the diagnosis of anterior cruciate and meniscal lesions. J Bone Joint Surg 71A:113–119
Goldberg AL, Rothfus WE, Deeb ZL et al 1989 Hyperextension injuries of the cervical spine. Skeletal Radiol 18:283–288
Golding SH, Wilson DJ 1988 The detection of soft tissue masses in limbs. Is CT reliable? Clin Radiol 39:345
Gompels BM, Darlington LG 1982 Evaluation of popliteal cysts and painful calves with ultrasonography. Comparison with arthrography. Ann Rheum Dis 41:355–359
Grover JS, Bassett LW, Gross ML et al 1990 Posterior cruciate ligament: MR imaging. Radiology 174:527–530
Harke HT, Clarke NMP, Lee MS 1984 Examination of the infant hip with real-time ultrasonography. J Ultrasound Med 3:131–137
Hartzman S, Reicher MA, Bassett LW et al MR imaging of the knee: part II. Chronic disorders 1987. Radiology 162:533–557
Herkowitz HN, Wiesel SW, Booth RE, Rothman RH 1982 Metrizamide myelography and epidural venography. Their role in the diagnosis of lumbar disc herniation and spinal stenosis. Spine 7:55–64
Herman LJ, Beltran J 1988 Pitfalls in MR imaging of the knee. Radiology 167:775–781
Hernandez RJ 1984 Concentric reduction of the dislocated hip. Computed tomographic evaluation. Radiology 150:266–268
Heuftle MG, Modic MT, Ross JS et al 1988 Lumbar spine post operative MR imaging with Gd-DTPA. Radiology 167–817–824
Hiltselberger WE, Witten RM 1968 Abnormal myelograms in asymptomatic patients. J Neurosurg 28:204–206
Holmes E, Rothman RH 1979 The Pennsylvania plan. An algorithm for the management of lumbar degenerative disease. Spine 4:156–162
Holt RG, Helms CA, Steinbach L et al 1990 Magnetic resonance imaging of the shoulder: rationale and current applications. Skeletal Radiol 19:5–14
Jackson RP, Cain JE, Jacobs RR et al 1989 The neuroradiographic diagnosis of lumbar herniated nucleus pulposus: a comparison of computed tomography (CT). Spine 14:1356–1361
Kransdorf MJ, Jelinck JS, Mose RP et al 1989 Soft tissues masses, diagnosis using MR imaging. AJR 153:541–547
Kulkarni MV, McArdle CB, Kopanicky D et al 1987 Acute spinal cord injury. MR imaging at 1.5T. Radiology 164:837–843
Kulkarni MV, Narvana PA, McArdle CB et al 1988 Cervical spine MR imaging using multislice gradient echo imaging. Comparisons with cardiac gated spin echo. Magnetic Res Imag 6:517–525
Laine HR, Harjula A, Peltokallio P 1987 Ultrasound evaluation of the knee and patellar regions. J Ultrasound Med 6:33–36
Lang P, Genant HK, Steiger P et al 1989 Three dimensional digital displays in congenital dislocation of the hip—preliminary experiences. J Paediatr Orthop 9:532–537
Lee CK, Rauschning W, Glenn W 1988a Lateral lumbar spinal stenosis: classification, pathologic anatomy and surgical decompression. Spine 13:313–320
Lee JK, Yao L, Phelps CT et al 1988b Anterior cruciate ligament tears: MR imaging compared with arthroscopy and clinical tests. Radiology 166:861–864
Levinsohn EM, Baker BE 1980 Pre-arthrotomy diagnostic evaluation of the knee. AJR 134:107–111
McAffee PC, Yuan HA, Fredickson BE, Lubicky JP 1983 The value of computed tomography in thoracolumbar fractures. J Bone Joint Surg 65A:461–473
Middleton WD, Reinus WR, Totty WG et al 1986 Ultrasonographic evaluation of the rotator cuff and biceps tendon. J Bone Joint Surg 68A:440–450
Middleton WD, Kneeland JB, Kellman CM et al 1987 MR imaging of the carpal tunnel. Normal anatomy and

preliminary findings in the carpal tunnel syndrome. AJR 148:307–316
Mikhael MA, Ciric I, Tarkington JA, Vick NA 1981 Neuroradiological evaluation of lateral recess syndrome. Radiology 140:97–107
Mink JH, Harris E, Rappaport M 1985 Rotator cuff tears: evaluation using double contrast shoulder arthrography. Radiology 157:621–623
Mink JH, Levy T, Crues JV 1988 Tears of the anterior cruciate ligament and menisci of the knee: MR imaging evaluation. Radiology 167:769–774
Mino DE, Palmer AK, Levinsohn EM 1985 Radiography and computerised tomography in the diagnosis of incongruity of the distal radio-ulnar joint. J Bone Joint Surg 67A:247–252
Mitchell DG, Levy I, Creus JV 1988 Tears in the anterior cruciate ligament and menisci of the knee: MR imaging evaluation. Radiology 167:764–774
Modic MT, Masaryk T, Boumphrey F et al 1986a Lumbar herniated disc disease and canal stenosis. Am J Neuro-Roentgenol 7:709–717
Modic MT, Masaryk TJ, Mulopulos GP et al 1986b Cervical radiculopathy: prospective evaluation with surface coil MR imaging, CT with metrizamide and metrizamide myelography. Neuroradiology 161:753–759
Montaldi S, Frankhouser H, Schnyder P, De Tritrolet N 1988 Computed tomography of the post-operative intervertebral disc and lumbar spinal canal: investigation of 25 patients after successful operation for lumbar disc herniation. Neurosurgery 22:1014–1022
Norman A, Nelson J, Green S 1985 Fractures of the hook of hamate. Radiographic signs. Radiology 154:49–53
Novick GS 1988 Sonography in paediatric hip disorders. Radiol Clin North Am 26:29–53
Pavlov H, Hirschy JC, Torg JS 1979 Computed tomography of the cruciate ligaments. Radiology 132:389–393
Pettersson H, Gillespy T, Hamlin DJ, et al 1987 Primary musculo-skeletal tumours examination with MR imaging compared with conventional modalities. Radiology 164:237–241
Pettersson H, Larsson EM, Holtas S et al 1988 MR imaging of the cervical spine in rheumatoid arthritis. Am J Neuro-Radiol 9:573–577
Polly DW, Callaghan JJ, Sikes RA et al 1988 The accuracy of selective magnetic resonance imaging compared with the findings of arthroscopy of the knee. J Bone Joint Surg 70A:192–197
Rafii M, Firooznia H, Bonamo JJ et al 1987 Athlete shoulder injuries: CT arthrographic findings. Radiology 162:559–564
Reicher MA, Bassett, LW, Gold RH 1985 High resolution magnetic resonance imaging of the knee joint: pathologic correlations 1985. AJR 145:903–910
Reicher MA, Hartzman S, Bassett LW et al 1987 MR imaging of the knee: I Traumatic disorders. Radiology 162:547–553
Resnick D, Andre M, Kerr R et al 1984 Digital arthrography of the wrist. A radiographic pathological investigation. AJR 142:1187–1190
Ross JS, Masaryk TJ, Schrader M et al 1990 MR imaging of the post operative spine. Assessment with Gadopentetate Dimegumine. AJR 155:867–872
Schnebel B, Kingston S, Watkins R, Dillin W 1989 Comparison of MRI to contrast CT in the diagnosis of spinal stenosis. Spine 14:332–337
Schonstrom NSR, Bolender NF, Spengler DA, Hansson JH 1984 Pressure changes within the cauda equina following constriction of the dural sac. Spine 9:604–607
Seeger LL, Gold RH, Bassett LW 1988a Shoulder instability: evaluation with MR imaging. Radiology 168:695–697
Seeger LL, Gold RH, Bassett LW, Ellman H 1988b Shoulder impingement syndrome; MR findings in 53 shoulders. AJR 150:343–347
Selby B, Richardson ML, Montana MA et al 1986 High resolution sonography of the menisci of the knee. Invest Radiol 21:332–335
Shuman WP, Rogers JV, Sickler ME 1985 Thoracolumbar burst fracture. CT dimensions of the spinal canal relative to post-surgical improvement. Radiol 145:337–341
Soble MG, Kaye AD, Guay RC 1989 Rotator cuff tear. Clinical experience with sonographic detection. Radiology 173:319–321
Standford W, Phelan J, Kathol MH et al 1988 Patellofemoral joint motion. Evaluation by ultrafast computed tomography. Skeletal Radio 17:487–492
Stockley I, Getty CJM, Dixon AK et al 1988 Lumbar lateral canal entrapment: clinical radiographic and computed tomography findings. Clin Radiol 39:144–149
Szypryt EP, Twining P, Wilde GP et al 1988 Diagnosis of lumbar protrusion—a comparison between magnetic resonance imaging and radiculography. J Bone Joint Surg 70B:712–722
Teplick JG, Haskin ME 1983 CT and lumbar disc herniation. Radiol Clin North Am 21:259–288
Thickman D, Axel L, Kiessel HY et al 1986 Magnetic resonance of avascular necrosis of the femoral head. Skeletal Radiol 15:133–140
Thiju CJP 1982 Accuracy of double contrast arthrography and arthroscopy of the knee joint. Skeletal Radiol 8:187–192
Thomas EA, Cassar-Pullicino VN, McCall IW 1991 The role of ultrasound in the early diagnosis and management of heterotopic bone formation. Clin Radiol 43:190–196
Tsuruda JS, Norman D, Dillon W et al 1990 Three dimensional gradient-recalled MR imaging as a screening tool for the diagnosis of cervical radiculopathy. AJR 154:375–383
Weekes RG, McLeod RA, Reiman HM, Pritchard DJ 1985 CT of soft tissue neoplasms. AJR 144:355–360
Wiesel SW, Tsourmas N, Feffer HL et al 1984 Positive CAT scans in asymptomatic patients. Spine 9:549–551
Wilson DJ, Gran DJ, MacLarnon JC 1984 Arthrosonography of the painful hip. Clin Radiol 35:17–19
Wilson DJ, McLardy-Smith P, Woodham CH, MacLarnon JC 1987 Diagnostic ultrasound in haemophilia. J Bone Joint Surg 69B:103–107
Wilson AJ, Totty WG, Murphy WA, Hardy DC 1989 Shoulder joint arthrographic CT and long term follow up with surgical correlation. Radiology 173:329–333
Zeinreich SJ, Long DM, Davis R et al 1990 Three-dimensional CT imaging in post surgical failed back syndrome. J Computer Assist Tomogr 14:574–580
Zinberg EM, Palmer AK, Coren AB, Levinsohn PJ 1988 The triple injection wrist arthrogram. J Hand Surg (Am) 13:803–809
Zlatkin MB, Reiche MA, Kellerhouse LE, Resnick D 1988 The painful shoulder: MR imaging of the glenohumeral joint. J Computer Assist Tomogr 12:995–1001
Zlatkin MB, Chao PC, Osterman AL et al 1989a Chronic wrist pain: evaluation with high resolution MR imaging. Radiology 173:723–729
Zlatkin MB, Iannotti JP, Roberts MC et al 1989b Rotator cuff tears: diagnostic performance of MR imaging. Radiology 172:223–229

5

Advances in diagnosis and treatment in closed traction lesion of the supraclavicular brachial plexus

R. Birch

The Medical Research Council special report on peripheral nerve injuries (Brooks 1954) is an example of a detailed and systematic study which has not been surpassed. In it, Brooks reviewed the outcome for 170 cases of open wound of the brachial plexus presenting to five designated peripheral nerve injury centres during and after World War II. He concluded that diagnosis at operation was difficult and that 'with the possible exception of lesions of the upper trunk, operative repair is valueless'. This view was supported at the SICOT meeting in Paris in the mid 1960s when surgeons with an interest in the field concluded that operations for diagnosis and for repair in traction and gunshot injuries of the brachial plexus were not worthwhile.

In the 1960s and early 70s many patients in the UK with complete lesions to the brachial plexus were treated by early amputation, glenohumeral arthrodesis and fitting with a prosthesis. Ransford & Hughes (1977) showed that only a small minority of patients actually used their prosthesis. Their paper showed how little could be done for those patients with the flail and painful arm.

Bonney (1954) in London persisted with earlier work on diagnosis and prognosis and Narakas & Verdan (1969) and Millesi (1968) applied microsurgical technique in the repair of lesions of the brachial plexus. Narakas, in particular, applied analytical and technical skills in the treatment of large numbers of patients and others were encouraged to return to the field after seeing these early results.

This review will attempt to define the significance of advances in understanding and in treatment of different aspects of lesions of the brachial plexus.

EPIDEMIOLOGY

Although individual units have accumulated much experience from large series, accurate information about the incidence, causation, social background and social consequences of brachial plexus injury is hard to find. This is deplorable, for these severe injuries occur in young motorcyclists at the outset of their working lives and there is permanent and painful disability in many. A survey of Fellows of the British Orthopaedic Association (Goldie & Coates 1991), requesting information about patients with closed traction lesion admitted during 1987, received 402 replies — 55% of those circulated. They uncovered 254 patients admitted with complete or partial lesion.

It seems reasonable to assume that between 300 and 350 patients suffer severe and permanent damage from closed traction lesion of the supraclavicular plexus every year in the UK. Rosson (1988) reviewed 106 patients injured in motorcycle accidents. He found that 91 were younger than 25 and 43 held only a provisional licence. Of the machines involved, over one-third had an engine capacity of 125 cc or less. In a separate study (Rosson 1987) of 102 motorcyclists presenting in 1985 to 1986 he found a mean age of 21 years, injury to the dominant arm in 65, and other severe injuries to the head, chest and viscera, or the other limbs in 51. Over one-third of his patients, followed for more than 1 year, remained unemployed, with severe pain in the injured limb in more than two-thirds. The recommendations from the RoyalCollege of Surgeons of England (Birch 1989) included limitation of the engine capacity of motorcycles and raising the age at which a licence was granted.

DIAGNOSIS

The extent of neural injury is obvious on clinical examination. The level of lesion may be more difficult to determine. Is the spinal nerve torn within the spinal canal, between the dorsal root ganglion and the spinal cord? If so, is there sparing of dorsal or ventral rootlets? Other difficulties include detection of injuries to nerves at more than one level and whether motor nerves have been torn directly from muscle. Certain clinical findings are particularly significant. Avulsion of the roots of the brachial plexus is likely in patients with Claude Bernard–Horner syndrome and pain. Fracture or dislocation of the first rib or the transverse process of the seventh cervical vertebra supports this diagnosis. Weakness of the trapezius, disturbance of sensation above the clavicle and paralysis of the ipsilateral hemidiaphragm indicate that the upper roots of the brachial plexus have been avulsed. In the worst cases there is swelling and deep bruising in the posterior triangle and radiographs may show that the cervical spine has been canted over, away from impact, or the upper limb appears to have been distracted from the chest. Complete avulsion is likely in these cases. Linear bruising along the course of nerve trunks in the arm implies rupture.

Bonney developed the concept of pre- and postganglionic injury, distinguishing between injuries to the spinal cord and those to peripheral nerves. In 1954 he described persistence of the axon reflex after injection with histamine and in 1958 he and Gilliatt recorded sensory action potentials from the median and ulnar nerve of a patient with complete preganglionic injury of the brachial plexus. These two investigations confirm that afferent axons remain myelinated if they are still in continuity with the dorsal root ganglion. Both investigations remain central in the physiological diagnosis of level of lesion.

Celli & Rovesta (1983) have developed refined and sensitive techniques of electrophysiological examination to determine the level of lesion and to distinguish between avulsion of the ventral and the dorsal rootlets. Dissatisfaction with their results in 234 patients operated on between 1971 and 1982 led them to supplement examination of the stump of the spinal nerve under the operating microscope with neurophysiological investigation (Celli et al 1974). They combined electromyographic examination of paravertebral muscles with pre- and intraoperative sensory-evoked potential recordings from 1980. They found a difference in 8 of 47 roots, indicating selective avulsion of a ventral or a dorsal rootlet.

This important work was developed at a time when imaging technique, using radiopaque medium, was inadequate to display intradural injury. Their approach remains of singular importance in attempting to quantify the state of the stump displayed at operation, and whether grafting to that stump is the correct course, or whether nerve transfer would be the better course. The impressive work of this unit is summarized in their paper of 1987.

Landi et al (1980) extended this work by recording cortical-evoked potentials through scalp electrodes from stimulation of nerve stumps displayed at operation. They compared preoperative with intraoperative somatosensory-evoked potentials with surgical findings in 15 patients. They found the investigation particularly valuable in determining the level of injury to the fifth cervical nerve. Jones (1987), Sugioka (1984) and Sugioka & Nagano (1989) report on detailed analysis of pre- and intraoperative neurophysiological records with the findings at operation.

The limitations of this mode of investigation are now clear. It is not quantitative. Intraoperative recording is sensitive to scarring about the exposed spinal nerve and sensory recording will not detect cases where there is isolated intradural injury to the ventral rootlets alone. Absence of sensory action potentials in preoperative work indicates that afferent nerve fibres have degenerated but will not distinguish between degeneration caused by postganglionic rupture and that following death of the neuron within an injured dorsal root ganglion.

IMAGING

Yeoman (1968) compared myelography with findings at operation and confirmed that the investigation is a useful one. He described the different radiological findings in preganglionic injury, and pointed out that meningoceles are more common for the eighth cervical and first thoracic roots. He also emphasized the importance of the tilting of the cervical spine as an indication of severity of lesion. Davies et al (1966) also compared radiological and operative evidence. However, myelography, particularly by oil-soluble media, was found to underestimate the severity of injury, particularly for the fifth and sixth cervical nerves. Nagano et al (1989) reviewed 90 cases where metrizamide was used in patients later explored, confirming that water-soluble media do allow more precise delineation of the spinal nerves within the spinal canal. David Sutton introduced computerized tomography (CT) scanning with contrast enhancement at St Mary's Hospital, London, in 1983 and Marshall and de Silva (1986) compared the CT scan with myelogram and the findings at operation in 16 cases. They showed that CT scan with contrast enhancement was a good deal more accurate, particularly for C5 and C6, than the standard myelogram and in some of their cases the dorsal and ventral rootlets could be plainly seen. This most useful technique has now been widely adopted. It is unfortunate that magnetic resonance imaging has, to date, proven unsatisfactory.

SURGICAL PATHOLOGY

Analysis of the findings at operations for diagnosis and repair from different centres is difficult because patterns of injury vary from series to series, reflecting differing indications for operation and reasons for referral. Two things are clear. All series report a high incidence of preganglionic injury of spinal nerves with the fifth and sixth cervical nerves being rather less vulnerable than the lower three. Complete avulsions form a significant proportion of operated cases (Tables 5.1 and 5.2).

Two features are particularly significant in determining (and also limiting) the possibilities of repair—the spinal cord and vascular injury.

The spinal cord

Bonney observed that preganglionic injuries of the brachial plexus are in fact injury of the spinal cord when in the course of hemi-laminectomy for diagnosis he noted atrophy of the spinal cord on the damaged side. Others who have performed hemi-laminectomy for diagnosis have observed that the ventral are more vulnerable than the dorsal roots (Alnot et al 1981, Privat et al 1982). The Brown–Séquard syndrome has been recorded in complete injuries of the brachial plexus and a careful examination of patients with complete lesions of the plexus will detect impairment of long tract function in as many as 10%. Flannery and colleagues (Flannery & Birch 1990, Flannery et al 1991) have drawn attention to two other important variations of injury to the spinal cord. Flannery & Birch described 2 patients who presented with paraparesis and great pain. They conclude that this was a variation of the central cord syndrome from compression of the spinal cord from haematoma. In both patients spontaneous recovery was good. Flannery et al (1991) recognized the importance of thoracic disc protrusion in the differential diagnosis of delayed affliction of the spinal cord. This possibility should be considered with a post-traumatic syrinx or direct tethering of the cord from the scar.

Vascular injury

Another notable observation is the incidence of vascular injury. This is higher in infra- than in supraclavicular injuries. Alnot & Bayon (1989) reported 22 ruptures of subclavian or of axillary

Table 5.1 Preganglionic injury to spinal nerves demonstrated at operation

C^4	C^5	C^6	C^7	C^8	T^1	Total and reference
1	22	39	68	53	43	Total 226 in 103 patients with complete lesion (Millesi 1987)
NR	50	118	151	162	152	Total 633 in 299 patients (Narakas 1989a)
3	52	58	57	51	50	Total 270 in 100 consecutive operations for diagnosis (Birch 1988–1990 unpublished data)

NR = Not recorded.

Table 5.2 Patterns of injury displayed at operation

Complete avulsion C5–T1	Avulsion of the lower roots of C7, C8 and T1. Rupture or LIC of upper roots of C5 and C6 (7)	Avulsion of the upper roots of (C5–C7), rupture or LIC of lower roots	Other combination of isolation ruptures or avulsion	Reference and total
14	64	6	16	Narakas (1989a): 100 consecutive operations
35	29	29	7	Birch (1988–1990, unpublished data): 100 consecutive repairs

LIC = Lesion in continuity.

artery in their first 100 operated cases. We have found 63 ruptures of the subclavian artery in 499 cases of supraclavicular lesion undergoing operation for diagnosis or for repair. Narakas (1987a) warns of the difficulties of later exploration as: 'immense technical difficulties arise because it is almost impossible to expose the plexus without damaging the vascular grafts or even a prosthesis if one has been used. In about one-third of our cases with early vascular and late nerve repair we found the vessel thrombosed and had to re-graft it'. We agree with the recommendation of Narakas against prostheses. The anastomotic site will not adapt to change in size and the surrounding haematoma as it becomes organized embeds the nerve in a fibrotic mass. We entirely agree with the recommendation of Alnot & Bayon (1989) that 'restoration of the continuity of a ruptured subclavian or axillary artery is desirable in all cases'.

ANATOMICAL STUDIES

Revival of interest in repair of traction lesions has led to much enquiry and two aspects are particularly notable.

Anatomy

Sunderland's massive study (1978) of the internal organization of nerve fibres within nerve trunks and of the reasons for the vulnerability of spinal nerves to traction stimulated Herzberg et al (1989) to a detailed and elegant study of the proximal intervertebral segments. They showed that transverse radicular ligaments protect C5–C7, but not C8 and T1. They point out that rupture of the upper three spinal nerves may be found only by dissection within the bony canal. Slingluff et al (1987) and Bonnel (1989) have considerably extended previous knowledge on the evolving pattern of nerve fascicles, their size, and their distribution along the course of the plexus. They have prepared detailed cross-sectional maps at different levels of the plexus. Their work offers the opportunity for more accurate matching of distal and proximal stumps.

Regeneration from the spinal cord

Bonney re-attached avulsed dorsal spinal rootlets to the spinal cord at operation in 1976 (personal communication). There was no recovery. Jamieson & Eames (1980) studied regeneration through re-implanted dorsal and ventral rootlets in dogs and presented histological and electrical evidence of regeneration of fibres from the anterior horn through the spinal nerve to skeletal muscle. Carlstedt and his colleagues (1990) at the Karolinska Institute, Sweden, have extended this work using rats and adult and newborn cats. They have proved that regeneration occurs through re-implanted lumbosacral ventral rootlets, re-innervating previously denervated muscle. They showed that synaptic reconnection occurred within the spinal cord itself and that the motor neurons had been reconnected in spinal cord segmental reflex circuits. They confirm that regeneration from the dorsal root in the adult animal does not occur and that nerve fibre ingrowth stops abruptly at the central–peripheral nervous system interface, *but they did demonstrate regeneration through the replanted dorsal root in the immature animals.*

These few studies of replantation of rootlets into the spinal cord are of fundamental importance and must act as a spur to further investigation and renewed clinical application.

TECHNICAL ADVANCES

We must acknowledge from the outset that the development or refinement of surgical techniques rests on advances in anaesthesia. Operations which were once hazardous and to be undertaken only in extremis are now standard. Prolonged and delicate work can be undertaken in confidence that circulation and ventilation are maintained and controlled. The discriminating use of neuromuscular blocking agents allows sensitive neurophysiological investigation at operation.

Incisions

The transverse supraclavicular approach, long favoured by Bonney, has been extended to the transclavicular approach (Bonney et al 1990) in which a bony flap, comprising the medial one-half of clavicle and a corner of manubrium sterni, is turned up on the sternomastoid muscle. The first costal cartilage is divided. The sternoclavicular joint is preserved. This approach affords unparalleled access to the whole of the brachial plexus and allows safe control of the great vessels at the root of the limb. It was developed to expose the cervicodorsal junction for treatment of tumour. It is now the exposure of choice in tumours of the brachial plexus and has been used in the display of neurovascular lesions above or behind the clavicle. A similar approach, ascribed to Duval, is described by Fiolle & Delmas (1921).

Instruments

There have been refinements in instruments and in sutures. The operating microscope has undoubtedly enhanced technical precision. Narakas (personal communication), who knows better than any, estimates that his results of nerve repair have been improved by 10% by microsurgical techniques. Fibrin clot glue (Young & Medawar 1940) was used extensively by Seddon and his school. It became unavailable in this country and its re-introduction (Egloff & Narakas 1983), in a more easily handled preparation, has substantially shortened the duration of operation and has probably improved the results of grafting and of nerve transfer.

RESULTS

Discussion of results of procedures is impossible without agreement on the mode of assessment. The Medical Research Council system (Seddon 1975) is useful in analysis of outcome for individual trunk nerves, but in measuring overall functional deficit of a limb it has proved inadequate. Narakas and his colleagues (Narakas 1989b) have devised a system for measuring functional return which considers in turn the shoulder, elbow, forearm and hand. Their system provides a useful measure of sensibility. This excellent mode is still being modified and has not yet been universally adopted. Until it is, comparison of results from different techniques of repair between different centres can only be superficial.

Direct suture

This is possible only in a few cases of open wounds, and then only if performed urgently. Direct suture has no place in the repair of traction lesions.

Conventional grafting

Repair of ruptures of C5 and C6 is followed by functional flexion of elbow and—usually imperfect—control of the shoulder in 60% of cases (Sedel 1987). The two most important reasons for failure are first, the extent of damage to the proximal stump and next, delay. The two are intertwined. Results from repair of the brachial plexus, as from repair of nerves anywhere else, deteriorate sharply with delay of over 3 months. Repair of traction lesion at more than 6 months from injury is, in the author's experience, hardly worthwhile. Useful return of hand function is found only in a tiny number of children, or adults where the lower trunk is transected by glass or the surgeon's knife, and then only when repair is effected within days of injury.

Vascularized ulnar nerve graft

Disappointment with results from conventional techniques spurred Jamieson to develop free vascularized ulnar nerve graft in cases of irreparable injury to C8 and T1. Before this Bonney had used the ulnar nerve, in suitable cases, as a two-stage pedicle graft following the technique of Strange (1947). Jamieson originally used the ulnar artery. The free vascularized ulnar nerve graft based on the superior ulnar collateral vessels was first used in London in 1981 in repair of an extensive defect of the median nerve following accidental injury to the suture line of the second stage of a pedicle operation. This modification was adopted because the ulnar artery is preserved and because the ulnar nerve is larger in the arm than in the forearm. Independently and at the same time Breidenbach & Terzis (1984) described and used this graft and Merle (1985) reported a detailed anatomical study with a clinical series. Much was hoped from this innovation, for it seemed that the problems of large defects, scarred bed and paucity of autograft could be overcome and that at last there was a chance of restoring useful function in the hand in patients with complete lesion of the plexus. In a review (Birch et al 1989) 63 patients were described. In a number of these, two or three strands of vascularized nerve graft were used to re-innervate the posterior cord and the median nerve. Of 42 cases with a minimum follow-up of 30 months, 9 were failures. Functional elbow flexion was restored in 32, but muscle transfer was necessary in 5 of these to achieve this. As to the hand, 10 adults regained crude hook grip with protective sensation, but true hand function with useful activity in intrinsic muscles and worthwhile sensation was regained in 1 patient only, a 3-year-old child. The harmfulness of delay was confirmed: in the 4 cases where interval from injury to repair exceeded 6 months, there was no functional recovery. Six of 23 cases operated upon between 2 and 6 months after injury failed; 14 of the 15 cases explored within 2 weeks of injury regained functional elbow flexion. This procedure undoubtedly has a useful place for treatment of unfavourable cases and also in patients where the potential for repair cannot be met by conventional grafting. The author believes that its best use is in conjunction with other modes of re-innervation of the upper limb and these will now be discussed.

Nerve transfer

The idea of transferring an uninjured nerve to the distal stump of an injured nerve is not new. Narakas (1987a) describes early work and points out that the principles of operations now performed were recognized decades ago. Seddon (1963) performed the first cases in which function was restored following intercostal neurotization of the musculocutaneous nerve via interposed ulnar nerve. Tsuyama's group adopted intercostal nerve transfer for patients with complete avulsion injury in 1965 and described their results in 179 patients (Nagano et al 1989). They divided the third and fourth ribs to allow gentle and adequate mobilization of the corresponding nerves and sutured these directly to the musculocutaneous nerve. Over 80% of their patients regained functional flexion at the elbow. These are extremely impressive results. The Tokyo group point out that delay is harmful and for patients presenting more than 10 months after injury they advise free muscle transplantation with intercostal transfer. This is an extensive and bold operation and their results are good.

Dolenc (1987) described the outcome in 150 patients operated upon between 1972 and 1983. He emphasizes the need for 'better use of the scarce axons of the intercostal nerve'. The present author agrees with Dolenc when he recommends that repair should be performed within days of injury, before Wallerian degeneration has occurred, for this allows recognition of the predominantly motor bundles of major peripheral nerves.

Kotani et al (1972) and Allieu (1989) independently used the distal part of the spinal accessory nerve in re-innervation of the upper limb, preserving rami to the upper fibres of the trapezius. Brunelli started using branches of the cervical plexus for transfer in 1977 and reviewed his results in 29 patients in 1987. He achieved important improvement in many of these and advises that the neurotization should be limited to a few well chosen muscles.

Detailed analysis of fibre counts and of the proportions of sensory and motor fibres has been done for all of those nerves used in transfer. Brunelli estimates that the number of motor fibres available from branches of the cervical plexus is about 4000. Estimates of myelinated nerve fibres for the accessory nerve range from 1700 to 2000 (Bonnel et al 1979, Alnot & Oberlin 1989). Holle and his colleagues (1989) present data for the intercostal nerves at different levels, from the paravertebral region (5500–8500 axons) to the lateral cutaneous branch (1000–1500 axons). It is remarkable that useful results are achieved using such slender nerves. The average axon count from analysis of 21 plexuses is over 18 000 and is about 5000 for the musculocutaneous nerve alone (Bonnel et al 1979, Slingluff et al 1987, Bonnel 1989)!

There is no doubt that recent work with nerve transfer represents a significant advance in treatment of traction lesion of the brachial plexus. The St Mary's and Royal National Orthopaedic Hospitals used nerve transfer only rarely until 1986. Since that time transfer of accessory to suprascapular nerve has been performed in over 70 patients and intercostal transfer to the lateral cord or musculocutaneous nerve in over 100. Some of the earlier results are particularly gratifying (Fig. 5.1). Relief of pain seems to be an important and unexpected bonus in a proportion of patients. This experience awaits detailed review, but it seems that useful functional gain is achieved for shoulder and elbow, with significant pain relief in over 60% of patients operated upon within 3 months from injury. In particular, success from a nerve transfer has greatly improved the prognosis for patients with irreparable injury to C5/6 and/or C7, but with preservation of C8 and T1. The results of reconstructive procedures for these patients have been disappointing.

RECONSTRUCTION

'Good nerve regeneration will result in far better function than musculotendinous transfers' (Narakas 1987a). This is particularly true for lesions of the brachial plexus. Injury to the spinal nerves causes loss of feeling and proprioception and the transferred muscles are usually weakened. Regeneration across a lesion in continuity is always imperfect which means that there is a poor motor for transfer. Cocontraction from disorderly regeneration is a common problem. The results are further

A

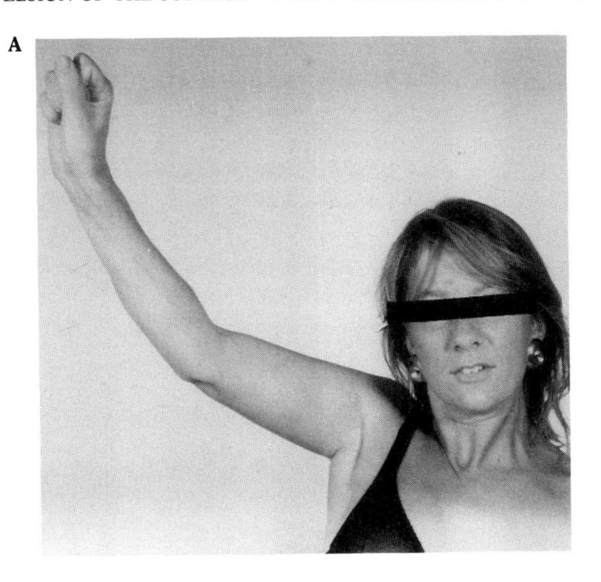

B

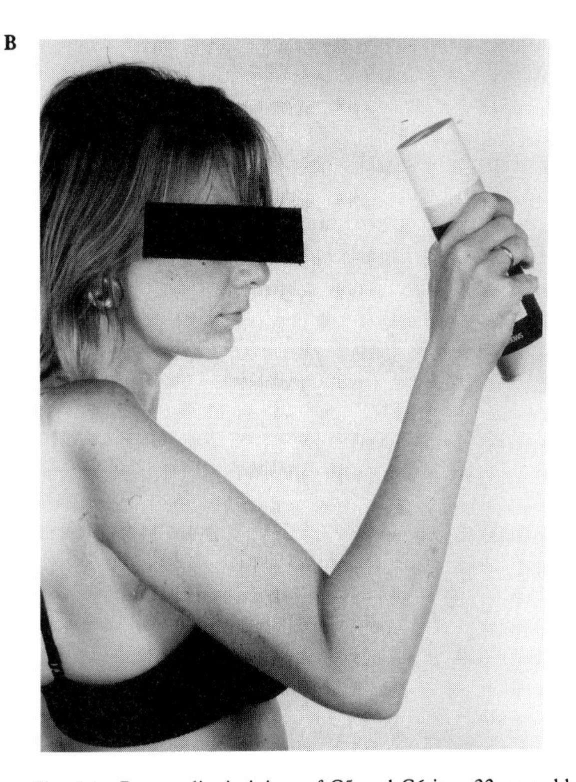

Fig. 5.1 Preganglionic injury of C5 and C6 in a 22-year-old woman. Repair was by accessory to suprascapular and by intercostals T3, T4 and T5 to musculocutaneous nerve at 6 weeks from injury. The sensory division of T4 was preserved. At 15 months pain, which had been severe, was abolished and the range of abduction and external rotation at the shoulder is shown (**A**). The range of flexion/extension at the elbow was full and she was able to lift weights of up to 5 pounds (**B**).

prejudiced by fixed deformity and contracture from injuries to the limb.

Shoulder

Ross & Birch (1991) reviewed 58 adults treated by arthrodesis, or muscle transfer, or external rotation osteotomy. The best results were from arthrodesis and results from transfer of latissimus dorsi were particularly poor. Ross & Birch point out that in patients with a complete supraclavicular lesion left untreated, 'at least sixty percent will fail to recover any shoulder activity and a further twenty percent will recover some power but little control'. Nagano and his colleagues (1989) describe the technique for glenohumeral arthrodesis by external fixation, an elegant technique developed by a unit which, having pioneered intercostal transfer to the musculocutaneous nerve, eschews accessory transfer for fear of weakening the thoracoscapular control. The Tokyo group favour glenohumeral arthrodesis in combination with intercostal transfer to restore elbow flexion. Sensible patients who are working, and who have irreparable lesion to C5 and C6, will regain useful function from glenohumeral arthrodesis. In the author's view the operation is hardly ever indicated in patients with a useless hand. In rare cases of paralysis of the thoracoscapular muscles from injury to the accessory and long thoracic nerves, scapulothoracic fusion, as described by Copeland & Howard (1978), is most useful.

Elbow

Alnot & Abols (1984) emphasized how serious the loss of elbow flexion is and pointed out that results from reconstruction were worse in patients with C5–C7 lesions that in those with only C5–C6 lesions. In their series of 44 patients, triceps to biceps transfer was the most successful. Sedel (personal communication) has particular experience with the Steindler flexoplasty and has good results from it. Marshall et al (1988) reviewed 50 patients and in this series, too, the triceps to biceps transfer proved the most effective. The author's experience from over 120 muscle transfers for elbow flexion is that triceps to biceps is the best but this is the operation which costs the patient most in loss of function. The Steindler operation often fails because of weakness of the superficial flexor muscles and there is a risk to the ulnar nerve. Pectoralis major transfer has proved particularly disappointing and the author has abandoned this operation. Transfer of latissimus dorsi is effective, but it is a lengthy and mutilating operation. Power from muscle transfer is weak unless the biceps muscle has had some recovery and results are far inferior, in range of motion and in power, compared to successful re-innervation of the musculocutaneous nerve.

Forearm and hand

Loss of extension of the wrist and fingers is a common problem following lesion to the brachial plexus. Flexor to extensor transfer is perhaps the most common of all reconstruction operations and yet little is written about it. Standard flexor to extensor transfer for high palsy of the radial nerve is assumed to be a reliable and a good operation. On the whole it is, although it can be difficult to re-train. In patients with injury to the sixth and seventh cervical nerves, however, pronator teres and flexor carpi radialis, with palmaris longus, are either paralysed or weak. The author's experience with some 150 flexor to extensor transfers in patients with lesions of the brachial plexus is that there are many unsatisfactory results. Lack of a good motor for wrist extension is an important cause of failure. Leffert (1985) has written at length on different modes of reconstruction and on the timing of operation and he speaks wisely of the indications for amputation. They are few. It is an operation, as with many other forms of reconstruction, which should be performed when the patient asks for it in a reasonable understanding of what the gain (or the loss) will be. Above all, patients must understand that amputation will not free them from pain and the operation is best advised for those who have returned to useful occupation, having adapted to their disability as best they can, but who find a flail and anaesthetic limb an impediment and even a hazard.

On reviewing more than 400 patients who have had reconstructive procedures, the writer is inclined to the heretical view that the patient with an intact fifth, sixth and seventh cervical nerve is far better off than the patient with eighth cervical and first thoracic nerves only. The former has normal shoulder, normal elbow flexion and normal sensation in the thumb, the index and the middle finger. There are spare extensors of the wrist available to restore flexion of the digits. Sucess following well timed nerve transfer weakens this view!

PAIN

Loss of a limb is bad enough—persisting severe pain within a useless arm is an abomination. Nearly all patients with preganglionic injury of a spinal nerve experience pain. It is worse in complete avulsion lesions and appears to be more severe if C8 and T1 are avulsed than if C5 and C6 are so injured. The important long-term study of Wynn Parry et al (1987), extending to 30 years, of 122 patients with preganglionic lesion showed that 48 experienced severe pain more than 3 years from injury. The description of pain is characteristic; there is a constant crushing or burning pain in the hand which is commonly described as feeling as if in a vice. Superimposed upon this are lightning shoots of pain passing down the whole arm, often of exquisite severity. Wynn Parry et al emphasize the effectiveness of distraction, of involvement in work or study, as a mitigating feature. This is a strong argument in support of their policy for rehabilitation which is to encourage patients to return to normal work and normal life as soon as possible.

Wynn Parry's unit has demonstrated that transcutaneous nerve stimulation, properly and patiently used, is effective in reducing pain significantly in some 50% of patients. They emphasize that a period of inpatient care is essential. Carbamazepine, an anticonvulsant, reduces the intensity and frequency of lightning pain in perhaps one-third. Occasional success has been described with acupuncture and hypnosis. A few patients find relief from cannabis.

There is good evidence that re-innervation of the limb, by graft or by nerve transfer secures important mitigation of pain in many patients. Bonnard & Narakas (1985) found that only 15% of patients had severe pain 2 years after neural repair. However pain relief following direct repair of ruptures is unpredictable and in some it seems that regeneration of nerves exacerbates the pain. The author has now seen some dramatic results from patients following successful intercostal transfer. In these, relief coincides with return of function and it appears that the operation of nerve transfer may prove to be of great importance in securing lasting and profound relief of pain.

There remains a group of patients who remain demoralized by extreme pain after all other modes of treatment have been exhausted. All units treating such patients know of those who have become hopelessly addicted to opiates and those who have killed themselves. For these, a direct approach to the central nervous system is the last resort. The record of interruption of spinal tracts in patients with chronic pain states is dismal. Thomas (1987, 1988) has reviewed his experience with thermocoagulation of the dorsal root entry zone (DREZ lesion) in over 50 patients. The operation was first performed by Syndou & Goutelle (1983) in 1974; they had had earlier experience with it in treatment of patients with pain from cancer. Nashold & Ostdahl (1979) continued with a modified technique. There is significant relief of pain in two-thirds of patients. In 10% there was a significant and lasting neural deficit, affecting the ipsilateral cervical cord.

This operation is an important addition which should be reserved only for those in intolerable pain after other treatment has been offered. The complications are severe. The patient should be advised of these risks by the doctor considering referral to a surgeon capable of carrying out the intervention. Few young patients will wish to proceed once these risks have been properly explained.

CONCLUSIONS

1. Certain clinical features allow early and accurate diagnosis of the level and extent of lesion. Diagnosis can be confirmed by appropriate neurophysiological investigations and by CT scan or myelography.
2. Repair of ruptures within the posterior triangle will achieve worthwhile function at the shoulder and elbow in about 60% of patients. The vascularized nerve graft is a little better.
3. Nerve transfer has radically improved the outlook for the shoulder and elbow in patients

with irreparable lesions of C5, C6, C7. When combined with conventional repair where possible, useful return of hand function can be expected in children and in a few adults.

4. Delay is utterly harmful. The earlier the repair is performed the better. Results deteriorate significantly with delay of over 3 months. In repairs after 6 months failure is the rule.
5. In neurovascular injury prompt restoration of arterial circulation is essential. Adequate exposure allows full display of the lesion. The timing of repair of nerves in such cases remains controversial; the writer holds firmly to the view that nerves should be repaired at that first operation.
6. Re-innervation of the limb secures significant pain relief in many patients.
7. A vigorous policy of rehabilitation directed to return to normal life is essential for psychological and physical well-being. Rehabilitation is the responsibility of the surgeon in charge of the case. Close supervision is necessary; judicious use of operations for reconstruction can assist in the process.
8. There are two promising fields for the application of basic work in clinical practice. There is greater understanding of the fine anatomy of the plexus and of peripheral nerve trunks, but use of this new work has scarcely begun. Some improvement in results can be anticipated from application of this work. Next, the clinical extension of earlier work on the replantation of avulsed spinal rootlets is overdue. This will require a safe and easy approach to the anterior and posterior parts of the spinal cord.

REFERENCES

Allieu Y 1989 Les neurotisations par le nerf spinal dans les avulsions du plexus brachial de l'adulte. In: Alnot JY, Narakas A (eds) Les Paralysies du plexus brachiale. Monographies du Groupe d'Etude de la Main. Expansion Scientifique, Paris, pp 173–179

Alnot JY, Abols Y 1984 Réanimation de la flexion du coude pars transferts tendineux dans les paralysies traumatiques du plexus brachial de l'adulte. Rev Chir Orthop 70:313–323

Alnot JY, Bayon P 1989 Lésions nerveuses et vasculaires associées dans les lésions traumatique du plexus brachial. In: Alnot JY, Narakas A (eds) Les Paralysies du plexus brachiale. Monographies du Groupe d'Étude de la Main no 15. Expansion Scientifique, Paris, pp 111–115

Alnot JY, Oberlin C H 1989 Les nerfs utilisables pour une neurotisation. In: Alnot JY, Narakas A, (eds) Les Paralysies du plexus brachiale. Monographies du Groupe d'Étude de la Main no 15. Expansion Scientifique, Paris, pp 37–42

Alnot JY, Jolly A, Frot B 1981 Traitement direct des lésions nerveuses dans les paralysies traumatique du plexus brachial chez l'adulte. Int Orthop 5:151–168

Birch R 1989 Brachial plexus and nerve injuries. Accident prevention—a social responsibility. Royal College of Surgeons of England, London

Birch R, Dunkerton M, Bonney G, Jamieson AM 1989 Experience with the free vascularised ulnar nerve graft in repair of supraclavicular lesions of the brachial plexus. Clin Orth Rel Res 237:96–104

Bonnard C, Narakas A 1985 Syndromes douloureux et lésions post-traumatiques du plexus brachial. Helv Chir Acta 52: 621–632

Bonnel F 1989 Anatomie du plexus brachial chez le nouveau—né et l'adulte. In: Alnot JY, Narakas A (eds) Les Paralysies du plexus brachiale. Monographies du Groupe d'Etude de la Main no 15. Expansion Scientifique, Paris, pp 3–13

Bonnel F, Allieu Y, Sugata Y, Rabischong P 1979 Bases anatomo-chirurgicales des neurotisation pour avulsion radiculeuses du plexus brachial. Anat Clin 1:291–296

Bonney G 1954 The value of axon responses in determining the site of lesion in traction lesions of the brachial plexus. Brain 77:588–609

Bonney G, Gilliatt RW 1958 Sensory nerve conduction after traction lesion of the brachial plexus. Proc Coll Med 51:365–367

Bonney G, Birch R, Marshall RW 1990 An approach to the cervico thoracic spine. J Bone Joint Surg 72B:904–907

Breidenbach W, Terzis JK 1984 The anatomy of free vascularised nerve grafts. Clin Plastic Surg 11:65

Brooks DM 1954 Open wounds of the brachial plexus. Peripheral nerve injuries. Medical Research Council special report. HMSO, London, pp 418–429

Brunelli G 1987 Neurotization of avulsed roots of the brachial plexus by means of anterior nerves of the cervical plexus. In: Terzis JK (ed) Microreconstruction of nerve injuries. WB Saunders, Philadelphia

Carlstedt T, Risling M, Linda H et al 1990 Regeneration after spinal nerve root injury. Restor Neurol Neurosc 1:289–295

Celli L, Rovesta C 1983 Intraoperative paravertebral muscular evoked potentials (PMEP) in treatment of traumatic root lesions of the brachial plexus. Communication, Brachial Plexus Meeting, London

Celli L, Rovesta C 1987 Electrophysiologic intraoperative evaluations of the damaged root in traction of the brachial plexus. In: Terzis JK (ed) Microreconstruction of nerve injuries. WB Saunders, Philadelphia pp 473–482

Celli C, Mingione A, Landi A 1974 Nuove acquisizione di tecnica chirurgica nelle lesioni del plesso brachiale. Indicazioni alla neurolisi, autoinnesti e trapianti nervosi. Communication LIX Congress, SIOT

Copeland SA, Howard RC 1978 Thoracoscapular fusion for facioscapulohumeral dystrophy. J Bone Joint Surg 60B:547–551

Davies ER, Sutton D, Bligh AS 1966 Myelography in brachial plexus injury. Br J Radiol 39:362–71

Dolenc VV 1987 Intercostal neurotization of the peripheral nerves in avulsion plexus injuries. In: Terzis JK (ed)

Microreconstruction of nerve injuries. WB Saunders, Philadelphia
Egloff DV, Narakas A 1983 Nerve anastamoses with human fibrin. Ann Chir Main 2:101–115
Fiolle J, Delmas J 1921 The surgical exposure of the deep seated blood vessels. Cumston CG (ed) Heinemann, London
Flannery MC, Birch R 1990 Acute compression of the cervical spinal cord: a complication of preganglionic injury to the brachial plexus. Injury 21:247–248
Flannery MC, Birch R, Bonney G 1990 Thoracic disc protrusions in a patient with preganglionic injury to the brachial plexus. Differential diagnosis of cord compression. Injury 21:246–247
Goldie B, Coates CJ 1991 A surgery of closed supraclavicular injuries of the brachial plexus. Br J Hand Surgery
Hara T, Atosaka Y, Tahahishi M et al 1985 Free muscle transplantation and intercostal nerve crossing as a reconstructive procedure for neglected brachial plexus injuries. Sei Kei Geha 36:1082–1090
Herzberg G, Narakas A, Comtet J-J 1989 Anatomie et rapports des racines du plexus brachial dans l'espace intertransversaire. In: Alnot JY, Narakas A (eds) Les Paralysies du plexus brachiale. Monographies du Groupe d'Etude de la Main no 15. Expansion Scientifique, Paris, pp 19–26
Holle J, Freilinger G, Sulzgruber C 1989 Anatomie chirurgicale des nerfs intercostaux. In: Alnot JY, Narakas A (eds) Les Paralysies du plexus brachiale. Monographies du Groupe d'Etude de la Main no 15. Expansion Scientifique, Paris, pp 46–48
Jamieson AM, Eames RA 1980 Reimplantation of avulsed brachial plexus roots: an experimental study in dogs: Int J Microsurg 2:75–80
Jones SJ 1987 Diagnostic value of peripheral and spinal somatosensory evoked potentials in traction lesions of the brachial plexus. In: Terzis JK (ed) Microreconstruction of nerve injuries. WB Saunders, Philadelphia, pp 63–472
Kotani PT, Matsuda H, Suzuki T 1972 Trial surgical procedures of nerve transfers to avulsion injuries of the plexus brachialis. Orthopaedic Surgery and Traumatology, Proceedings of the 12th Congress. S.I.C.O.T: 348, Tel Aviv
Landi A, Copeland SA, Wynn Parry CB, Jones SJ 1980 The role of somatosensory evoked potentials and nerve conduction studies in the surgical management of brachial plexus injuries. J Bone Joint Surg 62B:492–496
Leffert RD 1985 Brachial plexus injuries. Churchill Livingstone, New York
Marshall RW, de Silva RD 1986 Computerised axial tomography in traction injuries of the brachial plexus. J Bone Joint Surg 68B:734–738
Marshall RW, Williams DH, Birch R, Bonney G 1988 Operations to restore elbow flexion after brachial plexus injuries. J Bone Joint Surg 70B:577–582
Merle M 1985 Report of symposium on brachial plexus function and surgery. Peripheral Nerve Repair and Regeneration 1:59
Millesi H 1968 Zum Problem der Uberbruckung von Defecten peripherer Nerven. Wien Med Wochenschr 118:182–187
Millesi M 1987 Brachial plexus injuries, management and results. In: Terzis JK (ed) Microreconstruction of nerve injuries. WB Saunders, Philadelphia pp 347–360
Nagano A, Obinaga S, Ochiai N, Kurokawa T 1989a Shoulder arthrodesis by external fixation. Clin Orthopa 247:97–100
Nagano A, Tsuyama N, Ochiai N, Hara T, Takahashi M 1989b Direct nerve crossing with the intercostal nerve to treat avulsion injuries of the brachial plexus. J Hand Surg 14A:980–985
Nagano A, Ochiai N, Sugioka H et al 1989c Usefulness of myelography in brachial plexus injuries. J Hand Surg 14B:59–64
Narakas AO 1987a Traumatic brachial plexus injuries. In: Lamb DW (ed) The paralysed hand. Churchill Livingstone, Edinburgh, pp 100–115
Narakas AO 1987b Thoughts on neurotization of nerve transfers in irreparable nerve lesions In: Terzis JK (ed) Microreconstruction of nerve injuries. WB Saunders, Philadelphia, pp 447–454
Narakas A 1989a Lésions anatomo-pathologiques dans les paralysies traumatiques du plexus brachial. In: Alnot JY, Narakas A (eds) Les Paralysies du plexus brachiale. Monographies du Groupe d'Étude de la Main no 15. Expansion Scientifique, Paris, pp 69–90
Narakas AO 1989b Examen du patient et de la function des divers groupes musculaire du membre superior. Critères d'évaluation des résultats In: Alnot JY, Narakas A (eds) Les Paralysies du plexus brachiale. Monographies du Groupe d'Etude de la Main no 15. Expansion Scientifique, Paris, pp 49–64
Narakas A Verdan C 1969 Les greffes nerveuses. Z Unfall Berufskr 3:137–152
Nashold BS, Ostdahl RH 1979 Dorsal root entry zone lesions for pain relief. J Neuro Surg 57:59–69
Privat JM, Mailhe D, Allieu Y, Bonnel F 1982 Précoce hemilaminectomie cervicale exploratrice et neurotisation du plexus brachial. In: Simon L (ed) Plexus brachial et médicine de rééducation. Masson, Paris, pp 66–73
Ransford AO, Hughes SPF 1977 Complete brachial plexus lesions. J Bone Joint Surg 59B:417–442
Ross A, Birch R 1991 Reconstruction of the paralysed shoulder after brachial plexus injuries. In: Tubiana R (ed) The hand 4. SPAG, Paris
Rosson JW 1987 Disability following closed traction lesions of the brachial plexus sustained in motor cycle accidents. J Hand Surg 12B:353–355
Rosson JW 1988 Closed traction lesions of the brachial plexus—an epidemic amoung young motor cyclists. Injury 19:4–6
Seddon HJ 1963 Nerve grafting: 4th Watson Jones lecture of the Royal College of Surgeons of England. J Bone Joint Surg 45B:447–461
Seddon HJ 1975. Surgical disorders of the peripheral nerves, 2nd edn. Churchill Livingstone, Edinburgh
Sedel L 1988 Personal communication
Sedel L 1987 The management of supraclavicular lesion: clinical examination surgical procedures. In: Terzis JK (ed) Results in microreconstructon of nerve injuries. WB Saunders, Philadelphia, pp. 385–392
Slingluff CL, Terzis RK, Edgerton MT 1987 The quantitative microanatomy of the brachial plexus in man; reconstructive relevance. In: Terzis JK (ed) Microreconstruction of nerve injuries. WB Saunders, Philadelphia, pp 285–324
Strange FG St C 1947 An operation for nerve pedicle grafting. Preliminary communication. Br J Surg 34:423
Sugioka H 1984 Evoked potentials in the investigation of traumatic lesions of the peripheral nerve and the brachial plexus. Clin Orthop 184:85–92

Sugioka H, Nagano A 1989 Électrodiagnostic dans l'évaluation des lésions par elongation du plexus brachial. In: Alnot JY, Narakas A (eds) Les Paralysies du plexus brachiale. Monographies du Groupe d'Étude de la Main no 15. Expansion Scientifique, Paris, pp 123–129
Sunderland S 1978 Nerves and nerve injuries, 2nd ed. Churchill Livingstone, Edinburgh
Syndou M, Goutelle A 1983 Surgical posterior rhizotomies for the treatment of pain. Adv Technical Standards Neurosurg 10:147–185
Thomas DGT 1987 Dorsal root entry zone thermocoagulation. Adv Technical Standards Neurosurg 15:99–114
Thomas DGT 1988 Dorsal root entry zone thermocoagulation. In: Schmidek HH Sureet WH (eds) Operative neurosurgical techniques 2nd edn. WB Saunders, Philadelphia, pp 1169–1176
Wynn Parry CB, Frampton V, Monteith A 1987 Rehabilitation of patients following traction lesions of the brachial plexus. In: Terzis JK (ed) Microreconstruction of nerve injuries. WB Saunders, Philadelphia
Yeoman PM 1968 Cervical myelography in traction injuries of the brachial plexus. J Bone Joint Surg 50B:253–260
Young JZ, Medawar PB 1940 Fibrin suture of peripheral nerves. Lancet ii:126

6

Recent advances in flexor tendon surgery

J. W. Strickland W. F. Wagner

There have been considerable changes in the management of flexor tendon injuries in recent years. New tendon retrieval and repair methods following zone II flexor severance have been popularized and sheath preservation and closure havO been emphasized. Early post-repair mobility programmes have demonstrated their ability to improve gliding of the repaired tendon and the protocols used to achieve this motion have advanced to imparting near full passive or even active motion to the injured digit. Severe or untreated tendon injuries may be managed by free tendon grafting or staged flexor reconstruction and tenolysis has become a reliable final salvage for the adherent repair or graft. An active tendon prosthesis and chemical control of adhesion formation may be on the horizon. The evolution of highly sophisticated hand therapists and rehabilitation techniques has advanced the results of flexor tendon surgery well beyond previous expectations. This chapter will review many of the recent advances in flexor tOndon surgery including important supporting clinical and laboratory research.

FLEXOR TENDON REPAIR

The pioneering work of Verdan (1960) and Kleinert and associates (1969) established primary repair as the preferred method of treatments of acute flexor tOndon division within the digital sheath. It has also been demonstrated that, in most instances, it is better to repair both the flexor digitorum profundus and superficialis tendons rather than the profundus alone, as was thought to be wiser in the past (Verdan 1960, 1964, Kleinert et al 1981)

Suture materials and methods

In consequence of the universal improvement in the results of zone II flexor tendon repair following the use of early digital mobility programmes, there has been considerable effort to strengthen suture materials and repair techniques in an effort to allow more aggressive motion protocols with a lessened risk of rupture. Seradge (1983) gave further impetus to the search for a stronger repair when he noted that the results of tendon suture deteriorate when elongation or a gap at the repair site exceeds 3 mm.

In recent years, braided polyester fibre of 3-0 or 4-0 calibre has enjoyed the most popularity among hand surgeons, apparently because of its ease of handling and reduced tendency to slip (Strickland 1985a). The use of this material was supported in a study by Trail et al (1989) who demonstrated that braided polyester had adequate strength and minimal extension at failure. The authors found that monofilament polyglyconate had the highest tensile strength and best knot-holding ability of the currently used suture materials, although its use may be limited because it is both extensible and absorbable.

The Kessler grasping stitch first described by Kirchmayr (1917) or similar core suture methods have emerged as the most popular types of flexor tendon repair (Fig. 6.1). The Tajima modification (Urbaniak 1984), in which the suture knots are tied within the repair site, is particularly convenient because the suture can be placed in the tendon ends when they are identified and used to pass the tendon through the sheath and into position for repair without the need to damage (further) the tendon by instrumentation (Strickland 1985a), (Fig. 6.2).

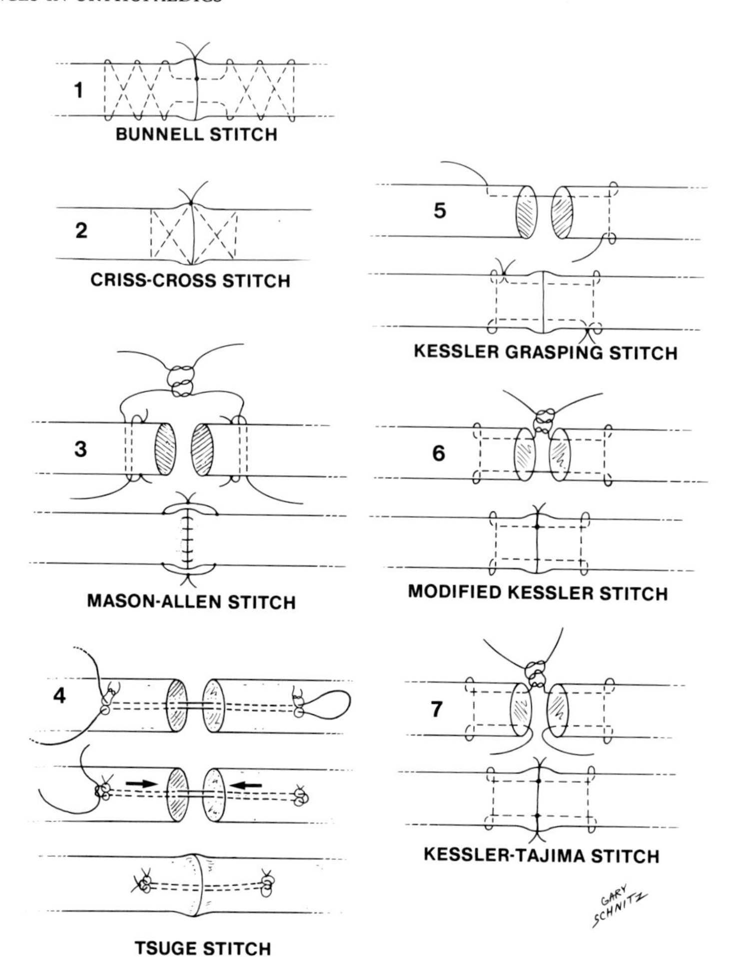

Fig. 6.1 Techniques for end-to-end tendon suture. (**1**) Conventional Bunnell stitch; (**2**) criss-cross stitch; (**3**) Mason–Allen (Chicago) stitch; (**4**) Tsuge looped intratendinous stitch; (**5**) Kessler grasping stitch; (**6**) modified Kessler stitch with single knot at the repair site; (**7**) Tajima modification of the Kessler stitch with double knots in the repair site.

Savage (1985) tested a complex six-stranded grasping technique of flexor tendon repair which he found to be three times stronger than the two Kessler repairs in vitro. He felt that the repair was strong enough to withstand early active digital motion. A subsequent clinical trial was initiated using this technique and the first results reported by Savage & Risitano (1989) were not appreciably better than other series in which conventional repairs and passive mobilization methods had been employed.

Wade et al (1986) evaluated the mechanical limitations of the modified Kessler technique and found that the peripheral running stitch was an important structural component of the suture. They stated that it was not merely a 'tucking in' stitch but essential to the prevention of early gap formation. The importance of the running suture was also described by Lin et al (1988) when they found that a running lock suture technique had greater tensile failure, strength and stiffness than traditional running suture methods. Wade et al (1989) reported that a horizontal mattress-type peripheral running suture provided a 93% increase in load at which a visible gap appeared, a 77% increase in load at 2 mm gap and a 89% increase in maximum strength

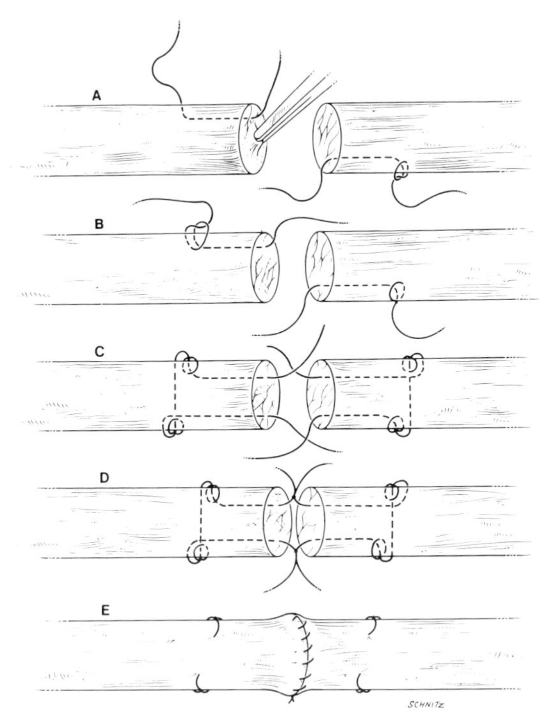

Fig. 6.2 The author's modification of the flexor tendon repair techniques described by Kessler and Tajima. Separate sutures are introduced into each tendon end at a distance of 0.5–1 cm. Approximately 25% of the diameter of the tendon is then grasped by a separate needle passage and locked on the side of the tendon. The suture is then passed transversely behind the knot across the tendon, where a second needle pass-and-lock suture is used to grasp the tendon side. Finally, the suture is passed behind the second knot and down the tendon to the tendon end. Following placement of a similar suture in the opposite end, the two tendon ends can be brought together, and the repair is usually tidied up by a circumferential running lock suture. (Modified from Strickland 1983.)

without adding bulk to the repair. Lister (1983) has emphasized that the epitendinous suture should be shallow and inverted to diminish the tendon bulk at the repair site.

Most surgeons now favour the Kessler method or one of its modifications in which the grasping feature is combined with end placement of the suture. This allows the knots to be buried at the tendon juncture site (Strickland 1983). Repairs are usually completed by the use of a running 6-0 non-absorbable monofilament suture and it would appear to be beneficial to use either the lock stitch or horizontal mattress methods to resist the appearance of gaps.

Partial tendon lacerations

Wray et al (1975) incited controversy about the need to repair partially severed flexor tendons. They concluded that partial flexor tendon lacerations should not be repaired and early active motion should be used unless bevelling of the laceration was present. They recommended that bevelled, partial tendon lacerations of less than 25% of the cross-sectional area could be either excised or repaired with a simple interrupted suture. To some extent, this work was supported by the experiments of Bishop et al (1986) who studied partial flexor tendon injuries in a canine model and concluded that lacerations of up to 60% of the cross-sectional area of a tendon are optimally treated with early mobilization without tenorrhaphy. Chow & Yu (1984) found that unsutured partially lacerated chicken tendons performed worse than those which were sutured. Kleinert (1976) and Schlenker et al (1981) have emphasized that untreated partial flexor lacerations can result in entrapment, rupture and triggering.

Despite these differing opinions, most hand surgeons probably neglect partial transverse flexor lacerations of less than 50% of the diameter of tendon and repair those which are greater. Flap or oblique lacerations are trimmed or repaired depending on their depth and configuration.

Flexor digitorum profundus tendon advancement

Wagner (1958) reviewed 27 patients with profundus tendon advancement and sited a number of common complications including flexion deformity of the repaired digit and hyperextension deformity in adjacent digits. These imbalances tended to progress as shortening became more extensive. Malerich et al (1987) felt that excessive advancement could also produce impaired grip strength and decreased flexion. In their anatomical study of the permissible limits of flexor digitorum profundus tendon advancement they suggested that the degree of tolerable tendon advancement was 1 cm. Considering the reasonably good results which can now be expected following zone I repair of the flexor digitorum profundus, it seems inappropriate to carry out tendon advancement with all of its pitfalls.

The procedure appears to be falling into disfavour with the majority of hand surgeons.

Sheath repair

Reviews of the the anatomy of the flexor pulley system by Lin et al (1989a) and Doyle (1988) indicate that while there are significant variations in the morphology of the first annular and cruciform (cruciate) pulleys, the modified descriptions provided by Doyle & Blythe (1975, 1977) are still appropriate for clinical use. To this system Manske & Lesker (1983) introduced the concept that the transverse fibres of the palmar aponeurosis serve as an additional proximal pulley which contributes approximately 7% to the biomechanical efficiency of the tendon sheath (Fig. 6.3). All authors (Doyle & Blythe 1975, Hunter et al 1980, Idler & Strickland 1986; Lin et al 1989b) have confirmed that the loss of the A^2 and A^4 pulleys produces the greatest loss of joint motion while the absence of A^3 alone results in a minimal biomechanical alteration. It has been further emphasized that since the A^2 and A^4 pulleys prevent bowstringing along the curved shafts of the phalanges, their loss necessitates increased tendon excursion before joint motion occurs.

In recent years, many surgeons have advocated preservation and repair of the flexor sheath at the time of tendon suture with the belief that the problems of tendon bowing, decreased range of joint motion, diminished flexion power, flexion contractures and pulley rupture could be greatly reduced (Lundborg & Rank 1978, Eiken et al 1980, Lister 1983). In theory, sheath repair improves tendon nutrition and diminishes the tendency for adhesion formation by blocking the ingrowth of perisheath tissues (Lister 1979, Kleinert et al 1981, Jaeger & Mackin 1984, Strickland 1985a). Repair of the sheath is often difficult and Lister (1983) has provided excellent technical advice on this procedure.

Although there is some evidence that sheath repair does favourably influence the recovery of tendon excursion (Eiken et al 1980, Peterson et al

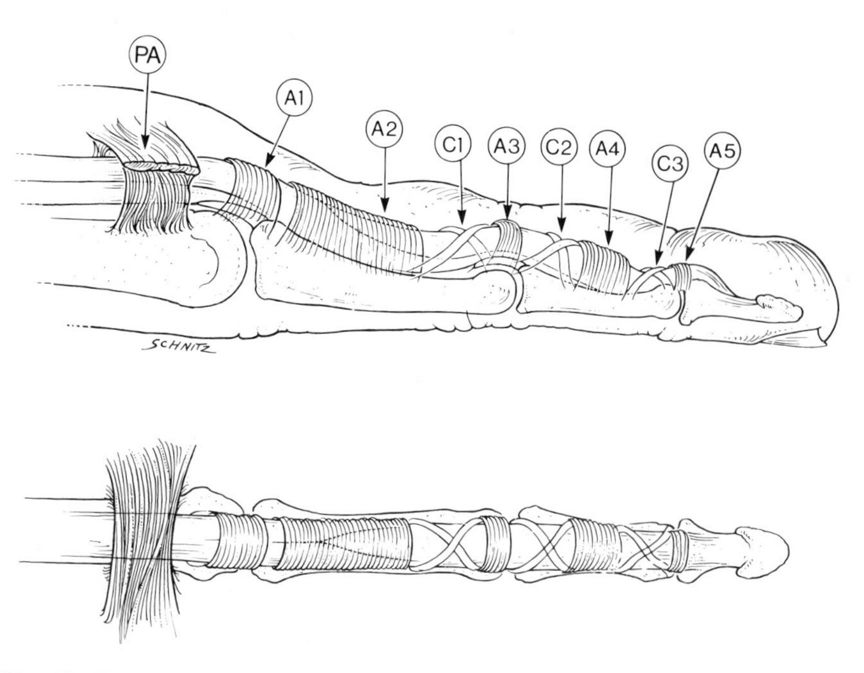

Fig. 6.3 The components of the digital flexor sheath are depicted in this drawing. The sturdy annular pulleys (A^1–A^5) are important biomechanically in keeping the tendons closely applied to the phalanges. The thin, pliable cruciate pulleys collapse to allow full digital flexion. A recent addition has been the palmar aponeurosis (PA) pulley which adds to the biomechanical efficiency of the sheath system. (Modified with permission from Idler 1985.)

1990), many laboratory and clinical studies have been inconclusive (Saldana et al 1987, Chow et al 1990, Gelberman et al 1990).

Tendon retrieval

Retrieval of the retracted proximal flexor tendon ends may be facilitated by 'milking' the proximal tendon into the repair site by flexing the wrist and fingers and massaging the palm and digit in a proximal-to-distal direction as advocated by Kleinert et al (1975). When this method fails, an excellent retrieval technique has been described by Sourmelis & McGrouther (1987), (Fig. 6.4). They recommend the use of a small catheter which is passed from the digital wound into the palm beneath the annular pulleys. The flexor tendons are left in situ in the sheath and, through a small palmar incision, the catheter is sutured to both tendons several centimetres proximal to the A1 pulley.

The catheter is then pulled distally where it will

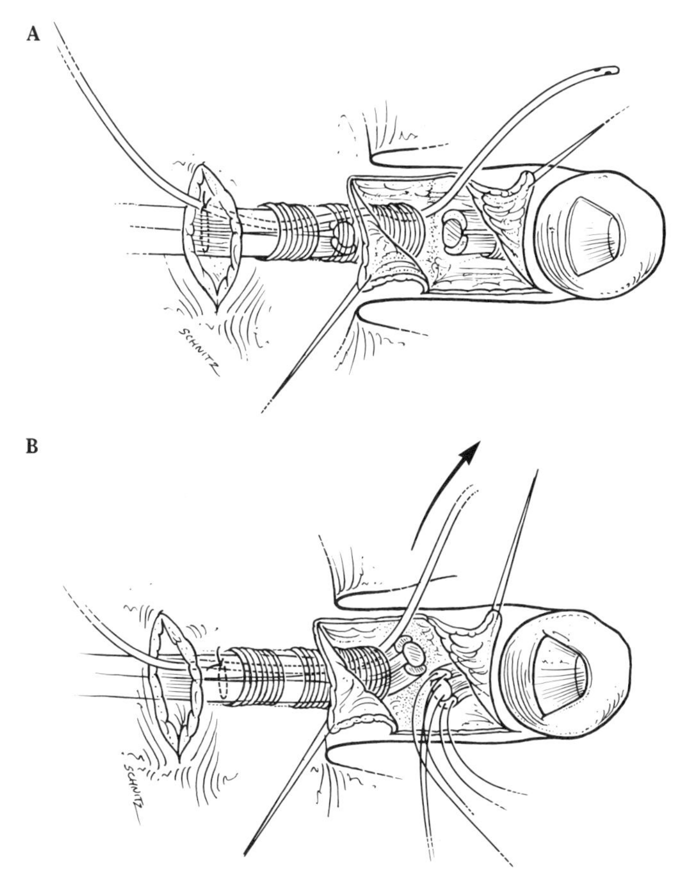

Fig. 6.4 McGrouther's method of retrieving retracted flexor tendons. **(A)** A polyethylene catheter is passed through the flexor tendon sheath alongside the proximal tendon stumps, which are left in situ. The catheter is sutured to both flexor tendons well proximal to the A^1 pulley and emerges in the cruciate–synovial window where the tendon stumps are to be delivered. **(B)** Distal advancement of the proximal flexor tendon stumps by traction on the polyethylene catheter. The suture can then be divided and the catheter withdrawn after the tendons have been transfixed by a transversely oriented 25-gauge hypodermic needle. Core sutures may then be placed in the profundus and superficialis. (Modified from McGrouther 1987.)

deliver the tendon stumps into the distal repair site. A hypodermic needle is then placed transversely across the A^2 annular pulley in order to maintain the tendons in the proper position and length. The connecting suture in the palm can then be divided and the catheter withdrawn.

In some instances, it may be better to identify the profundus and superficialis stumps in the A^1–A^2 interval or in the distal palm through a separate incision or a proximal continuation of the digital wound. Core sutures may then be placed in the proximal tendons and a rubber catheter, silicone infant gastrostomy tube or a suture passer is passed under the A^1–A^2 complex in order to advance them into the repair area (Strickland 1985a). Great care must be taken to retain the anatomical relationship of the tendons which existed at the level of injury before passing them back into the digit (Fig. 6.5).

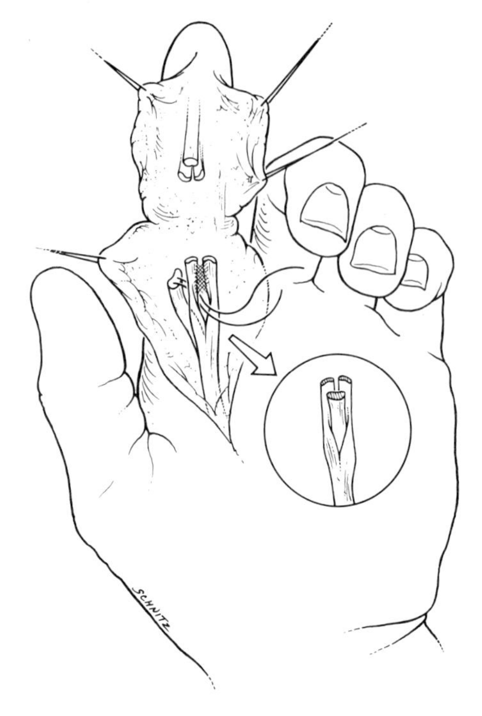

Fig. 6.5 The separated position of the two tendon ends in the distal palm following flexor tendon interruption and proximal retraction. Correct positioning of the profundus in the superficialis hiatus must be carried out prior to passage of the tendons distally into the digit. It is important to re-establish the anatomical relationship of the profundus and the superficialis tendon stumps so that they may be correctly repaired to the corresponding distal tendon stumps. In some cases, the profundus will have to be passed back through the hiatus created by the superficialis slips to lie palmar to Camper's chiasma and recreate the position of those tendons at the level of the tendon laceration. (Reproduced from Strickland 1985b.)

Technical points and pitfalls

Lister (1985) emphasizes the need to recognize the 'FDS spiral' when repairing that tendon. This anatomical transition occurs as the two slips of the flexor digitorum superficialis wind around the profundus over the proximal phalanx. If the superficialis laceration is sustained at the mid-point of this revolution, the proximal and distal ends will both rotate about 90° in different directions. Lister recommends that the opposing slips are derotated at the time of repair in order to prevent obstruction of profundus excursion.

Lister (1983, 1985) has also emphasized that every effort should be made not to violate the annular pulleys. This can usually be achieved by performing the repairs in the cruciate–synovial sheath 'windows' which can be more easily repaired or reconstructed following tendon suture. To accomplish this, small incisions are made in the C^1 cruciate synovial area or in the C^2 interval or both. By acutely flexing the distal interphalangeal joint, it is usually possible to deliver the distal profundus stumps into the wound. If at least 1 cm of the distal stumps can be exposed in this manner, the core sutures can be placed in the tendons. While most zone II repairs can be carried out in the C^1 cruciate–synovial interface, it may not always be possible to deliver 1 cm of the distal tendon into that interval. In those instances, it is necessary to make additional incisions in the C^2 cruciate synovial area of the sheath and then to flex the distal interphalangeal joint in order to expose enough tendon to allow suture placement (Fig. 6.6). The final repair can then be completed in either C^1 or C^2 windows depending on the distal level that can be achieved by the proximal tendon stumps. (Lister 1983, 1985, Lister & Tonkin 1986).

A final technical point to ease the passage of the tendon repair site underneath annular pulleys has been suggested by Lister (1988) and includes the closure of the overlying cruciate synovial sheath prior to extending the proximal and distal interphalangeal joints (Fig. 6.7). When the flexor tendon sheath cannot be repaired, annular pulleys may be grafted using a portion of the extensor

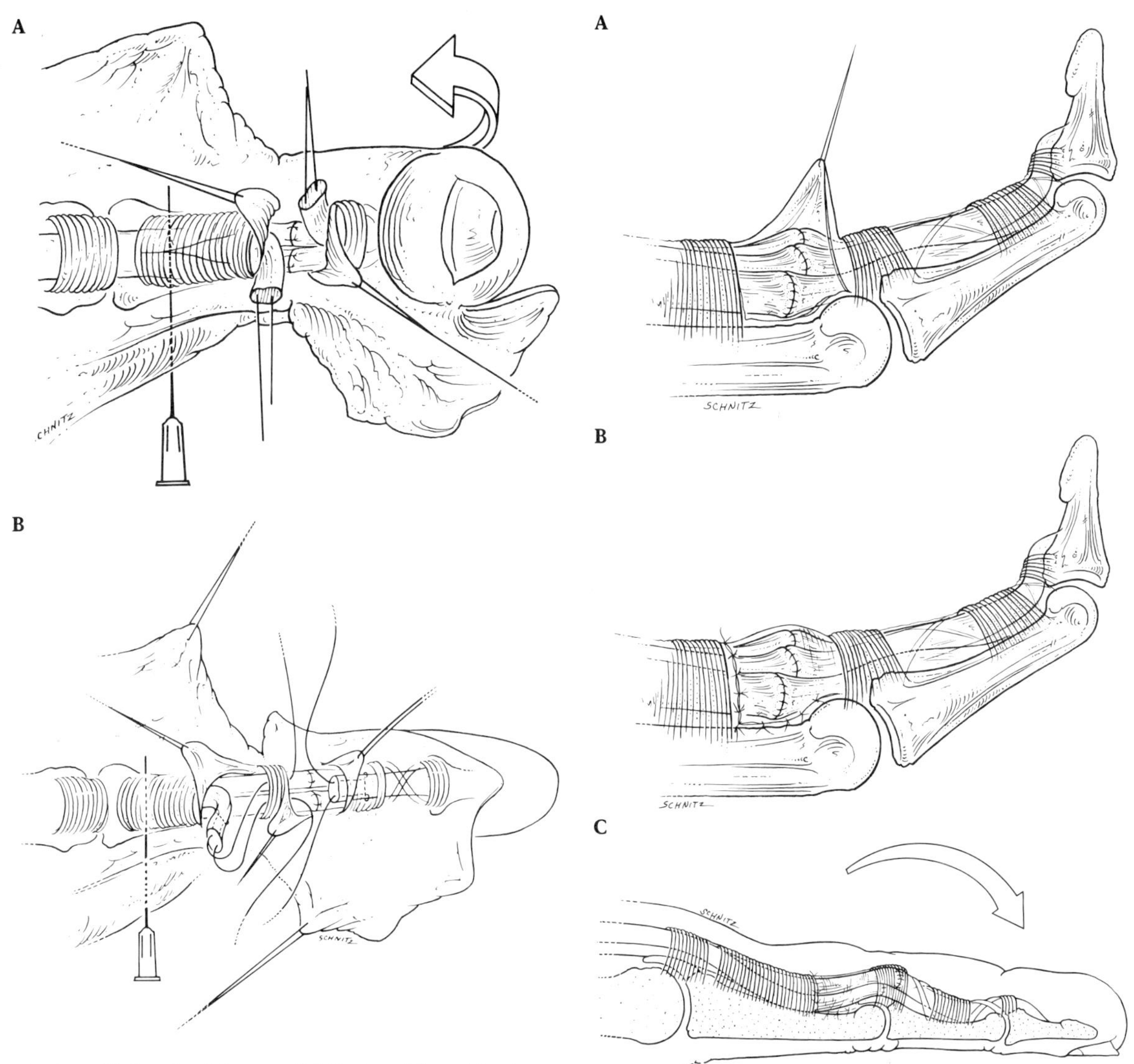

Fig. 6.6 **(A)** Repair of the superficialis first, followed by the profundus tendon, in the C[1] cruciate synovial interval with the distal interphalangeal joint in acute flexion. Restraint of the tendons at the distal level is assured by a transversely placed 25-gauge hypodermic needle through the A[2] pulley. **(B)** Profundus and superficialis repair on both the C[1] and C[2] cruciate-synovial intervals. Sutures placed in the proximal tendon stumps in the C[1] interval are completed in the C[2] interval when a sufficient length of the distal stumps cannot be delivered into the C[1] window.

Fig. 6.7 **(A–C)** closure of the C[1] cruciate–synovial window before extending the interphalangeal joint to facilitate delivery of the repair site beneath the A[3] annular pulley. Similar sheath closure in the C[2] cruciate synovial window may be required for more distal tendon interruption (From Lister, GD 1988, personal communication.)

retinaculum as recommended by Lister (1979, 1983). He also suggested that synovium taken from the extensor surface of the foot or hand or from an adjacent digital sheath could be used to repair the cruciate–synovial sections of the tendon sheath. Strauch et al (1985) and Saldana et al (1987) have described the use of autogenous vein patch grafts to close the sheath.

Post flexor tendon repair management

Following the publication of papers demonstrating the superior results of each movement after flexor tendon repairs (Duran et al 1976, Lister et 1977, Strickland & Glogovac 1980), almost all hand surgeons currently employ some type of early motion protocol. Experimental confirmation of the biological basis of these methods has been provided by the excellent laboratory studies of Gelberman et al (1980, 1981, 1982, 1983, 1986) which also indicated that, in the canine model, early passive motion increased the tensile strength of flexor tendor repairs at an earlier stage in the healing process while lessening adhesions and improving angular joint motion.

In the search for the most consistently effective method of imparting early motion stress to repaired flexor tendons, three general types of programmes, have evolved: active extention with rubber band flexion, controlled passive motion and controlled active motion. Some surgeons have employed combinations of these protocols and the use of a continuous passive motion machine has been reported (Bunker et al 1989).

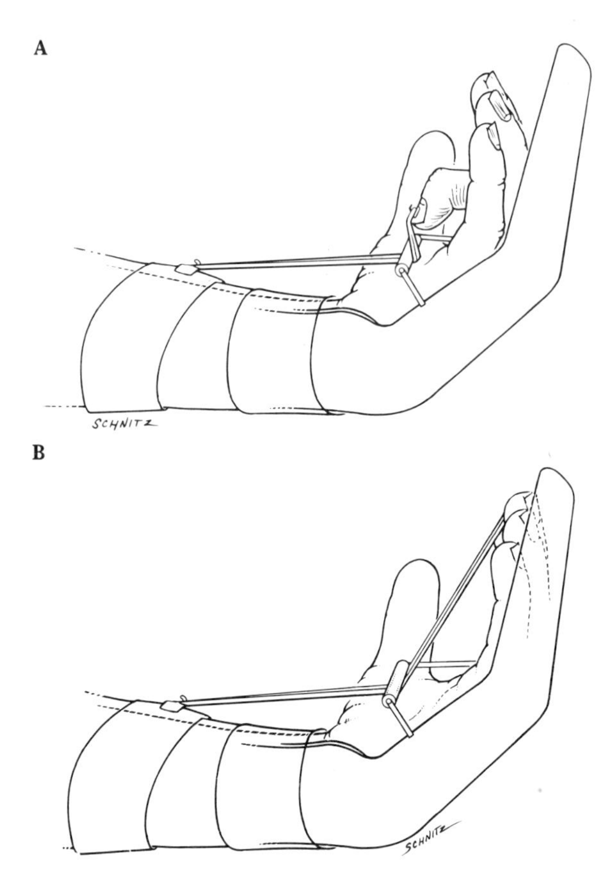

Fig. 6.8 The distal palmar bar under which the rubber band from the wrist to the fingernail of the digit is passed. (**A**) With digit in full flexion; (**B**) with the digit in nearly full extension. Various modifications of this splint are currently in use.

Active extension rubber band flexion method

The original controlled motion protocol developed by Kleinert and described by Lister et al (1977) permitted the patient actively to extend the finger within the limits of a dorsal splint. An elastic band anchored to a wrist band and attached to the fingernail was used to return the finger to a partially flexed attitude. This method has received several modifications (Slattery & McGrouther 1984, Chow et al 1987, Knight 1987, McCabe et al 1987) in an effort to provide less flexion at the wrist and increase the flexion at the metacarpophalangeal joints.

Almost all recent modifications of the active digital extension and rubber band flexion method of Kleinert now incorporate a distal palmar bar which gives the rubber band a more direct approach to the digital tip, resulting in near complete interdigital flexion as the rubber band contracts (Fig. 6.8). Cooney at al (1989) compared the Kleinert splint and one of its modifications with a distal palmar bar to a new splint that passively flexes and extends the digits by synergistic wrist extension and flexion. They found that the synergistic splint provided the largest tendon excursion in zone II and III, the greatest differential excursion between the flexor digitorum superficialis profundus tendons, and even greater excursion under physiological loading. They suggested that the new splint might increase repair excursion and strength with less resistance from adhesions. Chow et al (1990) modified the Kleinert splint in an effort to allow controlled active motion by using a single-core, coated elastic band attached to a proximal spring wire designed to decrease the tension imparted on the tendon during the last 20–30° of extension. The author believe that the new splint may also result in fewer flexion contractures.

Controlled passive motion method

Duran and colleagues (Duran et al 1975, Duran & Houser 1978) described their technique of controlled passive motion in which a posterior splint was applied immediately following surgery and specific limited passive exercises were then permitted at the proximal and distal interphalangeal joints in an effort to impart 3–5 mm of passive motion to the repaired tendons. The clinical effectiveness of a modified version of this method was reported by Strickland & Glogovac (1980) and the controlled passive motion method has subsequently evolved into protocols which encourage considerably more passive interdigital motion then was originally advised (Fig. 6.9). A retrospective study by Stone et al (1989) in which a modification of the Duran & Houser method was used postoperatively showed that an early onset of passive motion was associated with improved total active motion for isolated flexor digitorum profundus injuries at time of discharge from therapy. The proponents of the controlled passive motion protocol contend that it is less likely to result in flexion contractures than the rubber band flexion/active extension method. In addition, the involved digit is felt to be better protected between periods of exercise (Cannon & Strickland 1985).

Active mobilization

In an attempt to obtain better functional recovery, some surgeons have begun to employ early active motion following flexor tendon repair. Using various methods, Cullen et al (1989), Small et al (1989), and Savage & Risitano (1989) have reported recovery of function comparable to but not significantly better than passive motion protocols. The work of Savage (1988) would indicate that a position of wrist extension and metacarpophalangeal joint flexion

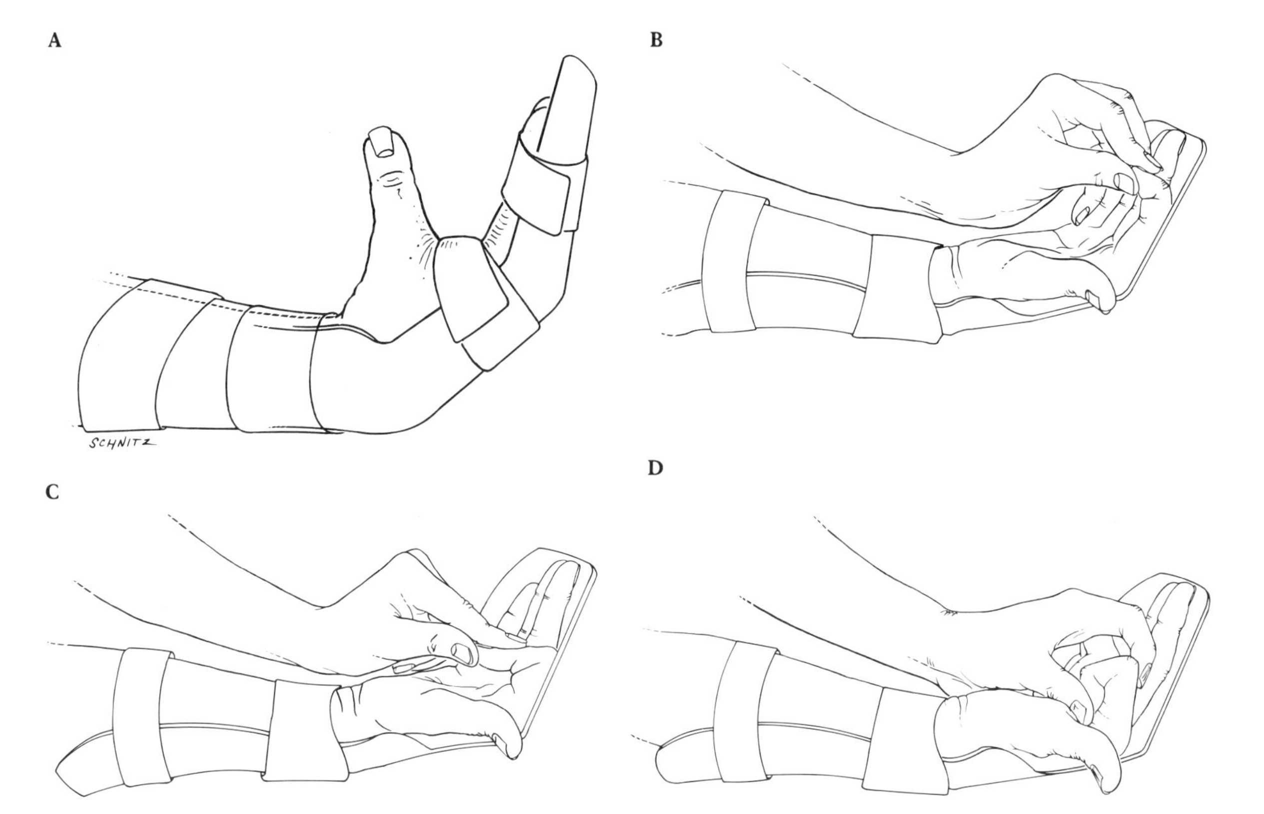

Fig. 6.9 The splint currently in use for the controlled passive motion method. **(A)** An Orthoplast dorsal blocking splint is used to hold the wrist in mild flexion, the metacarpophalangeal (MP) joints at about 45° and the PIP and DIP joints in nearly full extension. Velcro restraints are removed to allow **(B)** full isolated passive flexion of the DIP joint. **(C)** full isolated passive flexion of the PIP joint and **(D)** full passive flexion of the MP, PIP and DIP joints.

produces the least tension on the repaired tendon during attempts at active digital flexion.

Caveats for early mobilization programmes

Although it is convenient to have specific guidelines for early mobilization programmes, there are tremendous differences in the individual response to injury and surgery and a careful monitoring of the status of each patient is extremely important. Those patients who appear to be doing the best at early stage may, in fact, generate the greatest concern with regard to late tendon rupture (Strickland 1989a). Fingers which appear supple with minimal tissue reaction and a good active range of flexion at 3–5 weeks, in fact, could be placing greater stress on the immature tendon-healing at the repair site and be more prone to rupture than the patient whose finger remains swollen and reactive with dense fibrous tissue surrounding the tendon. Schneider (1985) accurately notes that 'in general, the better the patient's progress and range of motion, the slower the program is advanced for fear of rupture of the repair'. The finger which is not doing well at 3 weeks probably can be more aggressively approached with regard to active and passive range of motion exercises and dynamic splinting than can be the more supple mobile digit.

Despite the enthusiasm for early mobilization, there is still scepticism as to how much, if any, motion is really imparted to the flexor tendon repair, particularly during the first 3 weeks when the fibroblastic phase of tendon healing predominates. Manske (1988) in a review of flexor tendon healing stated that:

> although it is recognized that passive motion can move joints, it is not established that passive motion of the finger in fact moves a healing tendon through an effective range of excursion. It is likely that passive mobilization techniques have been successful because the muscle fibers are lengthened during digital extension, followed by active contraction of the muscle back to its resting length; in effect, the techniques are useful because the patient knowingly 'cheats' by spontaneous involuntary contraction of the muscle.

Complications

Wound breakdown and infection are potential complications following flexor repair in zone II, particularly when there has been crushing or extensive wounding of the involved digit. Rupture of one or both flexor tendon repairs is a significant complication. Leddy (1982) states that the 'preferred treatment is prompt re-exploration and repair'. While some authors (Schneider et al 1977) have implied that such ruptures cannot or should not be resutured, Allen et al (1987) reviewed 7 patients with ruptured flexor tenorrhaphies who underwent prompt surgical repair of the ruptured tendons and completed a second rehabilitation programme identical to that described for primary repair. Their results were felt to be comparable to those obtained by patients with uncomplicated primary repairs.

The most frequently cited late complications of the early postoperative mobilization programmes are those of flexion contractures at the proximal or distal interphalangeal joints or both. The protocols for the active extension/rubber band flexion, controlled passive motion, and active flexion all emphasize the need to extend the interdigital joints fully on a regular basis in an effort to abort such contractures. The active extension/rubber band flexion programme in particular has been implicated in the development of these deformities because the finger is kept in a flexed attitude between exercise periods. Prompt recognition of developing contractures, modification of the motion programme to permit greater extension and the judicious use of dynamic extension splints can help prevent or overcome these contractures.

Results

The student of flexor tendon surgery will be frustrated by the many variations in the methods of measurement and classification of results encountered in the literature. Despite the efforts of many authors to introduce assessment methods that demonstrate the results of various procedures, no universally accepted system has evolved. This lamentable absence makes it virtually impossible for the surgeon to compare reported results.

We have long advocated a simple formula for the assessment of digital performance after flexor tendon repair (Strickland & Glogovac 1980, Strickland 1985a, 1987c, 1989a) and continue to believe that it serves as an equitable method for the evaluation and comparison of results (Fig. 6.10):

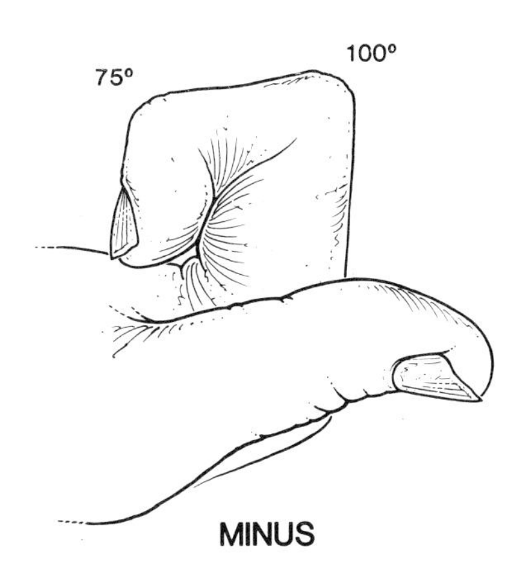

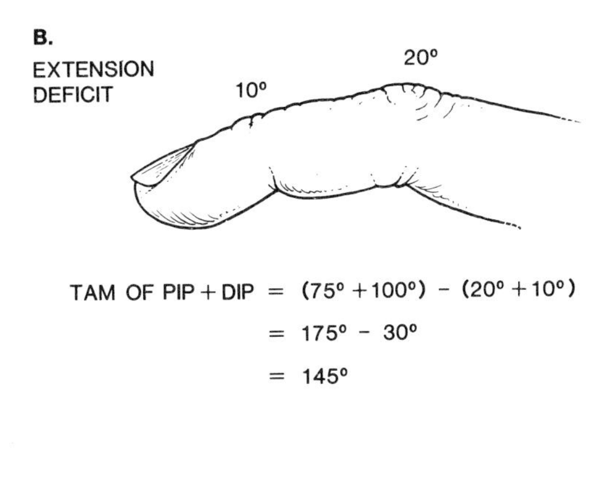

Fig. 6.10 The technique for measuring digital joint motion to be used in determining total active motion (TAM) and total passive motion (TPM) of the PIP joint. **(A)** Flexion is measured at the PIP and DIP joints while the patient attempts to make a complete fist. **(B)** Extension deficit at the PIP and DIP joints is measured. The combined extension deficit of the two joints is subtracted from the combined flexion to give the total active motion. Passive manipulation of the digit is carried out and the same formula is used to determine the total passive motion.

$$\frac{\text{PIP} + \text{DIP flexion}^{\star} - \text{extensorlag} \times 100}{175^{\circ}}$$

= % of normal PIP and DIP motion

*while attempting to make a complete fist

The percentage of normal results is then classified by the system suggested by the International Federation for Hand Surgeons as shown in Table 6.1.

While it is beyond the scope of this treatise to review all recent published results of flexor tendon repairs, a few notable papers will be discussed briefly.

The results of the use of a new dynamic splint in 36 patients have been published by Werntz et al (1989). Thirty-five of 46 fingers with zone II flexor tendon injury (76.1%) had excellent and 11 (23.9%) had good results using Strickland's modified criteria. Chow et al (1987) reported their results of regimen which included active extension against rubber band flexion as well as controlled passive extension and flexion following the repair of flexor tendons in the hand. Forty-four digits with a complete laceration of the flexor digitorum profundus and superficialis in zone II were treated. Using the 'Strickland formula', 36 fingers (82%) were rated excellent, 7 fingers (16%) were rated good and 1 finger (2%) was rated fair. None were rated poor and there was no statistical difference between the results of delayed primary repair and immediate primary repair. An additional multi-Army hospital study by Chow et al (1988), using essentially the same protocol and the 'Brooke Army Hospital modification of the Rubberband Passive Splint' also indicated superb recovery of function. That study included 66 patients (78 fingers) at multiple army hospital centres. Sixty-two fingers (80%) were rated excellent and 14 (18%) good with 2 (2%) fair and none poor. Bunker et al (1989) reported excellent results in 11 of 14 fingers (79%), good results in 1 (7%), and fair results in 2 fingers (14%) by the Buck-Gramcko scale when using a continuous passive motion machine following repair of zone II injuries. Using a six-strand method of

Table 6.1 Classification of flexor tendon results. Data from Kleinert & Verdan 1983

Classification	% of Return
Excellent	75–100
Good	50–74
Fair	25–49
Poor	0–24

repair and beginning active movements the day after repair, Savage & Risitano (1989) reported 52% excellent, 17% good, 22% fair, and 2% poor results by the Buck-Gramcko method in 23 zone II repairs. He reported no ruptures but did find 4% of repairs to have elongation and adherence.

While the majority of the efforts to assess the recovery of function following flexor tendon interruption concentrate on the return of interdigital flexion and extension, little emphasis has been placed on the return of digital strength. Gault (1987) studied 67 patients with 176 repaired flexor tendons who were reviewed for a mean follow-up interval 26.4 months. Grip strength averaged 74.5%, mean finger flexion pressure 76.8% and mean finger pinch pressure 74.7% of the opposite uninjured hand or digit. They concluded that grip strength was reduced after injury to tendons alone, particularly when there was concomitant damage to the median or ulnar nerves.

FREE TENDON GRAFTS

In those instances where flexor tendons sharply divided in zone I or II have not been or cannot be directly repaired, conventional free tendon grafting may still represent the best procedure for restoring finger function. In recent years there has been a disconcerting tendency to opt for immediate staged flexor tendon reconstruction when a digit is biologically suitable for a single-stage free graft.

Indications

The indications for conventional free tendon grafting have been well established. Pulvertaft (1975) stated that successful results from standard grafting methods are obtained only when certain rules are followed: the hand must be in good general condition without extensive scarring; passive digital joint motion must be good; there must be satisfactory circulation and at least one digital nerve must be intact. Schneider & Hunter (1982) have emphasized that the surgeon must decide whether a conventional free tendon graft or a staged reconstruction is most appropriate in a particular situation. Some patients will have have experienced failed primary surgery or previous efforts at flexor tendon reconstruction and the degree of scarring within the digit may preclude the realistic possibility of achieving a good result from free grafting.

Start and associates (1977) felt that the prerequisites for free tendon grafting with an intact superficialis tendon included a superficialis tendon that is normal; that the digit has full passive motion; that there is minimal soft-tissue scarring, and a patient who is between 10 and 21 years of age. Although generally in favour of free grafting for an isolated profundus division in selected cases, Pulvertaft (1960) expressed his concern when he stated: ‘it should not be advised unless the patient is determined to seek perfection and the surgeon is confident of his ability to offer a reasonable expectation of success without the risk of doing harm.’ In his early writings, Pulvertaft advised tendon grafting for the index and long fingers but felt that the ring and little fingers should have grafts only when the patient required specific action of those digits because of a special interest or occupation, as in the case of a musician or skilled technician. Pulvertaft (1984) later changed his thinking and advised that free tendon grafting is often appropriate in the small finger, particularly when the superficialis tendon is found to be weak. In such patients, the improvement of grip provided by the restoration of profundus function makes the procedure worthwhile. It can be seen that the late treatment of flexor digitorum profundus division or rupture with an intact superficialis tendon remains quite controversial. If the patient has full, strong function of the superficialis, the functional impairment to the involved digit may not be great. Since a tendon graft brings with it the risk of compromising existing function, a conservative approach with no treatment, tenodesis, or arthrodesis may be preferred to free grafting.

Technical points and pitfalls

Tubiana (1969, 1974) and Pulvertaft (1960) have detailed the principles of flexor tendon grafting which include that one graft should be placed in one finger; that an intact superficialis tendon is never sacrificed; that the graft should be of small calibre; and that its ends should be fixed away from the tendon sheath (Fig. 6.11). Tubiana also recommended the careful calculation of the tension of the graft and the sparing of at least one pulley to

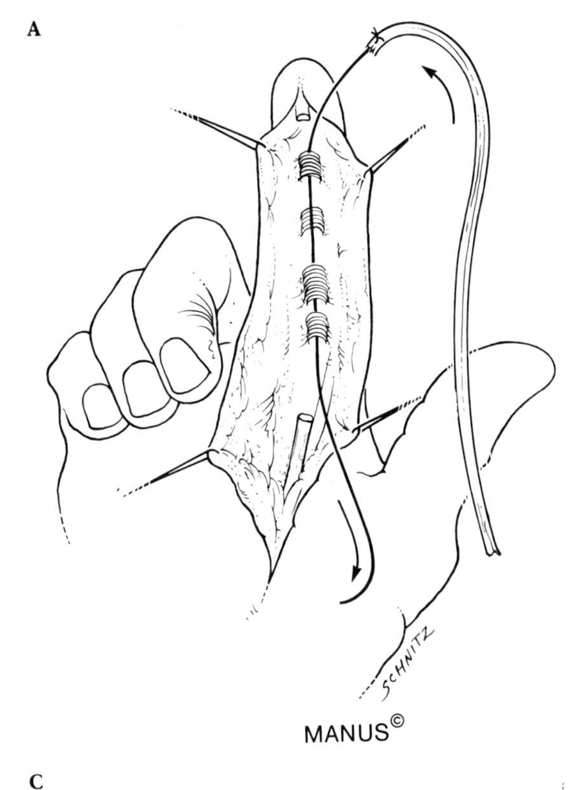

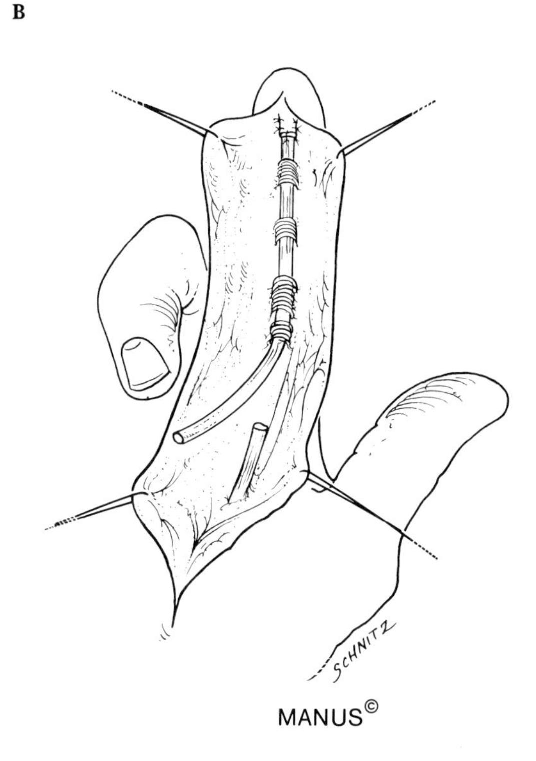

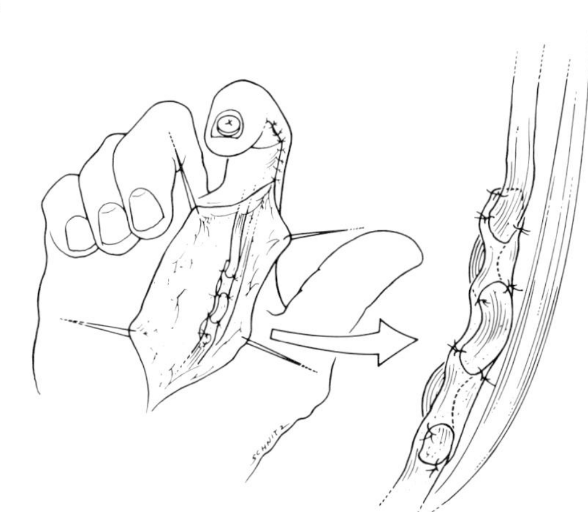

Fig. 6.11 Technique of the free tendon grafting. **(A)** and **(B)** Following preparation of a digital canal by excision of scar tissue and careful retention of annular pulleys, a free tendon graft is attached distally to a suture and passed from the base of the distal phalanx into the palm. The appearance of the tendon in the digital bed following completion of the distal juncture is shown. The method of distal juncture for adults is usually through a drill-hole in the distal phalanx, through which the tendon is drawn by a suture which is secured dorsally over the nail using a small sponge and button. The profundus stump is then sutured to the graft to secure the juncture. **(C)** Following closure of the digital wound, a Pulvertaft weave is completed in the palm under sufficient tension to flex the involved finger slightly more than its normal resting posture.

prevent bowstringing. While many surgeons, including Bunnell (1956), recommended excision of the majority of the flexor tendon sheath with retention of only small sections of the annular pulleys, it is now flet that one should strive to preserve as much of the sheath system as possible. Eiken et al (1980, 1981) have even suggested transplanting synovial tissue from the toes or wrists as the sheath autograft in order to close open sections of the fibro-osseous canal. The reconstruction of pulleys at the time of free tendon grafting is rarely advisable and in most instances, the finding of a deficient pulley system should serve as an indication to proceed with staged reconstruction.

There is some disagreement concerning which donor tendons should be chosen for free flexor tendon grafting. The palmaris longus, when available, probably has the most advocates although Pulvertaft (1984) favoured the plantaris, particularly when the superficialis was intact. Other tendons that may be employed as grafts include the extensor digitorum longus tendons to the second, third, and fourth toes; the extensor indicis proprius; extensor digiti quinti proprius; and the flexor digitorum superficialis tendon to the fifth finger (Kyle & Eyre-Brook 1954, White 1960).

Post free tendon graft management

While most surgeons are more reluctant to utilize early motion following grafts than they are following flexor tendon repairs, there is a growing effort on the part of some surgeons to utilize mobilization techniques similar to those employed following primary flexor tendon repair in an effort to mobilize tendon grafts. An article by Tonkin et al (1988) compared recovery of digital function following free tendon grafting with either a 3- or 4-week period of immobilization or with an immediate controlled mobilization postoperatively. The final motion obtained was independent of the postoperative management although the rate of graft rupture and of tenolysis was higher in the immobilization group. Chow et al (1987, 1988) indicate that the postoperative regimen which they have used so successfully following flexor tendon repair is equally effective for tendon grafts, although no results have been publised.

Complications

Many problems can develop following flexor tendon grafting including tendon adherence, joint contractures, graft rupture, bowstringing secondary to inadequate pulley preservation or restoration, recurvatum of the proximal interphalangeal joint, a graft that is too short or too long, and the lumbrical plus deformity described by Parkes (1971). While the management of most of these complications is apparent and specific for that condition, a ruptured graft is a semi-emergency. Rupture is more common at the proximal juncture than at the insertion and occasional mid-substance disruption can occur. As with tendon repair ruptures, prompt exploration repair stand the best chance of regaining reasonable function in this unfortunate situation.

Results

In 197k, Boyes & Stark assessed the results of 1000 consecutive free tendon grafts utilizing the method originated by Bunnell. This work will unquestionably serve as the definitive analysis of the performance of this technique. They found that factors which influOnced the recovery of function, in order of importance, were scar, joint involvement, age, nerve injury and the digit involved. An excellent study by McClinton et al (1982) serves as a classic review of the performance of 100 free grafts with an intact superficialis tendon. In their series the average active distal interphalangeal joint flexion was 48° following surgery and only 13 patients were considered to have an unsuccessful result. They concluded that, in properly motivated patients, tendon graft replacement of isolated profundus tendon injuries could give satisfactory results even in an older age group

Questions concerning the growth of autografted tendons have been well adressed by the work of Nishijima et al (1988), who found that chicken flexor tendon grafts demonstrated the same growth rate as control tendons. Although tendon growth was retarded compared to control tendons at 15 weeks after operation, it was not statistically different at 20 weeks. This experiment would appear to confirm the clinical impression which surgeons have long had—that flexor tendon grafts do grow and the rate of growth appears to be proportional to digital growth.

STAGED FLEXOR TENDON RECONSTRUCTION

Bassett & Carroll (1963) began using flexible silicone rubber robs to build pseudosheaths in badly scarred flexor tendons in the 1950s. Helal (1969, 1973) also used silicone rubber tendons clinically as early as 1966 for two-staged flexor reconstruction. The implant and method currently used by almost all hand surgeons have largely resulted from the work of Hunter and associates (Hunter 1965, 1984, Hunter & Salisbury 1970, 1971, Hunter & Schneider 1975, 1977). The procedure has proven to be an extremely important addition to the armamentarium to the hand surgeon for reconstructing flexor tendon function in the badly damaged digit. Numerous reports (e.g. Honnor & Meares 1977, LaSalle & Strickland 1983) have now been published that attest to the excellent performance of the technique in otherwise difficult or unsalvageable situations.

Indications

Staged flexor tendon reconstruction is reserved for badly damaged or previously operated digits with significant scarring and a deficient or damaged pulley system. As with conventional free tendon grafting, the digit must be in biological equilibrium without reactive scar and must have satisfactory passive movement, sensation and circulation.

To achieve optimal results, one must carefully follow the advice provided by the developers of the technique (Hunter & Schneider 1975, 1977). Schneider & Hunter (1982) emphasize that this procedure should only be carried out after multiple factors have been taken into consideration. The patient should be informed of the complexity of the problem, the length and magnitude of the surgery, and the need for extensive postoperative therapy. Not all patients' digits will be candidates for this lengthy and demanding procedure and, in some cases, arthrodesis or even amputation may be a more practical approach. It is emphasized that patients with severe neurovascular impairment are poor candidates for staged tendon reconstruction.

Technical points and pitfalls (Fig. 6.12)

Stage 1

While most surgeons prefer to implant the silicone rod from the distal foream to the digital tip, others prefer to carry staged tendon reconstruction from the digital tip to the palm. In those instances in which the palm has not been involved in the original or subsequent surgery, this technique may

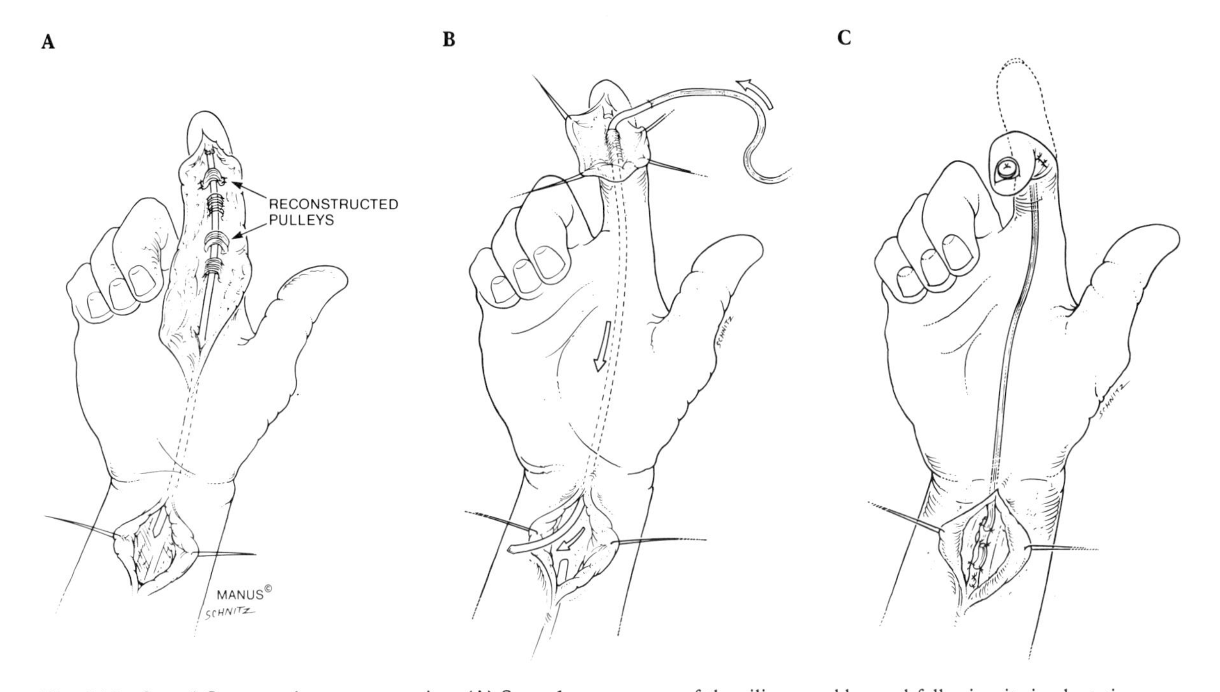

Fig. 6.12 Staged flexor tendon reconstruction. **(A)** Stage 1: appearance of the silicone rubber rod following its implantation. Pulleys have been reconstructed over the proximal and middle phalanges and the implant has been left free to glide proximally. **(B)**

be satisfactory (Rowland 1975, Strickland 1987b). Schneider (1985) now recommends the use of an implant that closely corresponds to the size of the expected graft. A 4-mm implant is frequently appropriate and it should be threaded through the remaining pulleys in such a manner that free gliding of the implant occurs with passive digital motion. After the definitive implant is placed in the digital bed its distal insertion is secured. There are currently two techniques available for the distal implant juncture, and surgeons must make their own decision on this point (Schneider & Hunter 1982, Schneider 1985). One design (Holter-Houser) has a metal end-piece on the implant, which may be fixed to bone beneath the profundus stump with a 2-mm Woodruff self-tapping screw. Direct suture of the silicone rod to the retained profundus stump is probably carried out more frequently than the more demanding anchorage necessitated by the use of the terminal screw. After placement of the implant has been completed, any deficiencies in the annular pulley system should be overcome by pulley reconstruction.

Stage 2

At approximately 3 months, when full resolution of the digital scars and the best possible passive motion has been obtained it is appropriate to proceed with the second stage of the reconstructive process. The replacement of the silicone-Dacron implant by a free tendon graft may be carried out by utilizing the terminal portions of previous stage 1 digital and distal forearm incisions. Unfortunately, the palmaris longus is usually not of sufficient length to serve as a good tendon graft for the staged reconstruction technique involving the forearm to the digital tip. When present, the plantaris tendon makes a better graft for this procedure because of its small size and long length. The tendon graft is attached to the distal end of the implant and pulled proximKlly through the pseudosheath into the proximal incision. Distal and proximal connections and graft tension are essentially the same as those employed for conventional free tendon grafting.

Post staged graft management

Although Schneider (1985) and his associates now favour an early protected motion programme initiated at 3 days following the second-stage grafting procedure, many surgeons feel that 3–4 weeks of immobilization are more appropriate, given the salvage nature of the procedure and the drastic effect rupture would have on the already complicated effort to return tendon function.

Complications

Complications after staged tendon reconstruction may include synovitis around the rod, infection or wound breakdown, and disruption of the distal implant–bone or tendon juncture after stage 1. Stage 2 complications include rupture of the graft, a graft that is too loose or too tight, the development of an intrinsic plus phenomenon, or flexion deformities at the distal or the proximal interphalangeal joint, or both (Chamay & Gabbiana 1978). Finally, adhesions of the graft may prevent successful recovery of digital motion and may require tenolysis (LaSalle & Strickland 1983). The complications of either stage of the reconstructive process may severely compromise the end-result and must be dealt with accordingly.

Results

In 1971, Hunter & Salisbury presented their preliminary results after staged flexor tendon reconstruction. LaSalle and Strickland (1983) confirmed the value of the technique as the best reconstructive option for severely damaged digits when they reported the recovery of an excellent or good result in 39% of the digits which underwent the procedure. They further found that the results were upgraded to 65% in the excellent or good category following tenolysis in 47% of patients undergoing the procedure. Subsequent studies by Wehbe et al (1986) evaluating the Philadelphia experience, found 150 fingers to have returned a total active motion of 176° and a mean grip strength of 79% compared to a preoperative 102° and 20% respectively. Complications included a flexion contracture of varying degrees in 41% of the fingers, rupture of the tendon graft in 14% and an infection in 4%.

Amadio et al (1988) evaluated 130 fingers in 101 patients treated with staged flexor tendon reconstruction between 1973 and 1984. Overall, a 54%

good or excellent result was achieved utilizing a total active motion percentage method although only 19% had a final total active motion of greater than 180° in the proximal and distal interphalangOal joints. Their complications included infection in 15%, rupture in 4%, amputation in 4% and reflex sympathetic dystrophy in 1%. Sixteen per cent of their patients required tenolysis after stage 2. They found that factors associated with a poor result included zone I or II injury in patients younger than 10 years.

Versaci (1970), Honner (1975), and Wilson et al (1980) all presented promising results of the use of staged flexor tendon grafts for isolated profundus injury. A dissenting experience, however, was reported by Sullivan (1986): only 7 of 16 cases achieved a satisfactory result. Five major complications occurred in 4 patients. The author concluded that the overall results were no better than the results obtained for single staged flexor tendon grafting through an intact superficialis. Sullivan believed that there was no advantage of staged flexor tendon grafts over unstaged grafts for isolated profundus loss.

FLEXOR TENOLYSIS

Tenolysis may be indicated following flexor tendon repair or grafting when the passive range of digital flexion significantly exceeds active flexion. The decision to carry out the procedure should be based on serial joint measurements which indicate that there has been no appreciable improvement for several months despite a vigorous therapy programme and the conscientious efforts of the patient.

Indications

The prerequisites for tenolysis as established by Fetrow (1967), Hunter et al (1982) Schneider & Hunter (1975), Schneider & Mackin (1978, 1985) should be closely adhered to. All fractures should be healed and wounds must have reached equilibrium with soft, pliable skin and subcutaneous tissues and minimal reaction around scars. Joint contractures must have been mobilized and a normal or near-normal passive range of digital motion achieved. While some controversy persists with regard to the proper timing for the procedure, it is now generally accepted that tenolysis may be considered 3 months or more after repair or graft providing the other criteria for the procedure had been satisfied and there has been no measurable improvement in active motion during the preceding 4–8 weeks (Strickland 1985c, 1987c). Satisfactory sensation and muscle strength should be regained and the patient must be carefully informed as to the objectives, surgical techniques, postoperative course, and pitfalls of the procedure.

Technical points and pitfalls (Fig. 6.13)

While the technique of flexor of tenolysis following failed tendon repairs or grafts is well known to hand surgeons, there have been some helpful contributions to this procedure in recent years. Schneider and associates (Schneider & Hunter 1975, 1982, Schneider & Mackin 1978, 1984, Schneider & Mackin 1985) made popular the use of local anaesthetic supplemented by intravenous analgesia and tranquillizing drugs for tenolysis. They contend that the method best allows the patient to demonstrate the completeness of the lysis by actively flexing the involved digit during surgery (Fig. 6.14). They also believe that it is important to allow the patient to observe the improved digital motion

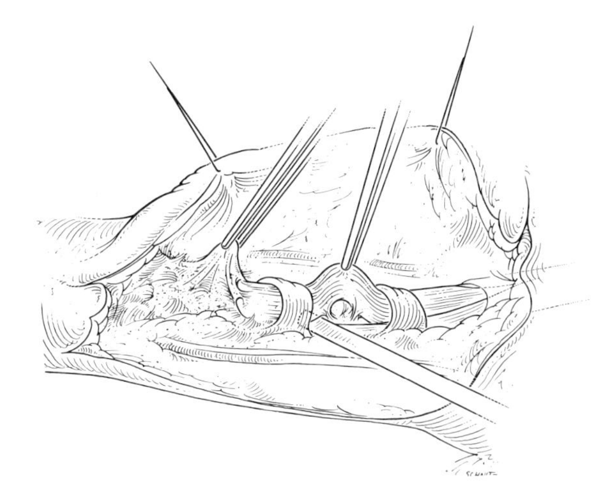

Fig. 6.13 Digital tenolysis of adherent flexor tendons. Careful release of adhesions beneath the pulleys is facilitated by the use of small knifeblades and elevators.

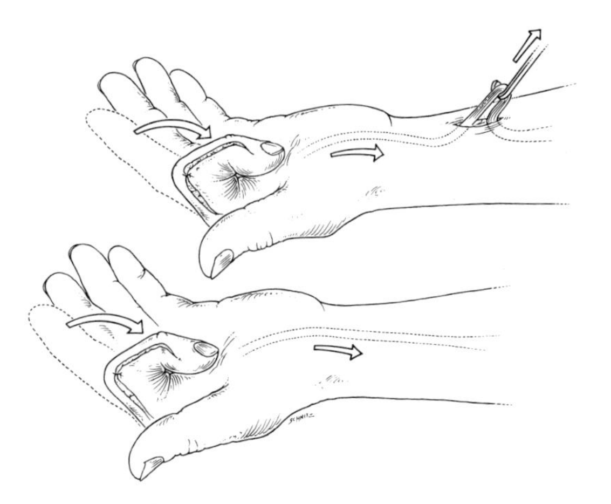

Fig. 6.14 Tenolysis is concluded when a complete release by all restraining adhesions has been achieved by either (**top**) a proximal traction check through a separate wrist incision or, preferably, by the active participation of the patient under local anaesthetic (**bottom**). (Reproduced with permission from Strickland 1985c.)

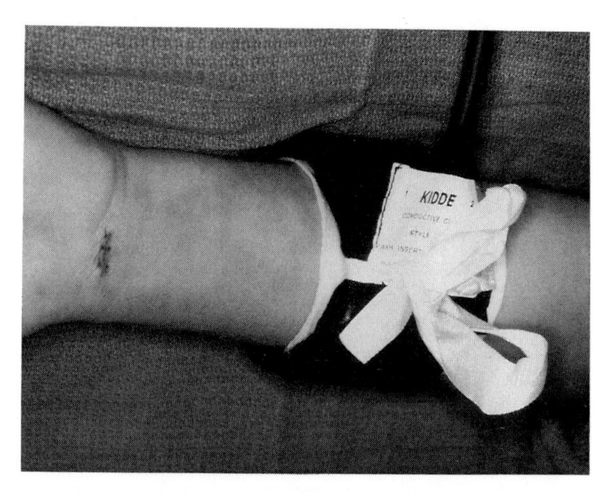

Fig. 6.15 A sterile paediatric pneumatic tourniquet applied to the mid forearm may be of considerable value during the tenolysis procedure. Its use often permits continued function of the extrinsic flexor musculature and can provide relief from the upper arm tourniquet discomfort while maintaining a bloodless field. The tourniquet is removed prior to the application of the dressing with or without reinflation of the proximal tourniquet. (Reproduced with permission from Strickland 1985c.)

during surgery in order to provide motivation for the maintenance of that motion during the rigorous postoperative therapy programme. Most surgeons now agree that the advantage of local anaesthesia and active participation are enormous and recommend its use whenever possible. The use of a sterile paediatric tourniquet applied to the mid-forearm has proved to be an effective method of dealing with the problems of muscle paralysis and tourniquet pain (Strickland 1985c, 1987c; Fig. 6.15). During tenolysis, it is important for the surgeon to make every effort to maintain the majority of each of the annular pulleys in order to prevent the biomechanical sequelae of pulley deficiency and the possibility of pulley rupture. Hunter et al (1982) have emphasized the importance of critically assessing the quality of the flexor tendons at the time of surgery. They state that if 30% of the tendon width has been lost or if the continuity of the tendon is thought to include a segment of scar tissue, it is questionable whether or not tenolysis should be carried out and it may be better to proceed with a staged reconstruction.

Various mechanical barriers have been employed to limit the reformation of peritendinous adhesions following tenolysis. There is conflicting opinion as to the usefulness of these materials. The most common indications for silicone interposition at present are in cases of repeat tenolysis in which the reformation of adhering scar tissue over a long distance would seem to be almost inevitable (Strickland 1985c, 1987c).

The use of local or systemic steroid preparations in an effort to modify the quality and quantity of tendon adhesions following tenolysis has provoked considerable debate. It is probably best to reserve the use of this medication for patients who have shown a propensity for the rapid and aggressive reformation of scar tissue or for those who are undergoing repeat lysis. In those instances, several millilitres of triamcinolone may be locally administered at the time of wound closure (Strickland 1985c, 1987c). One should be wary of the possibility of delayed wound healing or infection when using steroids in conjunction with this procedure. Several recent studies have examined the effect of other pharmacological agents on adhesion formation. Kulick et al (1986) have indicated that ibuprofen may reduce adhesion formation around flexor tendons and Szabo & Younger (1990) showed that pre- and postoperative subcutaneous injections of indomethacin significantly improved angular rotation in a rabbit model.

Post-tenolysis management

Although some authors have advocated immediate motion following flexor tenolysis, others have recommended starting therapy in several days or as soon as soft tissue healing permits. The rapid formation of new adhesions can probably best be discouraged by initiating finger movement within the first 12 hours following flexor tenolysis whenever possible. In those instances where the quality of the lysed tendon is in question, a frayed tendon programme has been suggested (Cannon & Strickland 1985, Strickland 1985c, 1987c) and involves passively manipulating the digit into the fully flexed position and then asking the patient actively to maintain that flexion (Fig. 6.16). If the digit retains its flexed position following the removal of the manipulating finger, muscle contracture and tendon movement have been confirmed. In this manner, the tendon moves through its maximal excursion but with much less likelihood of rupture.

Complications

Rupture of the tendon is an infrequent but catastrophic complication. When this occurs, the surgeon must decide whether the appropriate option for that patient is an immediate repair, or whether the patient's previous surgery and the status of the flexor tendon system mitigate against an effort at repair. In some instances, the additional surgical insult may be too great and it may be better to allow the finger to rest and to proceed at a later date with a staged flexor tendon reconstruction programme or simply abandon the effort to restore function and settle for arthrodesis or amputation.

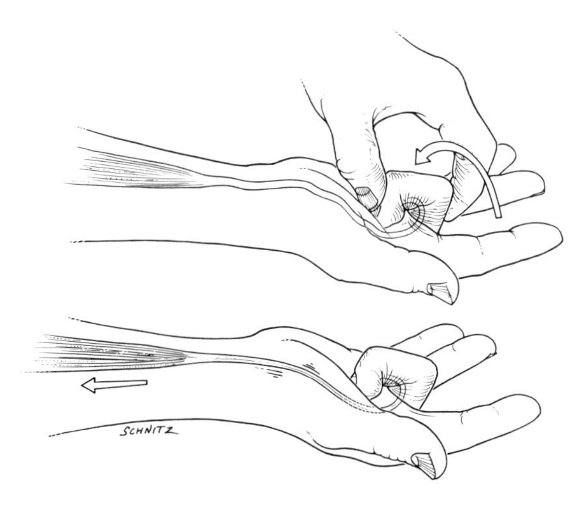

Fig. 6.16 Frayed tendon programme: technique of postoperative mobilization of the digit following flexor tenolysis. **(top)** Full passive flexion of all three digital joints is carried out, followed by active attempts to maintain flexion **(bottom)**. Tendon excursion is the same as that produced by active digital flexion with less tensile loading. This technique is particularly valuable for patients with somewhat stiffened joints or tendons of poor quality. (Reproduced with permission from Strickland 1985c.)

Results

The results of flexor tenolysis have been analysed utilizing a formula and a classification system compatible with that employed for other flexor tendon procedures (Whitaker et al 1977, Strickland 1985c). The findings of these studies indicate that tenolysis can be expected to return at least 50% of the preoperative discrepancy between active and passive motion at the proximal and distal interphalangeal joints in 65% of the digits that undergo the procedure. An additional 15% returned fair function, whereas 20% failed to benefit appreciably from the operation. A rupture rate of 8% remains disconcerting and is a calculated risk that must be explained to the patient prior to surgery.

FLEXOR PULLEY RECONSTRUCTION

While the restoration of a four-pulley system may ensure the best functional recovery, at least A2 and A4 need to be preserved or rebuilt if maximum efficiency is to be restored. Reconstructed pulleys must hold the tendon as close to the underlying bone as possible without restricting its gliding and it has been suggested that the pulley should be reconstructed just distal to the metacarpophalangeal and proximal interphalangeal joint at the bases of the proximal and middle phalanges (Schneider 1985).

Technical points and pitfalls

A number of methods have been advocated for the reconstruction of deficient annular pulleys at the time of flexor tendon grafting, staged reconstruction or tenolysis (Fig. 6.17). Pulleys may be reconstructed by the use of a slip of the superficialis tendon, by encircling tendon grafts around or through the phalanx or woven through the retained rim of a previous pulley (Kleinert & Bennett 1978), or by the use of a strip of the extensor retinaculum from the dorsum of the wrist (Lister 1979). In some instances, parallel slits in the palmar plate may be effectively developed into pulleys during the first stage of tendon reconstruction using a belt loop procedure as advocated by Karev (1984, Karev et al 1987). Cadaver studies by Lin et al (1989b) showed that while no pulley reconstruction method provided a normal tendon excursion–joint motion relationship, repair of the A2 and A4 pulleys was most effective in restoring joint motion. They further reported that only reconstruction using a double- or triple-loop tendon graft had a load to failure that most closely approximated an intact pulley.

The use of the synthetic material expanded polytetrafluoroethylene has shown favorable histological results in a primate model but needs to be further evaluated for strength properties that would correspond to human pulleys (Dunlap et al 1989). Other artificial materials used to recreate pulleys have included knitted Dacron arterial graft (Wray & Weeks 1974) and silicone rubber sheeting (Fig. 6.14; Bader et al 1968).

PERMANENT ACTIVE TENDON IMPLANT

A prototype active tendon implant developed by Hunter is now being used clinically in several centres. While the implant is not yet meant to be implanted permanently, in most instances it is replaced only at the time of failure and many have been in place for several years. Hunter et al (1988) evaluated the results of 45 active flexor tendon implants which were placed in scarred tendon beds of digits. The implant was constructed of silicone rubber with a Dacron core terminating in a loop proximally and a metal plate distally. Modification of the implant during the period of study was felt to

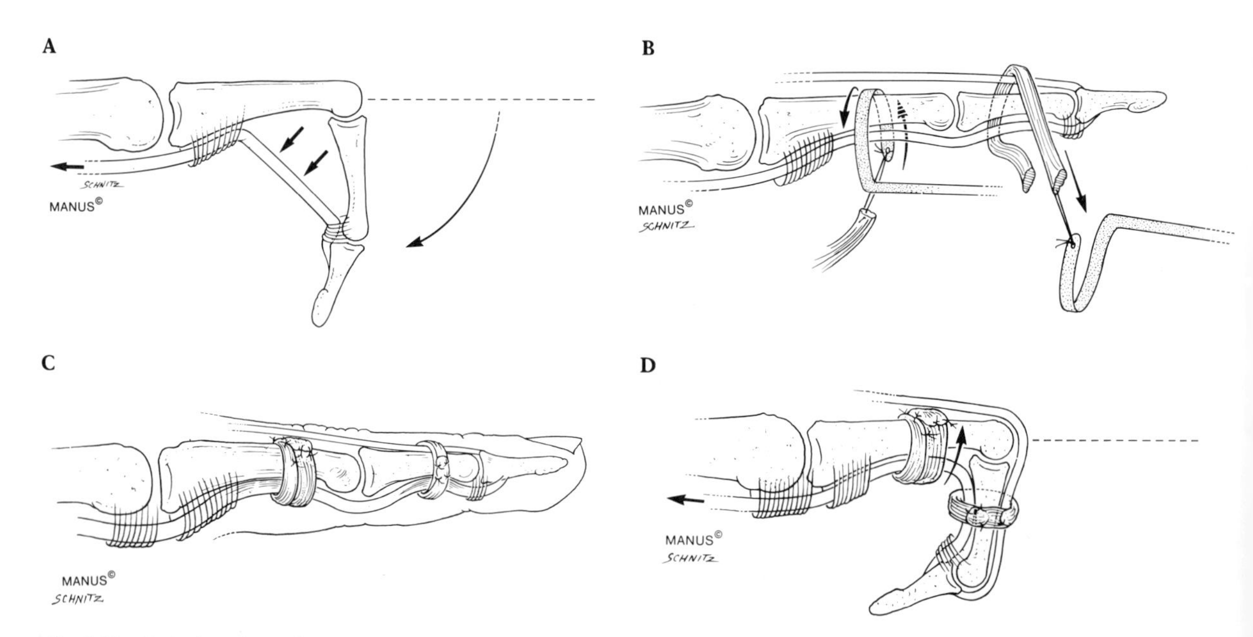

Fig. 6.17 Technique for pulley restoration using circumferential tendon grafts. **(A)** Marked bow-stringing and tendon inefficiency resulting from the loss of annular pulleys from the proximal A^2 to the A^5 level. Note the vertical displacement of flexor tendon and the need for increased tendon excursion to produce digital flexion. **(B)** The use of a circumferential ligature carrier beneath the extensor tendon at the mid proximal phalanx or over it at the middle phalanx to prepare a channel for the passage of a tendon graft. **(C)** Appearance of the pulley grafts after the juncture site has been rotated either to the side or dorsum of the digit. The proximal phalanx pulley has been reconstructed by two tendon loops to give a wider pulley restoration. **(D)** Improved mechanics of the flexor tendon following the restoration of annular pulleys over the proximal and middle phalanges.

have improved its reliability on longevity. Improvement and total active motion averaged 72° during implant functioning (stage 1) in a group of digits that before operation were classified as 78% Boyes grade 5 (salvage). The complication rate during stage 1 was 11% (5 out of 45). Of the 27 digits evaluated after implant replacement by tendon autograft (stage 2) there was an overall improvement of 62° total active motion with 70% of the digits being Boyes grade 5. The authors believe that the study demonstrates the feasibility of an active tendon implant and the possibility of a permanent prosthesis. Problems in developing permanent fixation between the implant and the host tissues remain to be solved although strides are being made.

REHABILITATION

It is probable that the emergence of sophisticated hand therapy has been more valuable for the recovery of function after flexor tendon repair and reconstruction than in any other area of hand surgery. They judicious use of splinting to overcome joint contractures, improve muscle strength, and maximize the function of adjacent uninjured digits is extremely valuable. Throughout the management of patients with flexor tendon injuries, the therapist must have a thorough understanding of the pathological anatomy, the findings at surgery, the quality of the flexor tendons, the presence or absence of portions of the flexor sheath system, and the realistic goals of any surgical procedure. One cannot overemphasize the need for close co-operation and understanding between patient, surgeon and therapist and the need to approach each patients as a separate person with unique requirements, limitations and goals.

KEY POINTS FOR CLINICAL PRACTICE

Flexor tendon repair has advanced to a stage where a satisfactory recovery of digital flexion and extension may be achieved providing certain suture methods and postoperative protocols are employed and the patient is co-operative throughout the protracted course of healing and rehabilitation which is usually required. The use of delicate, meticulous operative techniques for tendon surgery remains as important today as it was when emphasized over 50 years ago by Sterling Bunnell (Bunnell 1918). The surgeon carrying out acute flexor tendon repair or one of the reconstructive procedures for the flexor system must fully appreciate both the normal and pathological anatomy of the involved hand as well as the complexities of the surgical methods he or she is about to employ.

Suture methods which can resist the forces of early motion programmes and minimize gap formation are currently used by most surgeons and the Kessler grasping technique or one of its modifications has becomes the most popular. It has been further demonstrated that the epitendinous peripheral running stitch at the repair site is of considerable importance for gap prevention and the running lock stitch or horizontal mattress methods are probably the best.

There has been little conclusive evidence that repair of the flexor sheath at the time of tendon suture actually enhances the final result and the decision remains one prejudiced by the experience and training of the surgeon. Preservation of the annular pulleys, however, is of the utmost importance if the biomechanical integrity of the flexor system is to be maintained.

The institution of a closely monitored postoperative controlled motion programme has now been well demonstrated to improve the strength of the repair at an earlier time period while lessening adhesions and improving angular joint motion when compared to those methods which immobilize the repaired tendon for 3 or more weeks. When employing the active extension/passive rubber band flexion protocol, it appears that the new splints using a distal palmar bar to maximize composite digital flexion are the most effective. Proponents of passive early motion methods now advocate full flexion at all three digital joints and continuous passive motion machines, when modified for flexor tendon repairs, have improved results somewhat. Active motion programmes have been carefully applied by some but, to date, have not been shown to be superior to other more conservative methods. All early mobilization programmes now emphasize the need regularly and fully to extend the involved digits to minimize flexion contractures.

There is still a definite use for conventional free tendon grafting, which was the work-horse procedure for tendon surgeons several decades ago. While the techniques have not changed, the use of magnification and better instrumentation may help today's surgeons approach the excellent results achieved by our predecessors who accomplished this procedure with artistic skill.

When previous flexor tendon procedures have failed or there is significant damage or scarring of the digit, the staged reconstruction methods may be of tremendous benefit in restoring a functional digit. The indications and technical advice offered by Hunter and Schneider and colleagues (Hunter 1984, Schneider 1982, 1985, Schneider & Hunter 1982, Hunter & Schneider 1977) for this procedure must be closely adhered to and the complications are considerable. None the less, considering that it is usually employed as a salvage option in a badly damaged digit, the method is of great value.

Tenolysis is often required when previous repairs or grafts lack sufficient excursion to allow active digital motion commensurate with the digit's passive potential. The procedure is best done with the patient awake in order to demonstrate when the tendons have been completely extricated and the use of interpositional barriers and adhesion-limiting medications may have some occasional value. Early postlysis motion should be initiated and programmes that lessen the tensile demands on the lysed tendon may help prevent rupture.

The need to preserve or reconstruct pulleys at the time of flexor tendon surgery has been emphasized, and several techniques using tendon grafts, extensor retinaculum or synthetic materials have been shown to be effective in improving the biomechanical efficiency of the pulley-deficient digit.

The use of an artificial active tendon remains somewhat experimental although encouraging results have been tendered by the developers of the implant. In the future, it seems reasonable that a biologically inert gliding implant will be devised which is capable of achieving strong proximal and distal junctures with host tissues.

The maturation of hand rehabilitation specialists has been one of the greatest adjuncts of the recovery of digital function after flexor tendon disruption. The experience hand therapist can carefully tailor and alter programmes which can be of enormous benefit to the patient attempting to regain passive and active motion after these difficult injuries.

SUMMARY

It can be seen that tremendous recent strides have been made in the management of flexor tendon injuries. Although scientific investigation has provided a biological basis for many of the techniques which are currently in use, much has been left to trial and error. There remains much to be done in an effort to determine the best method of tendon repair, the best protocol and most advantageous timing for imparting motion stress to the repaired tendon and what, if any, chemical agents might be administered to effect the contradictory need for tendon healing without adhesions.

REFERENCES

Allen BN, Frykman GK, Unsell RS, Wood VE 1987 Ruptured flexor tendon tenorrhaphies in zone II: repair and rehabilitation. J Hand Surg 12A:18–21
Amadio PC, Wood MB, Cooney WP, Bogard SD 1988 Staged flexor tendon reconstruction in the fingers and hand. J Hand Surg 13A:559–562
Bader KF, Sethi G, Curtin JW 1968 Silicone pulleys and underlays in tendon surgery. Plast Reconstr Surg 41:157–164
Bassett CAL, Carroll RE 1963 Formation of tendon sheaths by silicone rod implants, Bone Joint Surg 45A:884–885
Bishop AT, Cooney WP, Wood MB 1986 Treatment of partial flexor tendon lacerations: the effect of tenorrhaphy and early protected mobilization. J Trauma 26:301–312
Boyes JH, Stark HH 1971 Flexor tendon grafts in the fingers and thumb. A study of factors influencing results in 1000 cases. J Bone Joint Surg 53A:1332–1342
Bunker TD, Potter B, Barton NJ 1989 Continuous passive motion following flexor tendon repair. J Hand Surg 14(B):406–411
Burnell S 1918 Repair of tendons in the fingers and description of 2 new instruments. Surg, Gynecol, Obstet 126:103
Bunnell S 1956 Surgery of the Hand, 3rd ed. JB Lippincott Philadelphia
Cannon NM, Strickland JW 1985 Therapy following flexor tendon surgery In: Strickland JW (ed) Symposium on flexor tendon surgery, Hand clinics. WB Saunders, Philadelphia, pp 147–166
Chamay A, Gabbiana G 1978 Digital contracture deformity after implantation of a silicone prosthesis: light and electron microscopic study. J Hand Surg 3:266–270
Chow SP, Yu OD 1984 An experimental study on incompletely cut chicken tendons—a comparison of two methods of management. J Hand Surg 9B:121–125
Chow JA, Thomes LJ, Dovelle SW et al 1987 A combined regimen of controlled motion following flexor tendon repair in 'no man's land.' Plast Reconstr Surg 79:447–453
Chow JA, Thomes LJ, Dovelle S et al 1988 Controlled motion rehabilitation after flexor tendon repair and grafting. A multi-centre. J Bone Joint Surg 70B:591–595
Chow JA, Stephens MS, Ngai WK et al 1990 A splint for

controlled active motion after flexor tendon repair. J Hand Surg 15A:645–651
Cooney WP, Lin GT, Kai-Nan A 1989 Improved tendon excursion following flexor tendon repair. J Hand Ther 2:102–106
Cullen KW, Tolhurst P, Lang D, Page RE 1989 Flexor tendon repair in zone 2 followed by controlled active mobilisation. J Hand Surg 14B:392–395
Doyle JR 1988 Anatomy of the finger flexor tendon sheath and pulley system. J Hand Surg 13A:473–484
Doyle JR, Blythe WF 1975 The finger flexor tendon sheath and pulleys: anatomy and reconstruction. In: AAOS symposium on tendon surgery in the hand. CV Mosby, St Louis, pp 81–87
Doyle JR, Blythe WF 1977 Anatomy of the flexor tendon sheath and pulleys of the thumb. J Hand Surg 2:149–151
Dunlap J, McCarthy JA, Manske PR 1989 Flexor tendon pulley reconstructions—a histological and ultrastructural study in non-human primates. J Hand Surg 14B:273–277
Duran RH, Houser RG (1978) Management of flexor lacerations in zone 2 using controlled passive motion postoperatively. In: Hunter JM, Schneider LH, Mackin EJ, Bell X (eds) Rehabilitation of the hand CV Mosby, St Louis pp 105–114
Duran RH, Houser RG, Stover MG 1975 Controlled passive motion following flexor tendon repair in zones 2 and 3. In: AAOS symposium on flexor tendon surgery in the hand. CV Mosby, St Louis
Duran RJ, Houser RG, Coleman CR, Postlewaite DS 1976 A preliminary report on the use controlled passive motion following flexor tendon repair in zones II and III. J Hand Surg 1:79
Eiken O, Holmberg J, Ekerot L et al 1980 Reconstruction of the digital tendon sheath. Scand J Reconstr Surg 14:89–97
Eiken O, Hagberg L, Lundborg GN 1981 Evolving biologic concepts as applied totendon surgery. Clin Plas Surg 8:1–12
Fetrow KW 1967 Tenolysis in the hand and wrist. J Bone Joint Surg 49A:667–685
Gault DT 1987 A review of repaired flexor tendons. J Hand Surg 12B:321–325
Gelberman RH, Jayasanker M, Gonsalves M, Akeson WH 1980 The effects of mobilization on the vascularization of healing flexor tendons in dogs. Clin Orthop 153:283–289
Gelberman RH, Amifl D, Gonsalves M et al 1981 The influence of protected passive mobilization on the healing of flexor tendons: a biochemical and microangiographic study. Hand 13:120–128
Gelberman RH, Woo SLY, Lothringer K et al 1982 Effects of early intermittent passive mobilization on healing canine flexor tendons. J Hand Surg 7:170–175
Gelberman RH, Vande Berg JS, Lundborg GN, Akeson WH 1983 Flexor tendon healing and restoration of the gliding surface. J Bone Joint Surg 65A:70–80
Gelberman RH, Botte MJ, Spiegelman JH, Akeson WH 1986 The excursion and deformation of repaired flexor tendons treated with protected early motion. J Hand Surg 11A:106–110
Gelberman RH, Woo SLY, Amiel D et al 1990 Influences of flexorsheath continuity and early motion on tendon healing in dogs. J Hand Surg 15A:69–77
Helal B 1969 Silastics in tendon surgery. Hand 1:120–121
Helal B 1973 The use of silicone rubber spacers in flexor tendon surgery. Hand 5:85–90
Honner R 1975 The late management of the isolated lesion of the flexor digitorum profundus tendon. Hand 7:171–174
Honnor R, Meares A 1977 A review of 100 flexor tendon reconstructions and prostheses. Hand 9:226
Hunter JM 1965 Artificial tendons. Early development and application. Am J Surg 109:325
Hunter JM 1984 Staged flexor tendon reconstruction. In: Hunter JM, Schneider LH, Mackin EJ, Callahan AD (Eds) Rehabilitation of the hand, 2nd edn. CV Mosby, St Louis, pp 288–313
Hunter JM, Salisbury RE 1970 Use of gliding artificial implants to produce tendon sheaths: techniques and results in children. Plastic Reconstr Surg 45:564–572
Hunter JM, Salisbury RE 1971 Flexor-tendon reconstruction in severely damaged hands: a two-staged procedure using a silicone-dacron reinforced gliding prosthesis prior to tendon grafting. J Bone Joint Surg 53A:829–858
Hunter JM, Schneider LH 1975 Staged flexor tendon reconstruction. Current status. AAOS symposium on tendon surgery in the hand. CV Mosby, St Louis, pp 271–274
Hunter JM, Schneider LH 1977 Staged flexor reconstruction. AAOS instructional course lectures, vol 26. CV Mosby, St Louis, pp 134–144
Hunter JM, Cook JF, Ochai N et al 1980 The pulley system. J Hand Surg 5:283
Hunter JW, Seinsheimer F, Mackin EJ 1982 Tenolysis: pain control and rehabilitation. In: Strickland JW, Steichen JB (eds) Difficult problems in hand surgery. CV Mosby, St Louis, pp 312–318
Hunter JM, Singer DI, Jaeger SH, Mackin EJ 1988 Active tendon implants in flexor tendon reconstruction. J Hand Surg 13A:849–859
Idler RS 1985 Anatomy and biomechanics of the digital flexor tendons. Hand Clin 1:6
Idler RS, Strickland JW 1986 The effects of pulley resection on the biomechanics of the proximal interphalangeal joint. Univ Penn Orthop J 2:20–23
Jaeger SH, Mackin EH 1984 Primary care of flexor tendon injuries. In: Hunter JM, Schneider LH, Mackin EJ, Callahan AD (eds) Rehabilitation of the hand, 2nd edn. CV Mosby, St Louis, pp 261–272
Kleinert H E, Verdan C 1983 Report on the Committee on Tendon Injuries. J Hand Surg 8:794–798
Karev A 1984 The 'belt loop' technique for the reconstruction of pulleys in the first stage of flexor tendon grafting. J Hand Surg 9A:923–924
Kerev A, Stahl S, Taran A 1987 The mechanical efficiency of the pulley system in normal digits compared with a reconstructed system using the 'belt loop' technique. J Hand Surg 12A:596–601
Kirchmayr L 1917 Zur Technik der Sehnenaht. Zentralbl Chir 44:27–52
Kleinert HE 1976 Commentary on 'Should an incompletely severed tendon be sutured?' The voice of polite dissent. Plastic Reconstr Surg 57:236
Kleinert HE, Bennett B 1978 Digital pulley reconstruction employing the always present rim of the previous pulley. J Hand Surg 3:297–298
Kleinert HE, Kutz JE, Ashbell TS, Martinez E 1969 Primary repair of flexor tendons in 'no man's land.' J Bone Joint Surg 49A:577
Kleinert HE, Kutz JE, Cohen MJ 1975 Primary repair of zone 2 flexor tendon lacerations. AAOS symposium on tendon surgery in the hand pp 91–104. C V Mosby, St Louis
Kleinert HE, Schepels S, Gill T 1981 Flexor tendon injuries. Surg Clin North Am 61:267–286
Knight SL 1987 A modification of the Kleinert splint for

mobilisation of digital flexor tendons. BJ Hand Surg 12B:179–181
Kulick MI, Smith S, Hadler K 1986 Oral ibuprofen: evaluation of its effect on peritendonous adhesions and the breaking strength of a tenorrhaphy. 11A:110–120
Kyle JB, Eyre-Brook AL 1954 The surgical treatment of flexor tendon injuries in the hand: results obtained in a consecutive series of 57 cases. Br J Surg 41:502–511
Lasalle WB, Strickland JW 1983 An evaluation of the two-stage flexor tendon reconstruction technique. J Hand Surg 8:263–267
Leddy JP 1982 Flexor tendons—acute injuries. In: Green DP (ed) Operative hand surgery. Churchill Livingstone, New York, pp 1347–1374
Lin GT, An KN, Amadio PC, Cooney WP 1988 Biomechanical studies of running suture for flexor tendon repair in dogs. J Hand Surg 13A:553–558
Lin GT, Amadio PC, An KN, Cooney WP 1989a Functional anatomy of the human digital flexor pulley system. J Hand Surg 14A:949–956
Lin GT, Amadio PC, An KN, Cooney WP, Chao EYS 1989b Biomechanical analysis of finger flexor pulley reconstruction. J Hand Surg 14B:278–282
Lister GD 1979 Reconstruction of pulleys employing extensor retinaculum. J Hand Surg 4:461–464
Lister GD 1983 Incision and closure of the flexor tendon sheath during tendon repair. Hand 15:123–135
Lister GD 1985 Pitfalls and complications of flexor tendon surgery. Hand Clin 1:133–146
Lister GD 1988 Personal communication
Lister GD, Tonkin M 1986 The results of primary tendon repair with closure of the tendon sheath. J Hand Surg 11A:767
Lister GD, Kleinert HE, Kutz JE, Atasoy E 1977 Primary flexor tendon repair followed by immediate controlled mobilization. J Hand Surg 2:441–451
Littler JW 1977 The digital flexor–extensor system. In: Converse JM (ed) Reconstructive plastic surgery, 2nd edn, vol 6. WB Saunders, Philadelphia
Lundborg G, Rank F 1978 Experimental intrinsic healing of flexor tendons based upon synovial fluid nutrition. J Hand Surg 3:21–31
Malerich MM, Baird RA, McMaster W, Erickson JM 1987 Permissible limits of flexor digitorum profundus tendon advancement—an anatomic study. J Hand Surg 12A:30–33
Manske PR 1988 Flexor tendon healing. J Hand Surg 13B:237–245
Manske PR, Lesker PA 1983 Palmar aponeurosis pulley. J Hand Surg 8:259–263
McCabe S, Lindsay M, Chesher S, Kleinert HE 1987 Muscle activity in a third-generation flexor tendon splint: an EMG study. American Society for Surgery of the Hand Annual Meeting, San Antonio
McClinton MA, Curtis RM, Wilgis EFS 1982 One hundred tendon grafts for isolated flexor digitorum profundus injuries. J Hand Surg 7:224–229
McGrouther DA 1987 Retrieval of the retracted flexor tendon. J Hand Surg 12B:109–111
Nishijima N, Ueba Y, Yamamuro T 1988 Growth of autografted tendons: an experimental study in vivo. J Hand Surg 13A:234–237
Parkes A 1971 The lumbrical plus finger. J Bone Joint Surg 53B:236–239
Peterson WW, Manske PR, Dunlap et al 1990 Effect of various methods of restoring flexor sheath; integrity on the formation of adhesions after tendon injury. J Hand Surg 15A:48–56
Pulvertaft RG 1960 The treatment of profundus division by free tendon graft. J Bone Joint Surg. 42A:1363–1380
Pulvertaft RG 1975 Indications for tendon grafting. AAOS symposium on tendon surgery in the hand. CV Mosby, Philadelphia, pp 123–131
Pulvertaft RG 1984 Tendon grafting for the isolated injury of the flexor digitorum profundus. Bull Hosp J Dis Orthop Inst Fall 44:424–434
Rowland SA, 1975 Palmar fingertip use of silicone rubber followed by free tendon graft. In: AAOS symposium on flexor tendon surgery in the hand. CV Mosby, St Louis, pp 145–150
Saldana MJ, Ho PK, Lichtman DM et al 1987 Flexor tendon repair and rehabilitation in zone II open sheath technique versus closes sheath technique. J Hand Surg 12A:1110–1113
Savage R 1985 In vitro studies of a new method of flexor tendon repair. J Hand Surg 10B:135–141
Savage R 1988 Influence of wrist position on the minimum force required for active movement of the interphalangeal joints. J Hand Surg 13B:262–268
Savage R, Risitano R 1989 Flexor tendon repair using a 'six strand' method of repair and early active mobilisation. J Hand Surg 14B:396–399
Schlenker JD, Lister GD, Kleinert HE 1981 Three complications of untreated partial laceration of flexor tendon—entrapment, rupture, and triggering. J Hand Surg 6:392–396
Schneider LH 1982 Staged flexor tendon reconstruction using the method of Hunter. Clin Orthop 171:164
Schneider LH (ed) 1985a Flexor tendon injuries. Little, Brown, Boston
Schneider LH (ed) 1985b Tenolysis. In: Flexor tendon injuries. Little Brown, Boston
Schneider LH, Hunter JM 1975 Flexor tenolysis. In: AAOS symposium on tendon surgery in the hand. CV Mosby, St Louis, pp 157–162
Schneider LH, Hunter JM 1982 Flexor tendon, late reconstruction. In: Green DP (ed) Operative hand surgery. Churchill Livingstone, New York pp 1375–1440
Schneider LH Mackin EJ 1978 Tenolysis. In Hunter JM Schneider LH, Mackin EJ, Bell JA (eds) Rehabilitation of the hand. CV Mosby, St Louis, p 229
Schneider LH, Mackin, EJ 1985 Tenolysis: dynamic approach to surgery and therapy. In Hunter JM, Schneider LH, Mackin EJ, Callahan AD (eds) Rehabilitation of the hand, 2nd edn. CV Mosby, St Louis, pp 280–287
Schneider LH, Hunter JM, Norris TR, Nadeau PO 1977 Delayed primary flexor tendon repair in no man's land. J Hand Surg 2:452–455
Seradge H 1983 Elongation of the repair configuration following flexor tendon repair. J Hand Surg 8:182–185
Slattery PG, McGrouther DA 1984 A modified Kleinert controlled mobilization splint following flexor tendon repair. J Hand Surg 9B:217–218
Small JO, Brennen MD, Colville J 1989 Early active mobilisation following flexor tendon repair in zone 2. J Hand Surg 14B:383–391
Sourmelis SG, McGrouther DA 1987 Retrieval of the retracted flexor tendon. Br J Hand Surg 12:109–111
Stark HH, Zemel NP, Boyes JH, Ashworth CR 1977 Flexor tendon graft through intact superficialis tendon. J Hand Surg 2:456–461

Stone RG, Spencer EL, Almquist EE 1989 An evaluation of early motion management following primary flexor tendon repair: zones 1-3. J Hand Ther pp. 223–230
Strauch B, De Moura W, Ferder M et al 1985 The fate of tendon healing after restoration of the integrity of the tendon sheath with autogenous vein grafts. J Hand Surg 10A: 790–795
Strickland JW 1983 Management of acute flexor tendon injuries. Orthop Clin North Am 14:827–849
Strickland JW 1985a Results of flexor tendon surgery in zone II. Hand Clin 1:167–180
Strickland JW 1985b Flexor tendon repair. Hand Clin 1:55–68
Strickland JW 1985c Flexor tenolysis. Hand Clin 1:121–132
Strickland JW 1986 Flexor tendon injuries, part 1: anatomy, physiology, biomechanics, healing, and adhesion formation around a repaired tendon. Orthop Rev XV:632–645
Strickland JW 1987a Flexor tendon injuries, part 3: free tendon grafts. Orthop Rev XVI:18–26
Strickland JW 1987b Flexor tendon injuries, part 4: staged flexor tendon reconstruction and restoration of the flexor pulley. Orthop Rev XVI:78–90
Strickland JW 1987c Flexor tendon injuries part 5: flexor tenolysis, rehabilitation and results. Orthop Rev XVI:33
Strickland JW 1987d Flexor tenolysis: a personal experience in: Hunter JM, Schneider LH, Mackin EJ (eds) Tendon surgery of the hand. CV Mosby, St Louis, pp 216–233
Strickland JW 1989a Flexor tendon surgery, part 1: primary flexor tendon repair. J Hand Surg 14B:261–272
Strickland JW 1989b Flexor tendon surgery, part 2: free tendon grafts and tenolysis. J Hand Surg 14B:368–382
Strickland JW, Glogovac SV 1980 Digital function following flexor tendon repair in zone 2: a comparison study of immobilization and controlled passive motion. J Hand Surg 5:537–543
Sullivan DJ 1986 Disappointing outcomes in staged flexor tendon grafting for isolated profundus loss. J Hand Surg 11B:231–233
Szabo RM, Younger E 1990 Effects of indomethacin on adhesion formation after repair of zone II tendon lacerations in the rabbit. J Hand Surg 15A:480–483
Tonkin M, Hagberg L, Lister G, Kutz J 1988 Postoperative management of flexor tendon grafting. J Hand Surg 13B:277–281
Trail IA, Powell S, Noble J 1989 An evaluation of suture materials used in tendon surgery. J Hand Surg 14B:422–427
Tubiana R 1969 Technique of flexor tendon grafts. Hand 1:108–114
Tubiana R 1974 Postoperative care following flexor tendon grafts. Hand 6:152–154
Urbaniak JR 1984 Replantation in children. In: Serafin D, Georigiade NG (eds) Pediatric plastic surgery, vol 2. St Louis, CV Mosby, p 1168
Verdan C 1960 Primary repair of flexor tendons. J Bone Joint Surg 42A:647–657
Verdan C 1964 Practical considerations for primary and secondary repair in flexor tendon injuries. Surg Clin North Am 44:951–970
Versaci AD 1970 Secondary tendon grafting for isolated flexor digitorum profundus injury. Plastic Reconstr Surg 46:57–60
Wade PJF, Muir IFK, Hutcheon LL 1986 Primary flexor tendon repair: the mechanical limitations of the modified Kessler technique. J Hand Surg 11B:71–76
Wade PJF, Wetherell RG, Amis AA 1989 Flexor tendon repair: significant gain in strength from the Halsted peripheral suture technique. J Hand Surg 14B:232–235
Wagner CJ 1985 Delayed advancement in the repair of lacerated flexor profundus tendons. J Bone Joint Surg 40:1241–1244
Wehbe MA, Mawr B, Hunter JM et al 1986 Two-stage flexor-tendon reconstruction. J Bone Joint Surg 68A:752–763
Werntz JR, Chesher SP, Breidenbach WC et al 1989 A new dynamic splint for postoperative treatment of flexor tendon injury. J Hand Surg 14A:559–566
Whitaker JH, Strickland JW, Ellis RG 1977 The role of tenolysis in the palm and digit. J Hand Surg 2:462–470
White WL 1960 Tendon grafts: a considerqtion of their source, procurement and suitability. Surg Clin North Am 40:403–413
Wilson RL, Carter MS, Holdeman VA, Lovett WL 1980 Flexor profundus injuries treated with delayed two-staged tendon grafting. J Hand Surg 5:74–78
Wray RC, Weeks PM 1974 Reconstruction of digital pulleys. Plastic Reconstr Surg 53:534–536
Wray RC Jr, Ollinger H, Weeks PM 1975 Effects of mobilization on tensile strength of partial tendon lacerations. Surg Forum 26:577–558

7

Assessment of adolescent acetabular dysplasia

A. Catterall

In recent years the realization that the end-result of total joint replacement in the young adult with osteoarthritis secondary to acetabular dysplasia is unsatisfactory has re-awakened interest in conservative surgery for this condition. The object of this surgery is to arrest the process or at worst delay the rate at which the deterioration may occur. To achieve this objective a better understanding must be achieved, not only of the biomechanics of the normal hip, but also of the indications for the various reconstructive procedures available to the orthopaedic surgeon. Assessment of the degree of instability present is fundamental to this objective.

A RÉSUME OF ACETABULAR DEVELOPMENT

In beginning a discussion on this subject it must be remembered that the hip joint is situated on the side of the ring of the pelvis and that the major growth centres for this ring lie in the floor of the acetabulum. Forces acting on the triradiate cartilage as the result of abnormal muscle tension, leg-length difference or hip incongruity may produce secondary changes in the acetabulum, both in depth and orientation.

When the cavity of the hip joint develops in the proximal part of the lower limb bud of the fetus the initial cavity is sufficiently deep that the femoral head is held captive within it. With time and growth the depth of the cavity of the acetabulum reduces so that it is at its shallowest at the time of birth (McKibbin & Ralis 1973). Following delivery the legs move into the position of extension and the cavity again deepens to produce its final overall shape by the age of 4 to 5 years. As growth continues important secondary centres of ossification appear in the anterior and anterolateral aspects of the articular cartilage of the acetabulum (Ponsetti 1978). These appear between the ages of 8 and 10 years and fuse at 15–18 years. Associated with these changes in depth are changes in orientation of the acetabulum. At birth there is 35° of anteversion which changes to 20° in the course of continued development.

Upper femoral development

At birth the whole of the upper end of the femur is in cartilage with the femoral head and greater trochanter formed as one continuous cartilagenous structure. The rate of growth in the growth plate on the medial side (femoral head) is twice as great as that in relation to the trochanter and this results in the appearance of the femoral neck in the course of the first year of life. Between 3 and 6 months of age there is a maturation of the blood supply to the femoral head. A branch of the medial circumflex artery takes over the major supply of this region via its medial and lateral retinacular vessels. This alteration is associated with the appearance of the upper femoral epiphysis between birth and 9 months of life, with a mean age of appearance of 6 months (Bertol et al 1982). Its presence splints the shape of the femoral head and its rate of enlargement is such that by the age of 9 it forms approximately 90% of the volume of the femoral head. This reflects the increasing forces passing through the femoral head as the child grows. Associated with this continuing growth there is a reduction in the neck–shaft angle and anteversion of the femoral neck from 145 and 35 to 120 and 20° respectively. The changes which are associated with avascular necrosis will obviously vary with the age

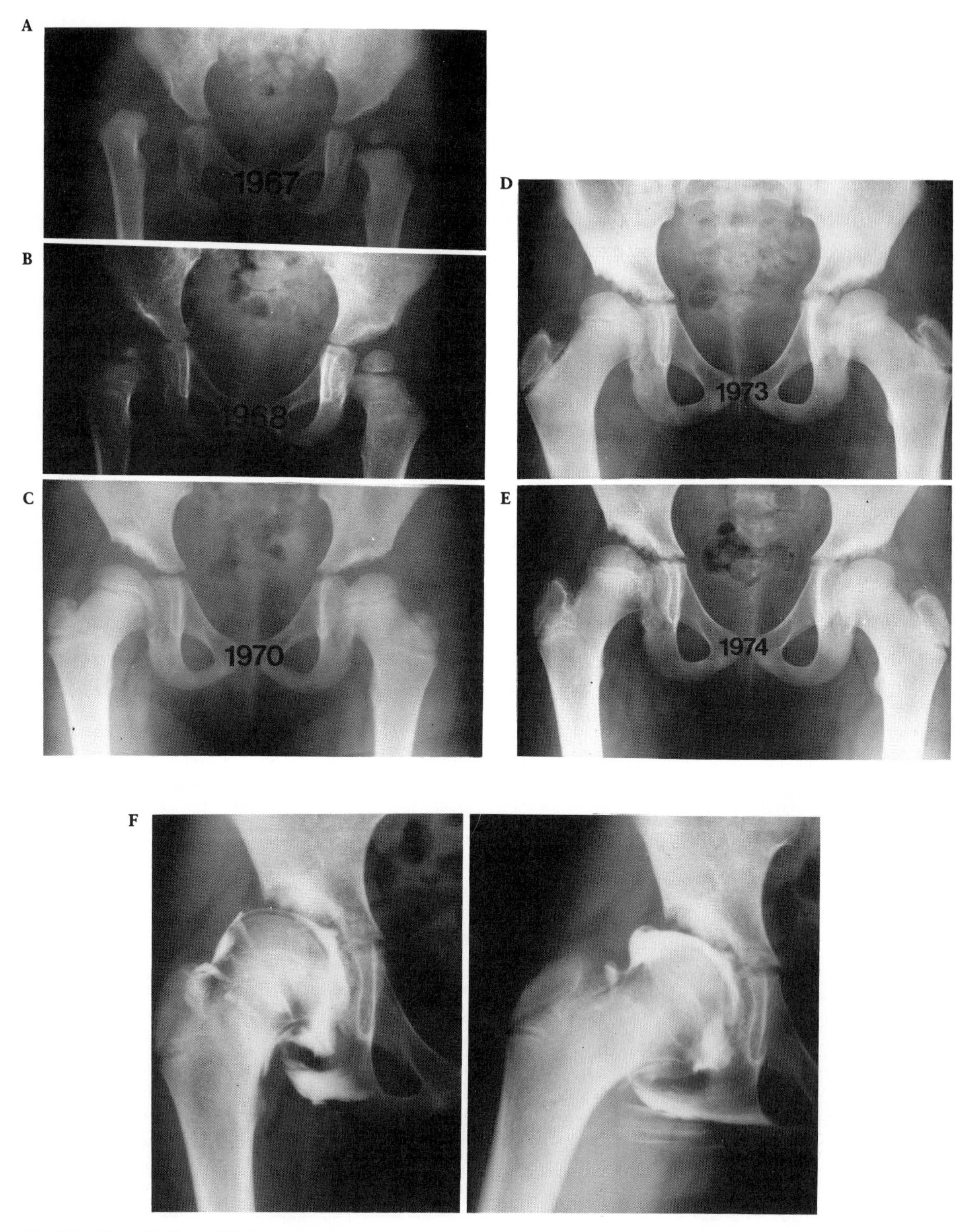

Fig. 7.1 (A) to (F) See p. 105 for explanation.

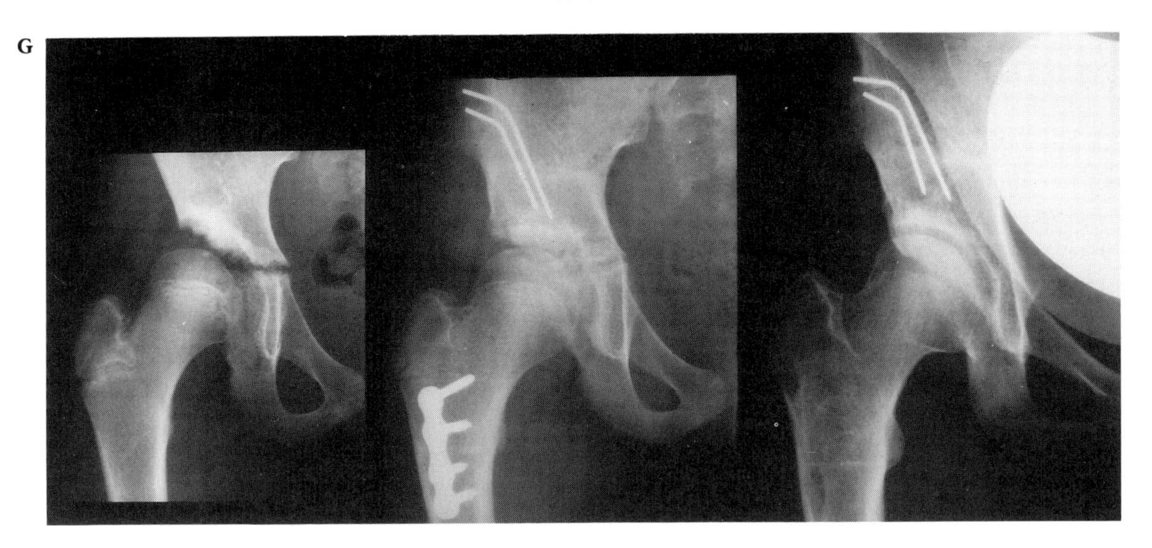

Fig. 7.1 (**A**) 1967. A child of 18 months with a congenital dislocation of the right hip. Treatment was by traction, and a frog plaster for 8 months. There is no acetabular tear drop on the dislocated side. (**B**) 1968. The hip is reduced and the tear drop has developed. This is equal to that on the opposite side; there is a marked residual acetabular dysplasia and a mild avascular change in the epiphysis on the reduced side. (**C**) 1970. There has been progressive improvement in the left hip with a reduction in the acetabular angle and in the width of the tear drop. On the right side the tear drop remains wide and there is no improvement in the acetabular dysplasia. Shenton's line is intact. (**D**) 1973. The left hip continues to improve. On the right there has been no improvement in the acetabular dysplasia and no reduction in the width of the tear drop. Shenton's line remains intact. There is persisting valgus in the femoral neck. Clinically the patient is starting to have discomfort and limp at the end of the day. (**E**) 1974. The patient's symptoms are beginning to deteriorate and there is a positive Trendelenburg test on the right side. The tear drop has widened and there is now a break in Shenton's line. More uncovering of the femoral head is present than in 1973. Treatment was advised. (**F**) Arthrography. This shows an eccentrically placed femoral head with congruency in flexion/abduction/internal rotation. This is a reducible subluxation suitable to a realignment procedure. (**G**) Sequential X-rays 2 and 5 years following innominate and femoral osteotomy. There is congruency between the femoral head and acetabulum with a normal neck shaft angle. Shenton's line is restored. Clinically she has resumed full activity and there is no residual aching or discomfort at the end of the day. (Reproduced with permission from Catterall 1982.)

at which the damage occurs and the area of the growth plate maximally affected. In the majority of cases there is an associated coxa magna with persistence of the femoral anteversion.

The hip joint

The normal growth changes already described will leave the femoral head relatively uncovered during the early years of growth and this is reflected in the CE angle which increases with time from 22° to greater than 30° at maturity. Loredo (1985) has measured the CE angle of Wiberg (1939) and can predict the measurement up to the age of 20 years by the formula: CE = 26.99 + age × 0.6. On the acetabular side the slope of the acetabular roof (Hilgenriener's angle; Hilgenriener 1986) reduces with time, partly as a result of ossification of roof and partly by a change in orientation of the acetabulumn. Radiologically this change in orientation is reflected by a progressive narrowing of the tear drop (Gilmour 1938, Catterall 1982).

Normal development of the hip joint following reduction of a dislocation is a progressive reduction in the slope of the acetabulum and its conversion to a dome-shape as the result of the appearance and later fusion of the secondary centres of ossification. The tear drop progressively narrows during this time. By contrast, when this development fails to occur the acetabulum remains sloping and the tear drop remains wide (Fig. 7.1). As the hip starts to decompensate there is a break in Shenton's line and a progressive widening of the tear drop. A coxa magna with valgus in the femoral neck may be associated with these changes (see Fig. 7.4b).

ABNORMALITIES WHICH MAY BE ASSOCIATED WITH ACETABULAR DEVELOPMENT

Abnormalities may occur at a number of sites; the lateral acetabular epiphysis; the femoral head, the femoral neck, and the congruity of the hip joint itself.

The lateral acetabular epiphysis

The importance of this structure in acetabular development has already been emphasized but a number of abnormalities may occur (Fig. 7.2). The epiphysis may fail to develop at the correct age, as a result of genetic or environmental influences such as loss of congruity of the joint. It may have been excised during the course of a limbectomy at the time of an open reduction (O'Hara 1990). As a result the lateral part of the femoral head is unsupported and this produces abnormal mobility of the overlying acetabular articular cartilage. These stresses inhibit the normal ossification of the acetabular roof and result in a secondary acetabular dysplasia with an unstable lateral segment (Figs 7.2 and 7.3). Secondarily the epiphysis may appear but fail to fuse. This again results in an unstable lateral segment. In both situations the abnormal mobility and pressures eventually result in a degenerative tear of this tissue which Dorrell & Catterall (1986) described as a tear of the acetabular labrum. Such patients present with initial aching related to exercise but with time the pain becomes suddenly sharp and mechanical, suggesting that the labrum itself is torn.

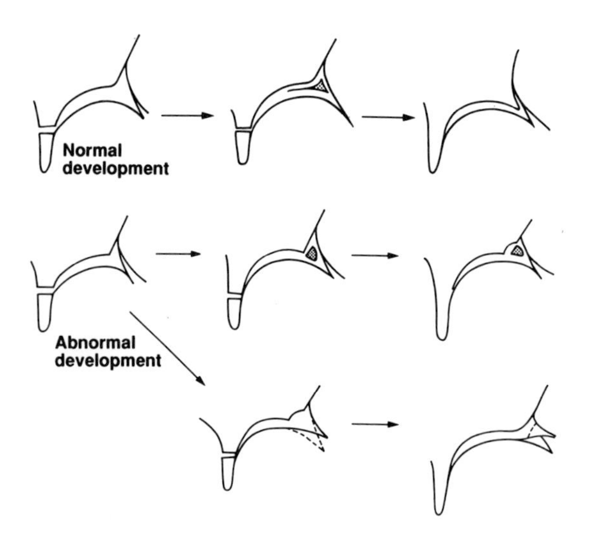

Fig. 7.2 The development of the lateral acetabular epiphysis and its variants.

The femoral head and neck

A number of changes occur in the femoral head and neck following treatment of dysplasia in the younger child. Operations on the upper femur, particularly if repeated and associated with minor changes of avascular necrosis, may result in a growth disturbance in which overgrowth is the predominant feature. This leads to a coxa magna without associated enlargement of the acetabulum, producing uncovering of the femoral head anterolaterally. This uncovering may be recognized clinically by palpation of the uncovered femoral head in the groin—the so-called Lump Sign of acetabular dysplasia. Ultrasound studies will confirm this uncovering. In many cases this overgrowth results in increasing valgus deformity of the femoral neck. This leads to a long leg on the involved side which forces the hip into adduction as the child stands and walks. The secondary acetabular dysplasia which ensues may be thought of as long leg dysplasia (Fig. 7.4).

Conversely the leg may be short. This may be the consequence of a surgical coxa vara or avascular necrosis where there has been involvement of the growth plate centrally or medially. The varus of the femoral neck limits the range of abduction present in the hip joint. It must be realized that for normal walking 10–15° of abduction must be present. To this should be added a further 10° for every 1 cm of shortening. If the amount of abduction is inadequate to meet this need then limp will occur and a secondary acetabular dysplasia may result with a progressive subluxation if this condition is not rectified in time. This syndrome may be best thought of as short leg dysplasia.

There are two consequences of these observations. Acetabular dysplasia when associated with the difference in leg length may be the consequence of long or short leg dysplasia. Secondly when treatment of acetabular dysplasia results in a difference in leg length, a secondary dysplasia in the opposite hip may occur.

A

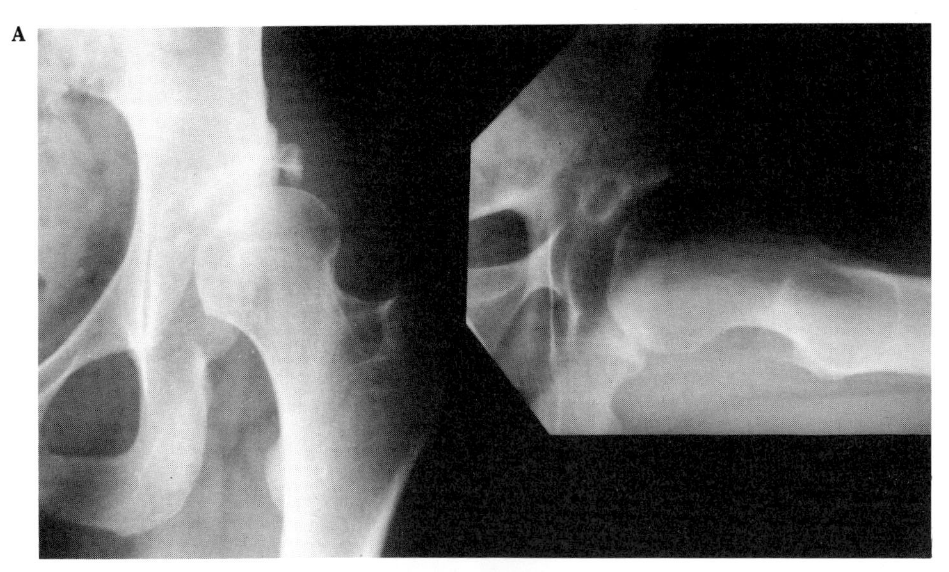

B

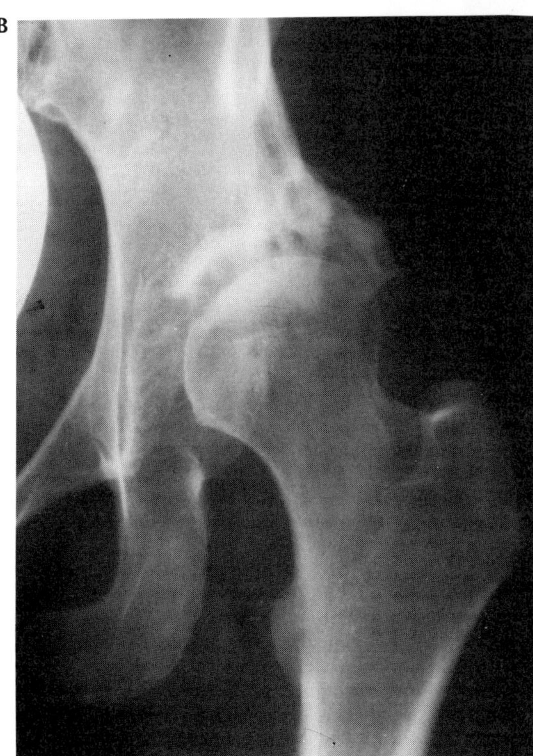

Fig. 7.3 (**A**) A 22-year-old woman. Four-year history of increasing discomfort which had recently become sharp in character. On clinical examination there was mild shortening, a prominent lump sign, and sharp mechanical pain when the hip was flexed and abducted, suggesting a torn acetabular labrum. Anteroposterior and lateral radiograph: the ununited acetabular epiphysis is noted. This could be seen to be unstable when the leg was moved into flexion and abduction. A medial acetabular cyst is noted. (**B**) Eighteen months following lateral shelf acetabuloplasty. Union of the lateral acetabular epiphysis is noted with an improved quality of the Sourcil and healing of the medium acetabular cyst. There is good incorporation and remodelling of the graft. Clinically function is now normal.

Congruity of the hip joint

This factor is probably the most difficult aspect of hip function to assess. A number of radiological observations may be made including the Sourcil (of the roof of the acetabulum) weight-bearing zone, the CE angle, lateral uncovering, superior joint space and Shenton's line (Fig. 7.5). In the normal hip there is a wide Sourcil or weight-bearing surface which is horizontally placed in relation to the loads applied to it. The CE angle alters with age but is

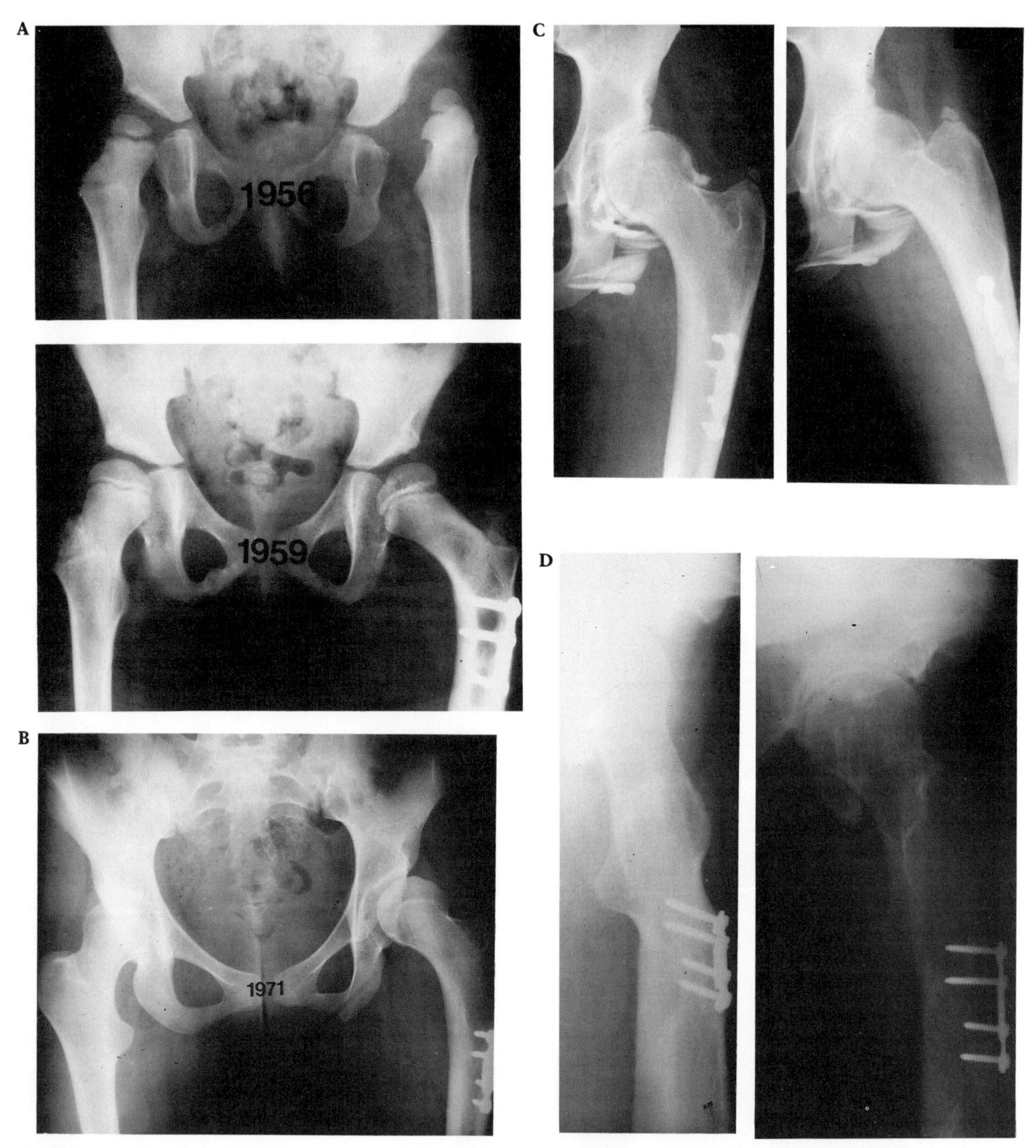

Fig. 7.4 (**A**) 1956. Child aged 20 months with a left congenital dislocation of the hip which was treated by open reduction and femoral osteotomy. The sequential X-rays show the pretreatment state and at 6 months and 3 years following operation. There is a stable reduction but a long femoral neck. Although movements were free, 2 cm of leg-length difference was noted; the left leg was long. (**B**) The standing radiographs at the age of 17 years showed a marked residual acetabular dysplasia with coxa magna and uncovering of the femoral head. Note the difference in the level of the ischial tuberosity confirming the presence of leg-length inequality. There is overgrowth in the length of the femoral neck compared with the opposite side. This is long leg dysplasia. (**C**) At arthrography there is good contact between the medial half of the femoral head and acetabulum but a difference in size between the two. The acetabular roof is apparently sloping. In abduction there is loss of contact between the femoral head and acetabulum medially (unstable movement). (**D**) The lateral radiographs show no improvement with position. Conclusion: this is an irreducible subluxation with unstable movement. (**E**) Eight years following a Chiari operation. The shortening induced by the operation has equalized the leg length. Adequate cover of the femoral head has been obtained and the stability produced has resulted in good long-term remodelling. (Reproduced with permission from Catterall 1982.)

E

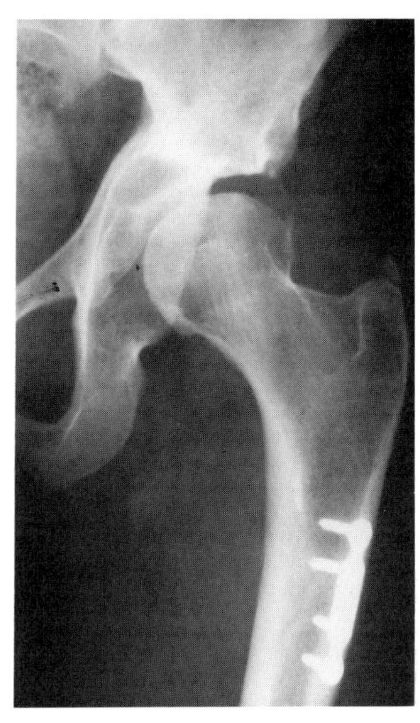

always greater than 25° in the mature adult. Loredo (1985) has shown that at a given age up to 20 years the CE angle = 26.99 + age × 0.6 (Fig. 7.6). There should be no lateral extrusion or uncovering of the femoral head. As congruity of the joint is lost the acetabulum usually becomes more sloping with a reduction in the area of weight-bearing in the acetabular roof and also the CE angle (Fig. 7.6). The sloping acetabulum allows a lateral shear force to be applied to the femoral head encouraging subluxation of the femoral head and therefore transferring the load-bearing surface to the lateral cartilagenous structures which will be subject to degenerative change with the time. *The principle, then, is established that a sloping acetabulum will not last in the long term.* In the early stages of a progressive subluxation Shenton's line may remain intact but an increasing break is suggestive of incongruity. Another important sign to note is the symmetry of the lateral and medial joint spaces. Narrowing of the superior joint space is an early feature of osteoarthritis but may also be associated with hinge abduction (Grossbard 1981, Quain & Catterall 1986) which, if allowed to persist, will lead to rapid deterioration in the wear of the joint surfaces (Cooperman et al 1983).

It is interesting to observe that where there is good congruity between the articular surfaces of the hip, knee and ankle the load across the articular cartilage is approximately 15–20 kPa/cm^2. The effect of these altered forces passing through the hip joint (Fig. 7.6) results in a 10-fold rise in the forces applied with a change of CE angle from 30° to 0°. This explains the rapid deterioration which may occur in such joints, and why conservative surgery must be performed early if it is to be undertaken.

ASSESSMENT

As with all difficult problems, the art of assessment begins with a good clinical history and examination followed by the assessments of plain radiographs which in many cases should include standing films.

Clinical history

Where previous treatment has been undertaken its nature and result must be assessed and the interval, if any, between the treatment and the onset of the present symptoms identified. The duration and nature of any pain are assessed. Aching related to activity suggests weak muscles and a hip that is beginning to decompensate. A persisting ache when associated with stiffness implies that the pain is coming from the joint, which may have early degenerative change. Sharp or mechanical pain superimposed on a background of aching suggests a more major derangement such as a tear of the acetabular labrum. The symptom of locking may be present with such a tear but is more commonly a symptom of osteoarthritis. The duration of limp in its relationship to exercise must be ascertained. Many patients will be aware of a difference in leg length; a change in leg length implies the onset of fixed deformity which is usually the signal for a more rapid deterioration in symptoms. A family history of hip abnormality may be found in many cases.

Clinical examination

Clinical examination is best considered in static and dynamic phases (Table 7.1).

The static phases

In the static phase the presence of any fixed deformity, flexion, adduction or rotation is identi-

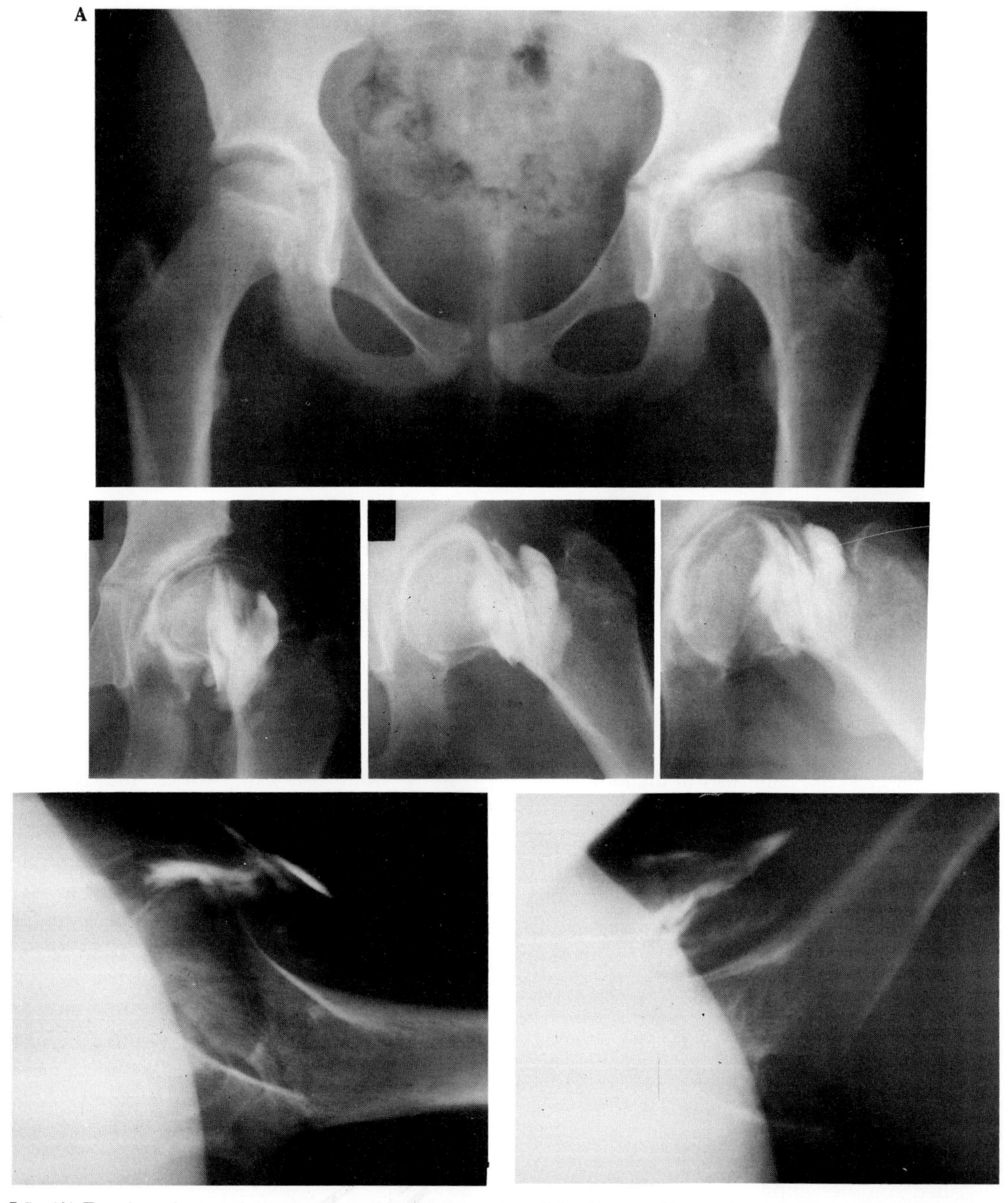

Fig 7.5 (**A**) Female patient aged 12 years. A congenital dislocation of the hip was diagnosed and treated conservatively at the age of 14 months. There was 2-year history of aching in the left hip with increasing limp for 1 year. Clinical examination revealed 2.5 cm of shortening and a prominent Lump sign. There was free flexion but abduction was only 20°; the Trendelenburg test was positive. The radiograph shows a residual acetabular dysplasia with evidence of a residual avascular change and a short femoral neck in normal alignment. There is a break in Shenton's line and the tear drop is wide. (**B**) Arthrogram. The anteroposterior radiograph in neutral, abduction and abduction with flexion. Note that in abduction alone the femoral head appears centred but is not in contact with the roof of the acetabulum. The congruous position is with the leg placed in the position of flexion, abduction and some internal rotation. (**C**) Arthrogram, lateral radiograph. In the neutral position there is marked uncovering of the femoral head antrolaterally and congruity is restored with the position of flexion and abduction. Note the degree of flexion required. Conclusion: this is a reducible subluxation requiring more than 30° of abduction and flexion to produce congruity. Re-alignment is required but if a femoral osteotomy were included this would induce further shortening. The patient therefore requires a triple innominate osteotomy because all the correction must be obtained above the hip.

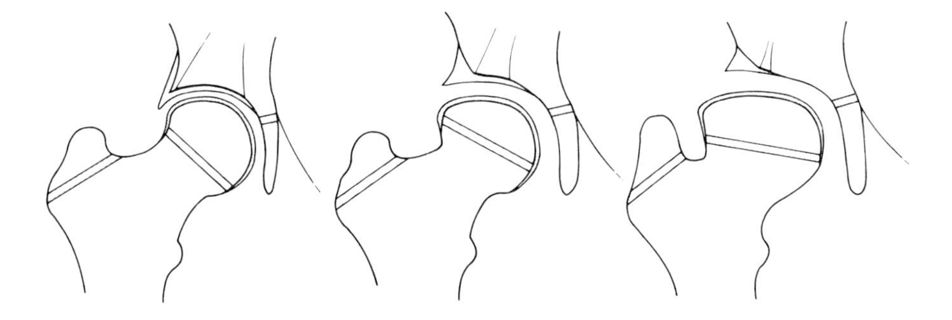

C.E. Angle = 26.99 + 0.6 x age

C.E. Angle	Kp / cm^2
35	18
20	59
5	225

Fig 7.6 Drawing of the appearance of a normal hip, a mild degree of acetabular dysplasia, and severe acetabular dysplasia with subluxation.

fied together with an assessment of leg length. A leg-length difference which is not attributable to fixed deformity implies true bony shortening. Subluxation, particularly when associated with a coxa magna, produces uncovering of the femoral head anterolaterally and this may be seen or felt as a lump below and medial to the anterior superior iliac spine. This is the lump sign of acetabular dysplasia.

The dynamic phase

In the dynamic phase, the examination continues with an assessment of the range of movement present from the position of fixed deformity, particularly in the plane of flexion and abduction. This range is recorded. As the hip flexes the position of the knee is observed. It may remain in the neutral position or be forced into abduction, suggesting femoral head deformity. As the hip is moved the lump is palpated to see if it reduces in size or remains prominent. The former implies a reducible subluxation while the latter implies a fixed subluxation. The Trendelenburg test is performed. On the non-weight-bearing side the leg remains in extension with the knee flexed and an immediate or delayed positive sign is looked for (Mitchell 1972). In the delayed test, as the patient stands on the involved leg the pelvis initially rises to produce a negative result but then falls again after a period of 20 to 30 seconds. Finally movements of the spine are checked for the presence of a scoliosis and mobility, particularly of the lumbar spine. Only at this stage is the patient asked to walk. As the patient walks the surgeon is watching for the influence of the fixed deformities and the Trendelenburg test on gait. If the gait differs from the features suggested by clinical examination, either the fixed deformities have been misjudged or other factors such as muscle weakness or a scoliosis producing pelvic obliquity have not been discovered in the assessment and re-examination is required.

Table 7.1 Sequence of examination for acetabular dysplasia

Static phase	Dynamic phase
Leg length	Range of movement
Fixed deformity	Trendelenburg test
Flexion	Immediate
Adduction	Delayed
The lump sign	Walking

Radiographic assessment

Plain radiographs taken in the lying and standing positions are now obtained with a shoot-through lateral (Smith Peterson view) of the involved hip. This will provide an understanding of the gross shape of the femoral head and acetabulum and the congruency of the joint. The position of the greater trochanter and its relationship to the centre of the head is noted. This assesses the efficiency of the abductor lever arm. In the normal hip the tip of the trochanter should be at the level of the centre of rotation of the femoral head and one full diameter lateral to it. The weight-bearing film will demonstrate the alteration in congruity as the patient stands and also the influence of any leg-length difference.

Conclusions of this primary examination

At the conclusion of this clinical history, examination and assessment of plain radiographs, the surgeon should have a clear understanding of the patient's problem, the rate of progress of the symptoms and hence the natural history of the hip disorder present. The nature of the fixed deformities and their influence on leg length will begin to orientate the assessment to suggest avenues of treatment. On the basis of this understanding further investigation may or may not be advised.

Further assessment and investigation

It is difficult in the present climate of the modern sophisticated techniques of computerized tomography (CT) and magnetic resonance imaging (MRI) scanning not to perform these techniques before using the simpler procedure of an examination under anaesthetic and arthrography. Both CT and MRI will provide information of the shape of the femoral head and acetabulum but are not in themselves real-time and hence do not give any form of dynamic assessment of the hip joint as it moves. This is best assessed with the patient anaesthetized so that dye may be injected into the joint and the hip moved without the influence of protective muscle spasm. There are now a number of reports of the value of CT and MRI images in assessment. However, the simplicity of an examination under anaesthetic and arthrography and the three-dimensional and dynamic information it provides makes it a most valuable assessment.

Examination under anaesthetic and arthrography

The object of this assessment is to identify the shape and relationship of the femoral head and acetabulum and how this changes as the hip is moved. Six types of movement are identified (Table 7.2). Stable but eccentric movement is observed either following Perthes' disease or as a consequence of avascular necrosis. There is uncovering of the femoral head, which is usually oval in shape. In abduction the femoral head rotates without hinging, but is never fully contained within the acetabulum. Uncovering the femoral head is not of necessity a cause of symptoms, provided the movement of the femoral head is congruous, as is often the case in the long-term follow-up of Perthes' disease. Such a hip has an extremely good prognosis in the short term, but osteoarthritis must be an inevitable long-term consequence. The onset of symptoms is difficult to predict.

A reducible subluxation is present when the femoral head is subluxated anterolaterally in the neutral position of weight-bearing but can be reduced when the leg is placed in flexion abduction and internal rotation (Fig. 7.6). By contrast an irreducible subluxation is present when there is uncovering of the femoral head which does not improve as the hip is moved. The movement of abduction is often associated with the loss of congruity within the femoral head and acetabulum (unstable movement or hinge abduction; Fig. 7.5). The concept of an unstable lateral segment has already been discussed but is recognized arthrographically by noting unstable movement of the articular cartilage on the outer aspect of the acetabulum. On occasions there may be a tear of the acetabular labrum (Dorrell & Catterall 1986) which may move in the same way as a torn meniscus in the injured degenerate knee. In a similar way an

Table 7.2 Examination under anaesthetic and arthrography

Types of movement
Stable concentric movement
Stable eccentric movement
Reducible subluxation
Irreducible subluxation
Unstable lateral segment
Unstable movement—hinge abduction

ununited lateral acetabular epiphysis may be observed moving vertically as the femoral head is positioned in abduction.

It must also be realized that this investigation should only be performed by the surgeon or surgical team who are going to undertake the management of the patient. It is ideally undertaken in the Department of Radiology, provided that facilities are available for the care of the anaesthetized patient. Video-recordings of the examination create the best record with still radiographs identifying the positive findings; the position of best fit or congruent position, and unstable movement or tears of the acetabular labrum. Video-recordings allow re-examination after the event and may be used for teaching or re-examination of case material if doubt exists about conclusions reached at the time of the examination.

Technique

The stages of the assessment are the logical extension of the clinical examination already described. The fixed deformities and the range of movement are noted after anaesthesia has been induced and compared with the preoperative state. Using sterile precautions radiopaque dye is now injected into the hip joint through a needle inserted anterolaterally, using the lump sign as the point of entry. As the dye is injected the hip is screened to be sure that the injection is not extra-articular. The amount of contrast injected should be sufficient to show the joint surface but not too great to obliterate the bone–articular cartilage interface. Once the dye has been injected the relationship between the femoral head and acetabulum in the neutral position is observed and then with the leg in the position of weight-bearing. This is usually achieved by placing the legs so that the feet are at the same level. This will often reveal considerable incongruity and suggest a cause for the patient's pain.

The leg is now moved in abduction. As this movement occurs the congruity of the hip joint is noted. In the normal hip the femoral head rotates in the acetabulum and a congruous relationship is maintained. When femoral head deformity is present, hinge abduction may be observed. In this unstable movement the outer aspect of the femoral head hinges on the lateral aspect of the acetabulum. Although this is classically seen in Perthes' disease (Quain & Catterall 1986), it is also seen as a consequence of avascular necrosis. In other cases, although the femoral head is normal the lateral aspect of the acetabulum is deficient, often with an ununited lateral acetabular epiphysis. This may be seen to move vertically up and down as the leg is moved into abduction and back to the neutral position. This suggests the diagnosis of an unstable lateral segment.

Radiographs now record the abnormality that has been noted and also the position of best fit. If unstable movement is present and hinge abduction is noted it will often be found that position of best fit or congruity between the femoral head and acetabulum is one of flexion, adduction and external rotation. By contrast, with the neutral or abducted position it will be noted that rotation in this position of stability is not associated with unstable movement of the femoral head.

THE REQUIREMENTS OF SURGERY

Before considering the details of assessment it is important to identify the objectives of reconstructive surgery (Table 7.3). This may be considered under a number of separate headings:

1. The time for remodelling is limited and therefore precise surgery is required.
2. Operations which restrict abduction will not last in the long term. The range of abduction must be adequate to compensate for any difference in leg length. Inadequate abduction may induce a secondary acetabular dysplasia.
3. A sloping acetabulum is unsatisfactory in the long term and reconstruction should make it horizontal and provide adequate cover and therefore stability for the femoral head.
4. If possible a normal abductor lever arm should be re-established.
5. Differences in leg length may prejudice the

Table 7.3 Objectives of surgery

Objectives of surgery
Precise operation
Maintain abduction and restore normal abductor lever arm
Equalize leg length
Restore horizontal position of acetabulum and adequate cover of femoral head

result, not only of the involved hip but also of the opposite clinically asymptomatic hip at the time of presentation.
6. Pain may be arising from structures other than the hip joint itself (for example, a neuroma on the lateral cutaneous nerve of the thigh).

Indications for operation

If the assessment which has been outlined suggests that the natural history of the hip abnormality is for progressive deterioration then treatment should be advised in an attempt to halt this.

Conservative treatment

Where the major problem is weakness of the abductor lever arm, because of either a short or varus deformity of the femoral neck, a graduated programme of abduction and hip extension exercises will often relieve the patient's symptoms. Hydrotherapy is sometimes of value. An arthrogram will show a stable joint with concentric movement. If symptoms persist transfer of the greater trochanter laterally and distally will relieve the patient's symptoms.

Operative treatment

In the majority of cases some form of surgical procedure will be required. The problem is whether the procedure should be above or below the hip joint, or on both sides. Treatment should be advised on the basis of the pathology demonstrated and the abnormality of movement present. Both will have been identified by the examination under anaesthetic and arthrography. The principles of treatment will depend on the abnormality present (Tables 7.4 and 7.5).

Reducible subluxation

Where a reducible subluxation is present the principle of management is to realign the hip joint so that it is stable in the neutral position of weight-bearing (Table 7.4, Fig. 7.6). In the majority of cases an acetabular realignment procedure is required as the primary pathology is acetabular dysplasia. In many cases there is an associated coxa valga so that the remainder of the realignment can be made in the femur. In general the 'rule of 30s' (Catterall, personal observation) should be followed. This rule states where more than 30° of realignment is required in one plane it is unlikely to be achieved in one stage. This rule has proved reliable because it is difficult to achieve more than 30° of flexion or abduction because of the configuration of the pelvis, and below the hip 30° of varus in the femoral neck will produce unacceptable shortening and an inefficient abductor lever arm. If, in a case of avascular necrosis (Fig. 7.7) there is shortening which contraindicates femoral osteotomy and a major correction is required, this may be achieved by a double or triple innominate osteotomy (Steel 1973, 1977, Tönnis 1982, 1990) or acetabular osteotomy (Eppright 1975, Wagner 1978a, b) so that all the realignment can be achieved in one stage.

Irreducible subluxation

Where there is no improvement in the congruity or stability of the joint with position, an irreducible subluxation is present. Realignment procedures are contraindicated because the deformity is fixed.

Table 7.4 Principles and methods of treatment according to arthrographic results

Arthrographic result	Principle of treatment	Method of treatment
Reducible subluxation	Realignment	Innominate + femoral osteotomy
Irreducible subluxation	Acetabular enlargement	Chiari operation or Lateral shelf acetabuloplasty
Ustable lateral segment	Lateral shelf stabilization	Lateral shelf acetabuloplasty

Table 7.5 Indications for femoral procedure according to arthrographic results

Arthrographic result	Method of treatment
Long leg dysplasia	Femoral shortening + varus
Concentric joint Weak abductors	Trochanteric transfer
Unstable movement (Hinge abduction)	Abduction/extension femoral osteotomy
Short neck dysplasia	Proximal femoral reconstruction

The principle of treatment, therefore, must be acetabular enlargement (Table 7.4, Fig. 7.4). This may be achieved by either a Chiari medial displacement osteotomy (Chiari 1974) or an augmentation lateral shelf acetabuloplasty (Wainwright 1976, Saito et al 1986, Catterall 1991). Both procedures will achieve cover of the anterior and lateral segment of the femoral head but are different in their operative technique. It is the author's practice to use the Chiari procedure where a fixed subluxation is present with the femoral head laterally displaced from the midline (Fig. 7.7). The long-term results of this procedure are satisfactory (Calvert et al 1987, Hogh et al 1987). When there is no serious lateral displacement or there is a deformity of the femoral head a lateral shelf will provide the cover and stabilization required without producing a localized area of weight-bearing, as might occur with a Chiari (Fig. 7.7).

An unstable lateral segment

The concept of an unstable lateral segment has already been defined. It is the best of the indications for lateral acetabuloplasty (Fig. 7.3). In many cases the femoral head is round and the problem is a deficiency in the lateral acetabular structures with either a failure or alternatively inadequate development of the lateral acetabulum. Buttressing these lateral structures will often permit their normal development.

Long leg dysplasia

The principle has already been established that at the end of treatment leg lengths must be equal. Where there is a long leg, part of the operative correction must be a shortening with adjustment of the neck-shaft angles to produce a congruous position in the femoral head and the acetabulum with the leg in the neutral position of weight-bearing (Table 7.5).

The weak abductor lever arm

When the femoral neck is short and the greater trochanter high, distal transfer of the trochanter has proved a very worthwhile procedure (Wagner 1978a,b, Lloyd-Roberts et al 1985). The transfer may be either distal or, more commonly, distal and lateral to re-establish the normal pull of the abductors. On occasions followng avascular necrosis there is an irreducible subluxation associated with a high trochanter and a Chiari operation is easily performed after elevation of the trochanter which is then re-attached in a lateral and more distal position.

Unstable movement (hinge abduction)

When the examination under anaesthetic and arthrography has demonstrated hinge abduction it will also have established the position for stable movement, which is usually in a variable degree of flexion, adduction and external rotation. A realignment/abduction/extension osteotomy with correction of this rotational anomaly will stabilize the hip joint and also has the advantage of increasing leg length and restoring a better abductor level arm. The results of this procedure have proved satisfactory (Bombelli 1976, Quain & Catterall 1986).

Short leg dysplasia

Often following avascular necrosis of the femoral head there is a combination of a short leg, high greater trochanter and hinge abduction. There may be an associated acetabular dysplasia. This is usually found where there is a varus deformity in the femoral neck. To overcome this problem a proximal femoral reconstruction is performed (Bombelli 1976). In this operation an abduction and extension wedge is removed with the proximal line of osteotomy oblique and at the level of the base of the femoral neck. At the same time the greater

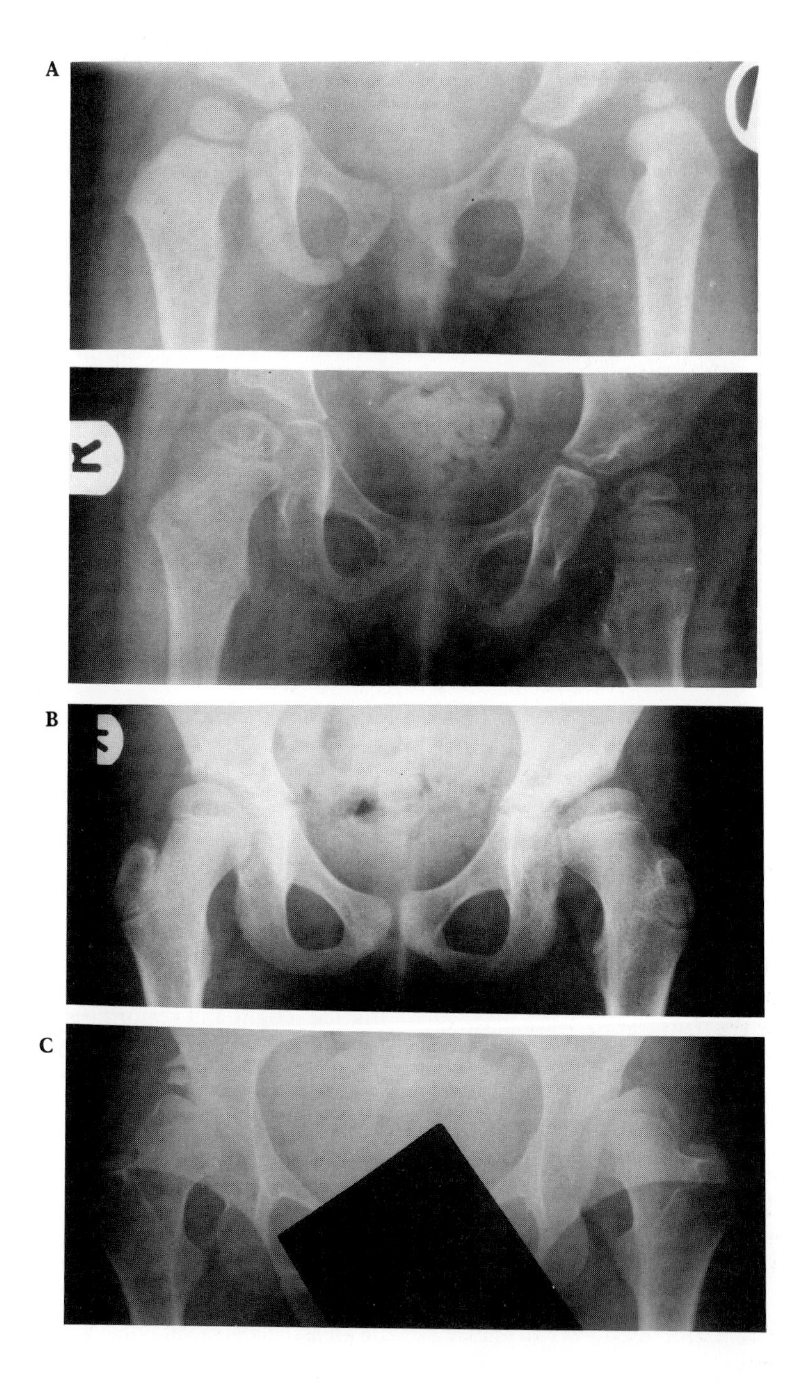

Fig. 7.7 (**A**) **Top** Child aged 20 months with congenital dislocation of the left hip treated by traction and 9 months in a frog plaster. **Bottom**: A year later there is evidence of avascular change in both hips. There is a persistent subluxation on the left side. No tear drop is present at this stage. (**B**) At the age of 8 years changes are present in both hips with a secondary acetabular dysplasia and subluxation on the right. The lateral acetabular epiphysis is present but not fused on this side. On the left the subluxation still persists with a marked break in Shenton's line. (**C**) At the age of 22 years both hips are symptomatic. On the left side there is an irriducible subluxation with uncovering and lateral displacement of the femoral head. On the right the lateral acetabular epiphysis remains ununited. There is a 'cocked-hat' deformity of the femoral head.

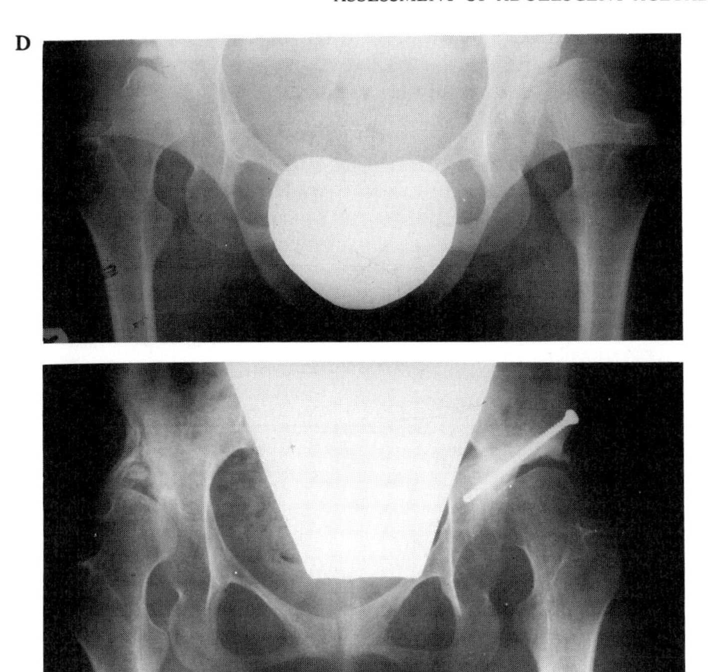

Fig. 7.7 (**D**) A Chiari operation was advised for the left hip and a lateral shelf acetabuloplasty on the right. The radiographs show the result 2 years postoperatively.

trochanter is detached and transferred laterally and distally. A 135° offset AO blade plate is inserted, leaving a 1–2 cm gap between the lateral aspect of the proximal fragment and the offset portion of the blade plate. As the osteotomy site is closed the femoral shaft is displaced laterally and downwards as the result of the oblique inclination of the osteotomy. This procedure improves the leg length and configuration of the femoral neck, restoring a normal abductor lever arm.

CONCLUSIONS

It must be accepted that no one procedure will successfully treat all presentations of this condition. However, an understanding of the pathology and careful clinical and radiological assessment should allow the surgeon to identify indications for the various operative procedures used in the management of these patients.

REFERENCES

Bertol P, MacNicol MF, Mitchell GP 1982 Radiographic features of neonatal congenital dislocation of the hip. J Bone Joint Surg [Br] 64:176–179

Bombelli R 1976 Osteoarthritis of the hip. Springer-Verlag, Berlin, pp 49–103

Calvert PT, August AC, Albert JS et al 1987 The Chiari pelvic osteotomy—a review of the long term results. J Bone Joint Surg 69B:551–555

Catterall A 1982 Acetabular dysplasia. In: Tachdjian MO (ed) Congenital dislocation of the hip. Churchill Livingstone, New York, p 479–499

Catterall A 1984 What is congenital dislocation of the hip? J Bone Joint Surg [Br] 66:469–470

Catterall A 1991 Pelvic osteotomies. In: Bentley G (ed) Operative surgery—orthopaedics. Butterworths, London

Chiari K 1974 Medial osteotomy of the pelvis. Clin Orthop Rel Res 198:55–71

Colton CL 1972 Chiari osteotomy for acetabular dysplasia in young adults. Bone Joint Surg (Br) 54B:578–589

Cooperman DR, Wallensten R, Stulberg SD 1983 Acetabular dysplasia in the adult. Clin Orthop 175:79–85

Dorrell JH, Catterall A 1986 The torn acetabular labrum. J Bone Joint Surg [Br] 68:400–403

Eppright RH 1975 Dial osteotomy of the acetabulum in the treatment of dysplasia of the hip. J Bone Joint Surg [Am] 57A:1172

Gilmour J 1938 Adolescence deformities of the acetabulum. Br J Surg 26:670

Grossbard GD 1981 Hip pain in adolescence after Perthes disease. J Bone Joint Surg (Br) 63B:572

Hilgenreiner 1986 Classic. Translation: Hilgenreiner on congenital hip dislocation. J Pediatr Orthop 6:202–214

Hogh J, MacNicol MF 1987 The Chiari pelvic osteotomy—a long term review of the clinical and radiological results. J Bone Joint Surg (Br) 69B:365–373

Lloyd-Roberts GC, Wetherill MH, Frazer M 1985

Trochanteric advancement for premature arrest of the femoral growth plate. J Bone Joint Surg [Br] 57B:21–24
Loredo J 1985 Estudo populacional do angulo CE de Wiberg e sua applcacao na pesquisa genetica da livaco congenita do quadril. Theses Campinas, San Paulo, Brazil
McKibbin B, Ralis Z 1973 Changes in the shape of the human hip joint during its development and their relationship to its instability. J Bone Joint Surg [Br] 55B:780
Mitchell GP 1972 The delayed Trendelenburg hip test. International Congress series 291. SICOT:
O'Hara JN 1990 Congenital dislocation of the hip—acetabular dysplasia in adolescence following limbectomy in infancy. Proc AAOS 113 (abstract)
Ponsetti IV 1978 Growth and development of the acetabulum in the normal child. J Bone Joint Surg (Am) 60A:575—585
Quain S, Catterall A 1986 Hinge abduction—its recognition and treatment. J Bone Joint Surg [Br] 69B:61–64
Steel HH 1973 Triple osteotomy of the innominate bone. J Bone Joint Surg 55: 343–350
Steel HH 1977 Triple osteotomy of the innominate bone. A procedure to accomplish coverage of the dislocated or subluxated femoral head in the older patient. Clin Orthop Rel Res 122:116–127
Saito S, Kakowka K, Ono K 1986 Tectoplasty for painful dislocation or subluxation of the hip. J Bone Joint Surg (Br) 68B:55
Tönnis D 1982 Triple osteotomy close to the hip. In: Tachdjean MO (ed) Congenital dislocation of the hip. Churchill Livingstone, New York, pp 565–566
Tönnis D 1990 A modified technique of the triple pelvic osteotomy. J Paediatr Orthop 1:141–149
Wagner H 1978a Experiences with spherical osteotomy for correction of acetabular dysplasia. In: Weil HH (ed) Acetabular dysplasia and skeletal dysplasias in childhood. Springer, Berlin, pp 131–146
Wagner H 1978b Femoral osteotomies for congenital dislocation of the hip. In: Weil HH (ed) Acetabular dysplasia, skeletal dysplasias in childhood. Springer, Berlin, pp 85–105
Wainwright D 1976 The shelf operation for hip dysplasia in adolescence. J Bone Joint Surg (Br) 58:159–163
Wiberg G 1939 Studies on dysplasia, acetabula and congenital dislocation of the hip with special reference to the complication of osteoarthritis. Acta Chirurg Scand 83 (suppl 58):1–135

8

Changes in the management of the child with Duchenne muscular dystrophy

G. A. Evans

One of the saddest conditions in children's orthopaedic practice is Duchenne's muscular dystrophy. It is a progressive degenerative process affecting skeletal and cardiac muscle without associated structural abnormality in the peripheral nervous system. The incidence varies both between and within different countries, with a range from 130 to 390 per million male births. It is genetically determined as an X-linked recessive disorder, with the abnormality located at the central area on the short arm of the X chromosome known as band p21. There is a high frequency of new mutations. The effect is complete absence of the protein dystrophin from the muscle cell in Duchenne, whilst Becker's dystrophy is characterized by reduced levels of the protein. At present there is no cure for the disease. For this reason there has been considerable pessimism and a relatively negative attitude in the past towards treatment of the secondary deformities. Such patients have frequently been under the care of paediatricians and have not been referred for orthopaedic attention, with the result that many surgeons are unaware that a problem exists.

The recent changes in the management of Duchenne's dystrophy can be described in general principles as follows:

1. *Improve the quality of life* while the patient is still walking, and also when confined to a wheelchair.
2. *Early treatment is easier* for the patient and associated with the least morbidity.

NATURAL HISTORY

An understanding of the nature and timing of the secondary orthopaedic problems is essential for appropriate treatment. There are two phases in the child's life (Fig. 8.1). During the first phase the child is able to walk. In 56% the onset of walking is delayed until at least 18 months (Emery 1987), whereas 97% of normal children are walking by this age (Neligan & Prudham 1969). The severity of the disorder and rate of functional deterioration can vary considerably between individual patients. On average a child's walking deteriorates progressively after 7 years and ceases at an average age of $9\frac{1}{2}$ years (Rideau 1984). Age alone is an unreliable index of disease progression (Sutherland et al 1981). The weakness is progressive but not linearly. For this reason the benefit of any suggested treatment has to

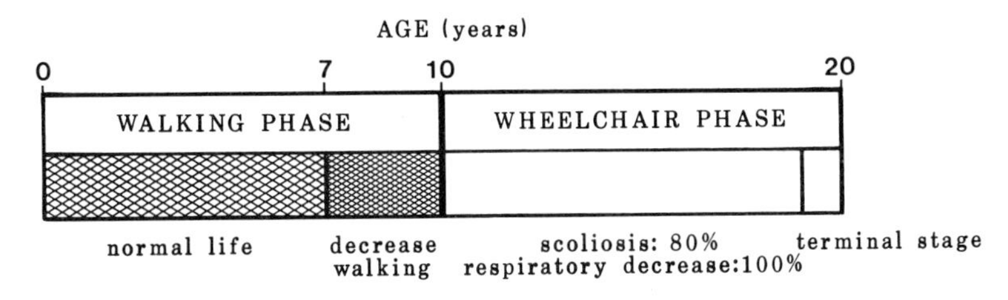

Fig. 8.1 The main phases and features of Duchenne dystrophy. (Redrawn with permission from Rideau et al 1981.)

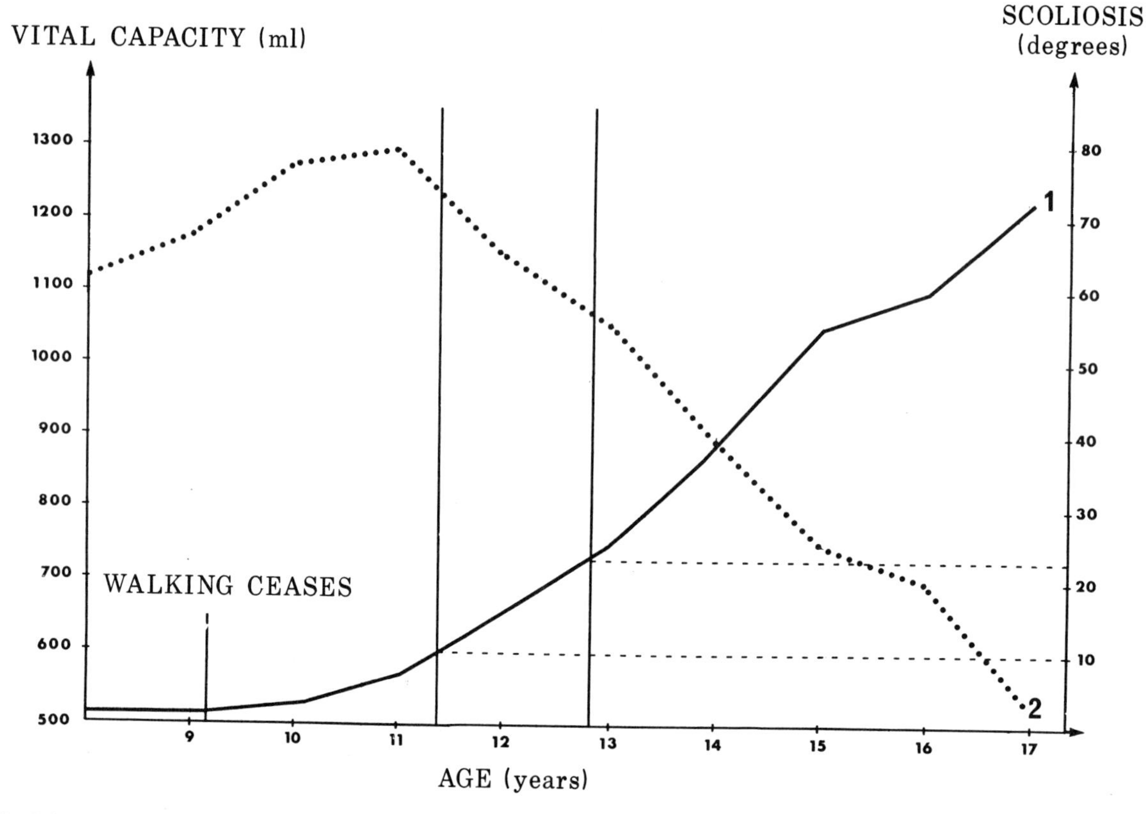

Fig. 8.2 The natural history of scoliosis (1) and absolute measurement of vital capacity (2) in the more progressive form. With a scoliosis of 10–23° the vital capacity is already deteriorating at a mean age of 12 years. (Redrawn with permission from Rideau et al 1981.)

be evaluated with considerable care. This loss of walking roughly coincides with a plateau in the previously rising values of lung function tests (Fig. 8.2).

The second phase of life is in a wheelchair, and is associated with progressive flexion deformities of hip, knee and elbows. Equinovarus deformity becomes severe and interferes with comfortable shoewear and tolerance for standing frames. The onset of a progressive deterioration of respiratory function 1 or 2 years after walking ceases is associated in the majority with a progressive scoliosis (Fig 8.2). Kurz et al (1983) estimated that there is a 4% deterioration of vital capacity for each year of life and a similar loss for every 10° increase of the scoliosis. Some patients are overweight, whereas others become very thin and atrophic. Most die of respiratory failure at a mean age of between 16 and 17 years, and 90% are dead by 20 years. The occasional patient dies suddenly and unexpectedly from arrhythmia secondary to cardiomyopathy. The age at death does not correlate significantly with the age of onset of symptoms but does correlate with the age of becoming confined to a wheelchair (Emery 1987). Some of the simple and more sophisticated measurements that can be undertaken to monitor the progression of the disease are listed in Table 8.1.

DIAGNOSIS

The first priority for the orthopaedic surgeon undertaking a general clinic is to have a *high level of awareness* of the diagnosis. In a survey of 83 families, Read & Galasko (1986) found that the diagnosis had been missed in every one of the 37 patients referred primarily to an orthopaedic surgeon. In the whole group there was a mean delay of 2 years during which time inappropriate treatment, difficulties in communicating with parents, much parental anxiety and further pregnancies occurred.

The clinical diagnosis may not be so obvious in

Table 8.1 Measurable parameters of the progression of Duchenne muscular dystrophy

Routine: Clinical examination	*Investigations*
Weight percentile	Forced vital capacity
Timed Gowers' test	Myometry (Hosking et al 1976)
Walking speed	Sitting spinal X-rays
Contractures	Cobb angle
	Kyphotic index (Cambridge & Drennan 1987)
	Electrocardiogram
Research: Gait laboratory	
Anterior pelvic tilt	Ultrasound to image muscle loss
Ankle dorsiflexion in swing	Nuclear magnetic resonance for muscle chemistry
Position of ground reaction force	
Cadence	
Double-stance period	

the very young. However, unlike the subtle presentation of many other conditions, muscular dystrophy has a simple screening test which can be performed at any clinic, namely the serum creatine kinase. This test should be undertaken on any child, especially young boys, with unexplained weakness, clumsiness or disturbance of gait, and on those unable to walk by 18 months of age. A degree of intellectual or speech impairment may be present which, when associated with hypotonia and clumsiness, leads to a mistaken diagnosis of cerebral palsy. All 'toe-walkers' should be screened for myopathy. In almost all cases there is a history of inability to run properly.

The diagnostic tests are as follows:

1. *Serum creatine kinase* levels in healthy newborn infants are often slightly raised to 200–300 iu and then drop and remain constant until an occasional second slight elevation during the adolescent growth spurt. In early Duchenne dystrophy the enzyme is raised up to 100 times greater than normal, but the levels drop around the time the boys become confined to a wheelchair, presumably due to the decrease in functioning muscle tissue and reduction of physical activity.

2. *Serum aldolase* is raised 10–20 times the normal range.

3. *Electromyography* is diagnostic of myopathy but not specifically of Duchenne dystrophy. At an early stage the action potentials are reduced in duration and amplitude with polyphasic potentials more frequent than normal. Later, with the loss of motor units, there is very little activity.

4. *Needle biopsy of muscle* was first advocated by Duchenne but has recently been developed into a reliable clinical investigation (Edwards et al 1973, 1980). Open biopsy under general anaesthesia is no longer required. Histology shows variation of fibre size, prominent rounded fibres which stain densely with eosin, necrosis with phagocytosis, and eventual fatty replacement. Histochemical staining shows that no particular fibre type is predominantly affected and there is no grouping of fibre types (Brumback & Leech 1984).

5. *DNA probes* have been used to identify the abnormal gene location at Xp21. These tests are particularly helpful in conjunction with the serum creatine kinase test in providing 95% accuracy of female carrier detection (Harper 1986), and for prenatal diagnosis from amniotic fluid cells at 16 weeks' gestation or chorion biopsy at 10 weeks' gestation.

6. *Dystrophin* measurement of muscle biopsies is likely to become a more widespread clinical tool.

The family

Having made the diagnosis it is important that the family are given the information in an appropriate manner. Parents require an open, sympathetic, direct and uninterrupted discussion of the diagnosis in private, with sufficient time for them to take in the news and for information to be repeated and clarified. Evasive, unsympathetic and hurried consultations can result in long-lasting adverse emotional responses (Woolley et al 1989). There are five sequential stages in the coping process (Falek 1977), although some parents may not progress through all the stages. These are:

1. Shock and denial.
2. Anxiety.

3. Anger and guilt.
4. Depression.
5. Psychological homeostasis.

In this respect it is helpful to work in conjunction with a paediatrician or physician with a special interest in the disorder. After careful consideration referral of the patient to a specialist multidisciplinary clinic will probably provide the greatest expertise for the child and family with a minimum of hospital attendances (Table 8.2).

Table 8.2 Outline of multidisciplinary team for muscular dystrophy and individual roles

Physician	Informs and supports family Controls weight Respiratory and cardiac care Terminal care Probably co-ordinator of multidisciplinary team
Geneticist	Confirms diagnosis Genetic counselling
Orthopaedic surgeon	Enhances independent walking Minimizes contractures of legs Prevents collapsing scoliosis
Family care officer	Ensures adequate facilities at home and school Supports family
Paramedical team	Physiotherapist, dietician, orthotist

WALKING PHASE

MECHANICAL DISORDER AND COMPENSATORY MECHANISMS

The sequence of changes is summarized in Table 8.3. The weakness progresses from proximal to distal. The initial weakness of the hip extensors is compensated by lumbar hyperlordosis, without apparent pelvic tilt, which moves the line of the ground reaction force behind the fulcrum of the hip joint (Sutherland et al 1981). In response to the later onset of slight weakness in the quadriceps the ground reaction force is also adjusted in front of the knee by a combination of anterior pelvic tilt and a foot-flat contact with the floor. This is in effect a dynamic equinus (Khodadadeh et al 1986). This mimics an instant during the normal gait cycle at the end of stance phase, when the heel rises off the floor and only the hip flexors and calf muscles are contracting (Fig. 8.3). There is loss of ankle dorsiflexion during swing phase in Duchenne dystrophy and hip flexion is increased to allow clearance of the foot. Flexion and abduction contractures of the hips, especially of tensor fascia lata,

Table 8.3 A simplified summary of the sequence of changes in the legs during the walking phase, and the timing of surgical options

Sequence of problems	Compensation	Secondary effect	Surgical options
Early weakness of hip extensors	Lumbar hyperlordosis moves ground reaction line behind the hip		
Early weakness quadriceps	Dynamic equinus and anterior pelvic tilt provides adjustable ground reaction anterior to knee	Loss of ankle dorsiflexion, but not fixed equinus initially	Early release of hip contractures ± elongation of heel cords while distal strength is still good
Increased weakness of hip extensors/abductors	Broader-based gait	Increasing hip flexor–abductor contracture	
Increasing fixed equinus		Progressive reduction of velocity, step length and cadence Decreasing support area under forefoot	
Marked weakness of hip and quadriceps Severe equinus (± varus)	Shoulder sway The adjusted position of hip and knee over the forefoot has to be very precise	Precarious gait which finally decompensates	or Late release of hip and calf contractures to allow long leg bracing

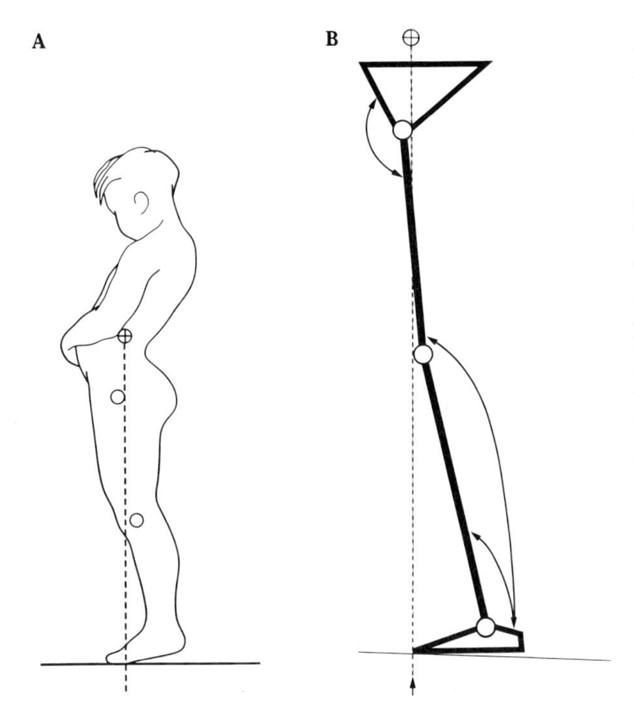

Fig. 8.3 (**A**) The characteristic standing posture in Duchenne dystrophy with the ground reaction force behind the hip and in front of the knee. This mimics stance phase in a normal limb when the heel starts rising (**B**). Hip and knee extensors are not required. The hip flexors and calf muscles are working, and in Duchenne muscular dystrophy these muscles develop contractures.

develop early and this is well before there is significant weakness and functional deterioration of gait (Vignos & Archibald 1960). It has been shown that 5- and 6-year-old boys have increased anteroposterior and lateral sway while standing (Barrett et al 1988). This is probably due to the continued slight adjustment required by the dynamic equinus. It is interesting that the early prescription of ankle foot orthoses reduces the range of anteroposterior sway but not its frequency, presumably by providing some stability. As the weakness increases it becomes progressively more difficult to get up from a sitting position on the floor (Gowers 1879). Progression of the disease can be monitored by the number of seconds taken to do this manoeuvre (Rideau 1986). It appears that the problem is due to a combination of muscle weakness and the constraint caused by the hip flexor–abduction contracture.

The calf muscle appears hypertrophied. It is true that the muscle is well preserved relative to other muscles in the leg but the hypertrophy is due to increase of connective tissue and fat (Jones et al 1983). The foot-flat gait or dynamic equinus gradually becomes a fixed equinus, presumably due to the relative lack of muscle growth alongside the growing tibia, as it is not being stretched normally while walking. The increasing connective tissue within the muscle may also be contributory. The equinus maintains the ground reaction force in front of the knee, and through or just behind the hip, so that even when the child is no longer able to rise from the floor he can still walk. At this stage release of the equinus contracture will result in loss of walking. Limited elongation of heel cord may provide improvement of stability without mechanical decompensation (Williams et al 1984), but prescription of a compensatory ground reaction ankle foot orthosis may be necessary.

As a result of progressive weakness and equinus the walking speed, step length, and the number of steps taken per minute (cadence) decrease (Sutherland et al 1981). The proportion of the gait cycle with both feet on the ground increases (double support time; Khodadadeh et al 1987). There is increasing shoulder sway. Eventually the equinus becomes so severe that the floor contact is limited to the metatarsal heads. This is a precarious balancing act, without the ability to adjust the position of the reaction force under the forefoot. There is loss of push-off and difficulty with clearance in swing. Minor degrees of fixed flexion at the knee will cause the body to collapse. Early varus posturing of the foot also makes it unstable. Confidence is lost and walking ceases. Contributory factors (Vignos & Archibald 1960) which may cause premature loss of walking are:

1. *Lower limb fractures* or general illness resulting in recumbency. It is imperative that lower limb fractures are treated by a technique which allows continued weight-bearing. This may involve internal fixation.
2. *Obesity.* This causes the muscle power to body mass ratio to decompensate earlier. Patients are given a high-protein and a low-fat and carbohydrate diet in order to maintain their weight according to percentile charts which have been specifically designed for this condition (Griffiths & Edwards 1988; Fig. 8.4).

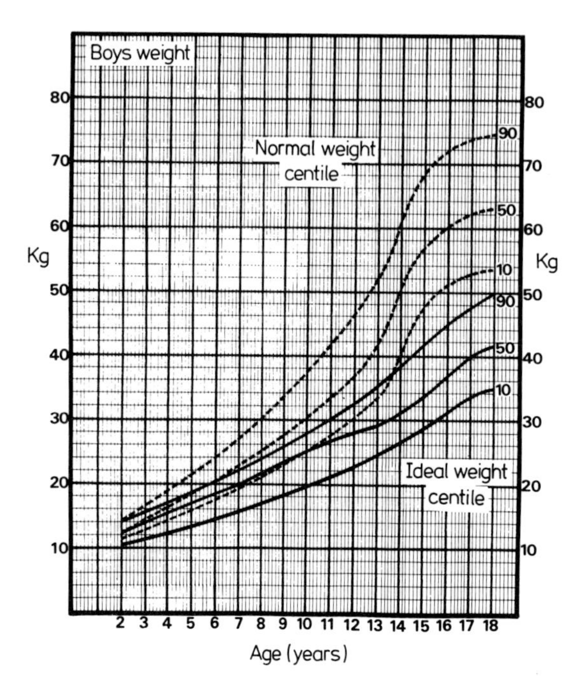

Fig. 8.4 Ideal weight centile chart for boys with Duchenne muscular dystrophy. (Reproduced with permission from Griffiths & Edwards 1988.)

3. *Convenience*: it is sometimes easier for a family to use a wheelchair prematurely in order to complete daily activities quickly.

4. *Emotional factors*. Some boys appear to lack motivation. There is a higher incidence of behaviour and emotional disturbances than in other physically handicapped children without cerebral involvement (Leibowitz & Dubowitz 1981). In addition, although there is considerable variation, the overall mean IQ is 1 s.d. below normal. This does not apper to be due to any lack of educational opportunity (Emery 1987). There is a suggestion that the impairment correlates with the cerebral atrophy observed on computerized tomography (Yoshioka et al 1980).

ORTHOPAEDIC MANAGEMENT

The objective is to prolong the walking ability with the minimum of imposition and potential morbidity for the patient. There appear to be three different approaches, each one claiming a limited benefit of not dissimilar magnitude. It is probable that none can alter significantly the progression of muscle weakness. In principle they aim to control or correct the secondary contractures and provide improved stability. The timing, duration and requirements of the three treatments are different.

Physiotherapy programme

Systematic passive stretching of muscle started early delays but does not prevent lower limb contractures. It also allows parental involvement. The daily regime is time-consuming, and overstretching probably causes additional muscle damage as well as producing a stressful relationship between child and parent. When undertaken by a physiotherapist this contact frequently becomes a significant psychological support for the child. The duration of benefit for walking is variable. Scott et al (1981) claimed the equivalent of a 2-year functional benefit but with parental compliance in only two-thirds of cases. Rideau (1985) found that the average prolongation of walking was only 8 months.

Night-splinting for equinus is of doubtful benefit. It may help if started before the development of the contracture, but about 60% fail to comply with the treatment (Scott et al 1981). Accurate fitting and repeated prescription with growth are additional problems. Active exercise against weight resistance may give a transient initial improvement of strength in the less severely affected patients (Vignos & Watkins 1966). There is no appreciable functional benefit from this and it is time-consuming and not cost-effective (Dubowitz et al 1984). Patients should be advised to take normal physical activity as far as possible.

For a patient nearing the end of the walking phase the daily use of a standing frame decreases the disuse element of muscle atrophy and minimizes the development of flexion contractures. It is suggested, in combination with the duration of independent walking and standing, that a minimum of 3 h standing daily is required (Vignos & Archibald 1960). This appears to be a useful prelude for those patients to be treated with long leg braces for continued walking.

Early release of contractures without bracing

This new approach has been advocated by Rideau (1984). The rationale is that contractures often progress more rapidly than loss of muscle strength (Vignos & Archibald 1960). All the lower limb contractures, especially of the iliotibial band, are corrected at an early stage when the muscles are still relatively strong. Rehabilitation is rapid, and independent walking is improved. It should be stressed that this option is still being assessed but early results are encouraging. The timing of the operation is usually between the ages of 4 and 6 years, when the timed Gowers' test is 5 seconds or less. Traditional teaching would not advise surgical intervention at this stage.

The specific bilateral releases described are as follows:

1. Proximal division of the superficial hip flexors: tensor fascia lata, sartorius and also rectus femoris if tight.
2. Division of the fascia lata transversely from in front of the hip to behind the greater trochanter.
3. Resection of the iliotibial band and the lateral intermuscular septum from the hip down to the knee.
4. Sliding lengthening of the Achilles tendon if there is an early calf contracture.
5. Closed distal tenotomy for a medial hamstring contracture if present.

The first three elements are performed through an oblique groin incision and a more distal longitudinal incision on the outer thigh. In early disease closed tenotomies in the groin, which are sometimes of value at a late stage when the fascia is obviously bowstringing, are not adequate. Postoperatively the patient remains in bed for 3 or 4 days for comfort and then mobilizes with weight-bearing, usually without the need for casts or splints. Hospitalization can be reduced to about 2 weeks at this early stage. The later the surgery is undertaken the longer the rehabilitation. If the timing is incorrect and the muscle weakness is such that the loss of the equinus results in decompensation, the situation can be retrieved by prescription of a polypropylene ankle–foot orthosis. However, the objective is early surgery, followed by freedom from both orthoses and the daily time-consuming physiotherapy programme.

As a result of this treatment there appears to be a functional benefit in the majority with regards to the ease of walking and one of my patients remarkably was able to 'run' for the first time. The timed Gowers' test sometimes improves and there is a delay of both the increasing Gowers' time and recurrence of hip contractures for approximately 3 years (Rideau et al 1986). In a study of 18 such patients undergoing similar surgery in a different centre the results were reproduced: 13 had significant functional benefit (Rideau et al 1987). In a series of 30 cases with an average follow-up of 4 years and 5 months there were no serious complications, 1 superficial wound infection and 4 hypertrophic scars. If in untreated cases the average age of cessation of walking is 9 years and 6 months, 20 of the treated cases are still walking at over 10 years of age (Rideau 1990). While it is not possible to undertake a statistical analysis of the results at this stage, the clinical impression is that independent walking and freedom are prolonged by approximately 2 years (Riccio 1990). Some patients, however, do not derive as much benefit (Giannini et al 1990). They probably suffer from the more progressive form of the disease. Further work needs to be undertaken to try to identify at an early stage those patients in whom the intervention will not be cost-effective.

Late surgery to facilitate bracing

The established surgical option is to correct severe contractures when independent walking is lost in order to make the lower limbs braceable. Lightweight ischial-bearing long leg braces with knee locks and fixed ankles are prescribed to allow a further period of therapeutic walking and limited independence. Only boys and families with adequate motivation derive such benefit functionally and being overweight is a disadvantage. The treatment is offered when independent walking has almost stopped, managing for approximately half an hour daily, and falls are frequent. The specific bilateral surgical procedures (Fig. 8.5) are as follows:

1. Division of the superficial hip flexors proximally—tensor fascia lata, sartorius and rectus femoris.
2. Transection of the fascia lata and iliotibial band at the hip and just above the knee.
3. Sliding lengthening of Achilles tendon.

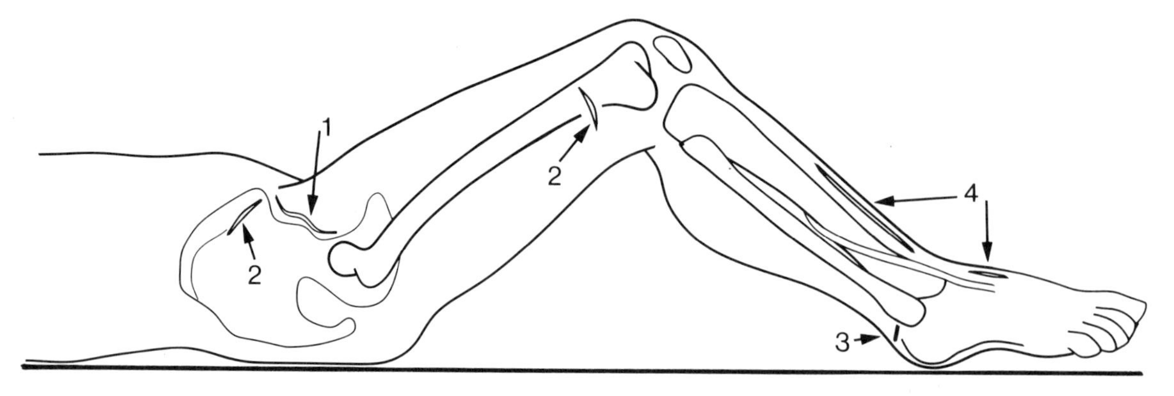

Fig 8.5 Late surgical releases to facilitate bracing can be performed percutaneously (1–3) and combined with transfer of tibialis posterior tendon (4).

4. Transfer of the tibialis posterior tendon through the interosseous membrane to the dorsum of the foot (intermediate cuneiform bone).

In most thin children percutaneous incisions can be used for release of the contractures (Siegel et al 1968), as they greatly reduce postoperative discomfort and help the early rehabilitation required. Although the tibialis posterior tendon may not be tight at this stage it will become so, resulting in severe equinovarus posture of the foot. Tenotomies only delay the deformity which can be corrected or prevented permanently by the tendon transfer at this stage (Drennan 1983). No further physiotherapy or splinting will be required for the ankle. Ordinary shoes or trainers can be worn, and the plantigrade foot will allow the use of a standing frame even when walking has ceased.

After the operation well-padded long leg casts are applied with the knee extended and feet plantigrade. Early mobilization is essential, regaining the erect position on a tilting bed the next day. If the patient can tolerate this he is encouraged to take a few steps and gradually progress from parallel bars to walking sticks. The casts are replaced by the custom-made orthoses usually at 4 weeks, although some centres do this much earlier. In general a pair of walking sticks helps confidence, and may prevent a heavy fall which can fracture an arm and destroy the willingness to continue brace-walking. This regime is of functional benefit, improves morale, and delays the onset of severe flexion contractures of hip and knee (Spencer & Vignos 1962, Eyring et al 1972). It is also claimed to delay the onset of scoliosis, (Heckmatt et al 1989), although this may possibly be due to the fact that the best therapeutic walkers are those with the slower progression of disease, including spinal deformity. Rapid deterioration of scoliosis was apparently prevented in the 22% of boys who were able to continue brace-walking throughout the pubertal growth spurt. The average prolongation of walking in this study of 93 patients was 21 months, with the longest being 6 years. In a separate study of 24 patients Capelli et al (1990) reported a mean prolongation of walking of 1.8 years (range 1–3.7 years). The factors which predict the duration of walking ability after bracing include the percentage of residual muscle strength, vital capacity, and a measurement of the total functional muscle mass by changes in the creatinine coefficient (Vignos et al 1983).

In conclusion, the relative merits of the treatment options have not yet been fully defined. All require patient compliance, especially the daily physiotherapy programme. The physiotherapy can complement surgical treatment, but appears to be an unnecessary routine after early surgical release. The best results of any treatment will be found in boys with the more slowly progressive disease. A choice has to be made with regards to the timing of surgery (Table 8.3). The merits of early surgery are the rapid rehabilitation and subsequent freedom from time-consuming physiotherapy and bracing. If the quantum of additional walking is similar to that after late surgery and bracing, then clearly the former is preferable. It is possible that late bracing may still provide some prolongation of walking even after the benefits of early surgery are lost. With time results will become statistically meaningful, and much work has also to be done on refining patient selection.

SITTING PHASE

The primary orthopaedic objective during this phase is to maintain a comfortable sitting position. However, it may also be possible to retard the development of severe flexion deformities of hip and knee which are uncomfortable while recumbent.

FLEXION CONTRACTURES

These may be helped by the regular use of a standing frame, if possible throughout the adolescent growth spurt. When walking ceases the standing frame is applied during school lessons, in order to minimize the imposition for other activities, and is usually tolerated for at least 2 h daily. It was initially surprising to find that the boys enjoyed the limited mobility provided by a swivel walker (Fig. 8.6), which was designed for myelomeningocele patients (Butler et al 1982), rather than using a static standing frame. With time the mobility in the swivel walker is lost and standing even in the static frame produces pressure symptoms under the feet or in front of the knees. The periods of standing gradually drop to half an hour, repeated twice daily, and finally the inconvenience is no longer cost-effective and the standing programme is abandoned. For the boys with rapid progression of weakness it does not alter the final deformity but is good for morale initially, whereas in those with a slower progression the protection throughout the growth spurt appears to reduce the deformity considerably. A lot of well-meaning time and effort can be expended by physiotherapists at this stage with passive stretching and application of intermittently

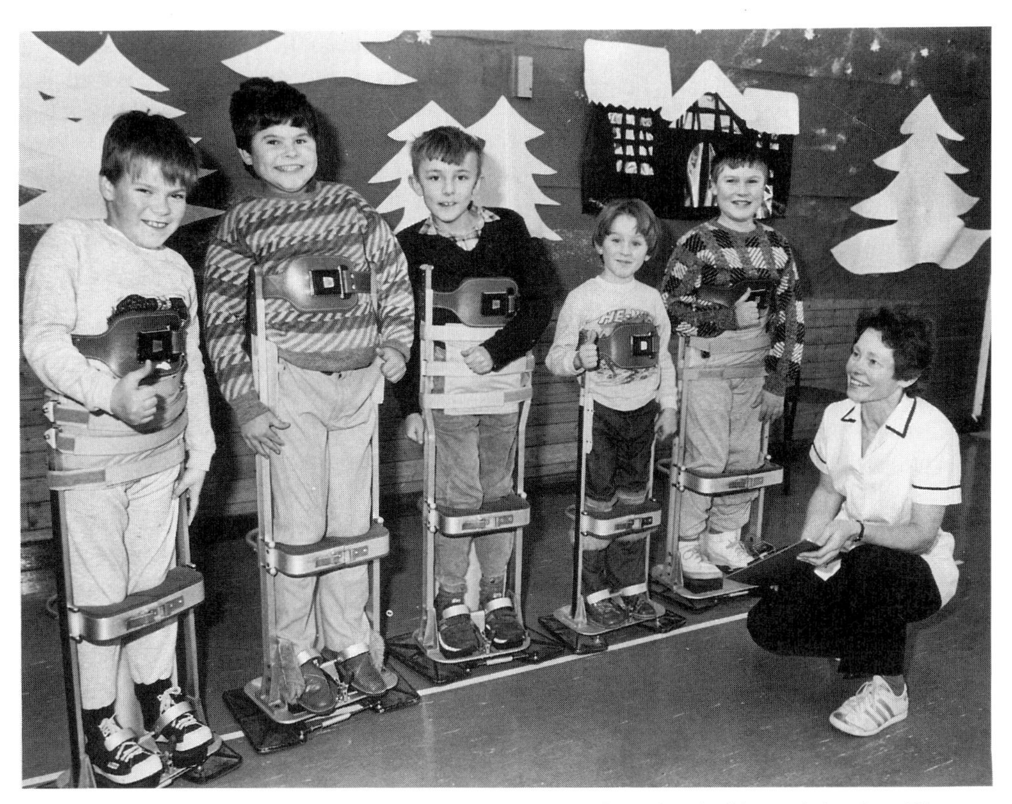

Fig 8.6 A standing programme at school using swivel walkers. (Reproduced with permission from The Shropshire Star.)

inflated pneumatic splints, with little tangible physical benefit in the longer term. Of course there are benefits for morale and the physiotherapist frequently becomes a major psychological support for the child. The standing programme and physiotherapy should be undertaken if compliance and morale are good but clearly should not become an additional burden for the child.

SCOLIOSIS

A collapsing scoliosis with pelvic obliquity develops in 95% of patients (Cambridge & Drennan 1987) 1 or 2 years after the loss of walking. Severe scoliosis makes comfortable sitting difficult so that frequent and elaborate adjustments of seating do not prevent pain and occasional skin breakdown. Untreated, some patients become bedridden years before death (Smith et al 1989). The direction of the curve is usually determined by asymmetrical contracture of the iliotibial band (Cambridge & Drennan 1987) but unfortunately early release of these contractures does not prevent or reduce the severity of scoliosis.

A small minority of patients develop a less severe extended double-curve pattern but there are no early distinguishing features (Smith et al 1989). The development of kyphosis while sitting is a prognostic indicator for the onset of scoliosis but despite initial optimism (Gibson & Wilkins 1975) early maintenance of the lumbar spine in extension rarely prevents severe deformity. Lumbar extension was frequently seen to coexist with scoliosis (Smith et al 1989). The adverse prognostic features for progressive scoliosis while seated are therefore:

1. Pelvic asymmetry due to hip contractures.
2. Lumbar kyphosis.
3. Excessive weight.

The objective for treating the scoliosis is to retain a comfortable sitting position. There are a large number of studies showing that prophylactic spinal bracing retards the development and progression of scoliosis but does not change the final outcome (Gibson et al 1978, Hsu 1983, Rideau et al 1984, Seeger et al 1984, Cambridge & Drennan 1987). The mechanical principle of a total-contact body orthosis is the application of three-point fixation to counter the effect of gravity. The pressure applied to the ribs approximately halves the measured respiratory function. It is also an imposition on the child to continue wearing such a device throughout the day for most of his remaining life. Eventually it is discarded when as a result of severe scoliosis it becomes uncomfortable and there is respiratory compromise. For these reasons spinal jackets are not the optimal treatment. They are reserved for families who do not wish their sons to have the alternative surgical option or in the rare case of rapid progression where the duration of benefit from surgery possibly will be negligible. Patients and families are given the opportunity before making a decision to meet boys and families who have already had surgical treatment.

The advance which has allowed surgical instrumentation of the spine in Duchenne dystrophy is the Luque segmental fixation (1982). The proven technique involves fixation of the Luque rods to the pelvis by the Galveston technique (Allen & Ferguson 1984) in order to correct or prevent pelvic obliquity (Fig. 8.7). It is important that the rods are bent to conform with the dorsal kyphosis and lumbar lordosis in order to maintain comfortable weight transfer through the ischial tuberosities and thighs while sitting. The segmental fixation is sufficiently secure to dispense with postoperative external supports and the patient is sat up in bed within 2 or 3 days and is back in a wheelchair within a week. During the operation the blood loss appears to be twice as much as for any other neuromuscular disorder requiring this procedure. There are increased risks associated with anaesthesia (Smith & Bush 1985).

Several different specific techniques have been developed applying the basic principles of segmental instrumentation. It is probable that formal facet excision and bone grafting of the dorsal spine are unnecessary, but this is done in the mobile lumbar segment so that a fusion mass relieves the stresses on the metal rods in the long term and protects against pelvic obliquity. It is generally agreed that instrumentation to the upper thoracic spine—usually T3—is necessary to prevent late deformity above a shorter fusion. Of interest, now that patients can live much longer with assisted ventilation, late lateral flexion deformities of the neck have been observed above the accepted high dorsal fusion (Rideau 1990). Although Sussman (1986) claims

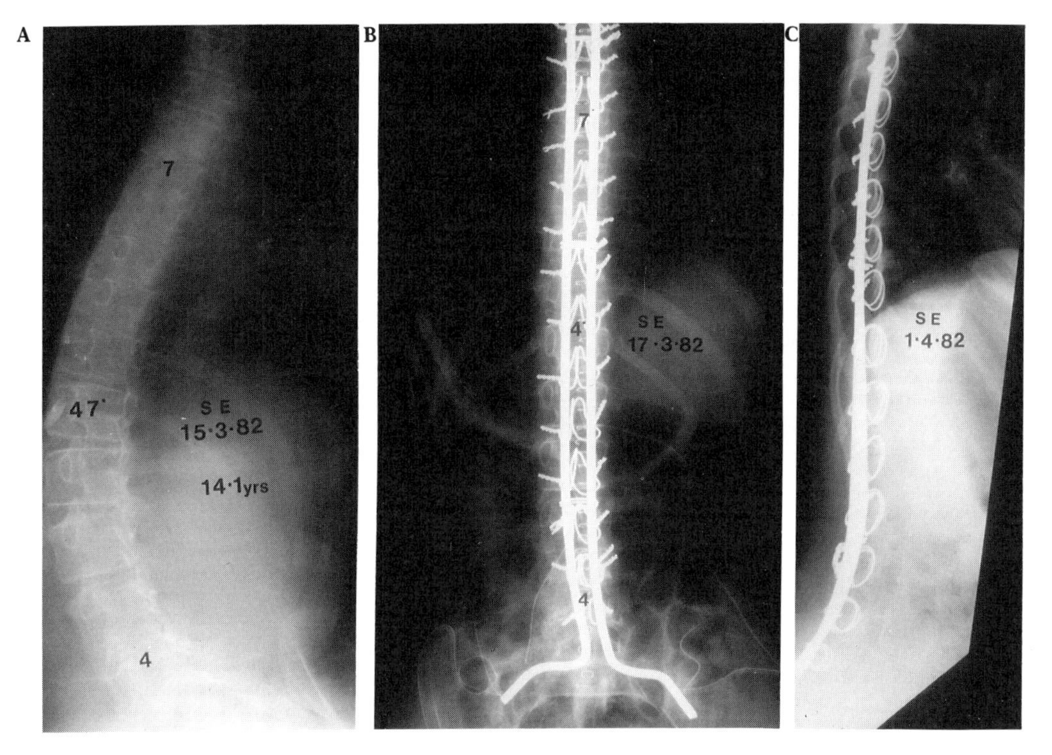

Fig 8.7 A collapsing scoliosis (**A**) treated surgically by Luque instrumentation (**B**). The lateral view (**C**) shows retention of the lumbar lordosis by contouring of the rods.

that fusion to the fifth lumbar vertebra is adequate in the short term, this needs to be confirmed in a longer review. A rectangular configuration of the rods, either at both ends (Dove 1986) or just the top end, may strengthen the instrumentation but in our experience these closed loops prevent longitudinal growth of the immature spine. The continued growth within this constraint produces rotational deformity (Mehdian et al 1989). In different circumstances this has been called the crankshaft phenomenon (Dubousset et al 1989). Accordingly a method of instrumentation without fusion has been developed at Oswestry by Mehdian et al (1989) with the objective of obtaining a rectangular configuration while still allowing growth. The rods are passed through two cannulated H bars. One is positioned distally and the other some 3 cm below the proximal end of the rods to allow for growth.

Appropriate timing is critical in order to provide greatest safety during the operation and the most efficient instrumentation. This can be determined by a combination of repeated measurements of vital capacity and sitting X-rays of the spine (Fig. 8.2). Based on the work of Rideau (1986), the absolute value of vital capacity reaches a plateau at or shortly after the cessation of walking. In patients with the most rapid progression of disease the vital capacity starts to decline a year or more later and coincides with rapid increase of scoliosis. There is, of course, a gradual deterioration in vital capacity expressed as a percentage of normal throughout this period (Fig. 8.8). The window of surgical opportunity is at the end of the plateau (Fig. 8.2) when the deformity is minimal and fully correctable at operation. Expressed as a percentage of normal, surgery is relatively safe at a vital capacity above 40% (Fig. 8.8), and prolonged postoperative ventilatory support is needed for a vital capacity below 35% (Smith et al 1989). The average scoliosis at a 40% vital capacity measures only 23° (Rideau et al 1984). The timing of surgery clearly has to be early and is almost prophylactic. If spinal bracing has been prescribed the curve will reach the operative range when the child is older and has greater respiratory deterioration, at which stage the operation is more dangerous. The definitive treatment for scoliosis is

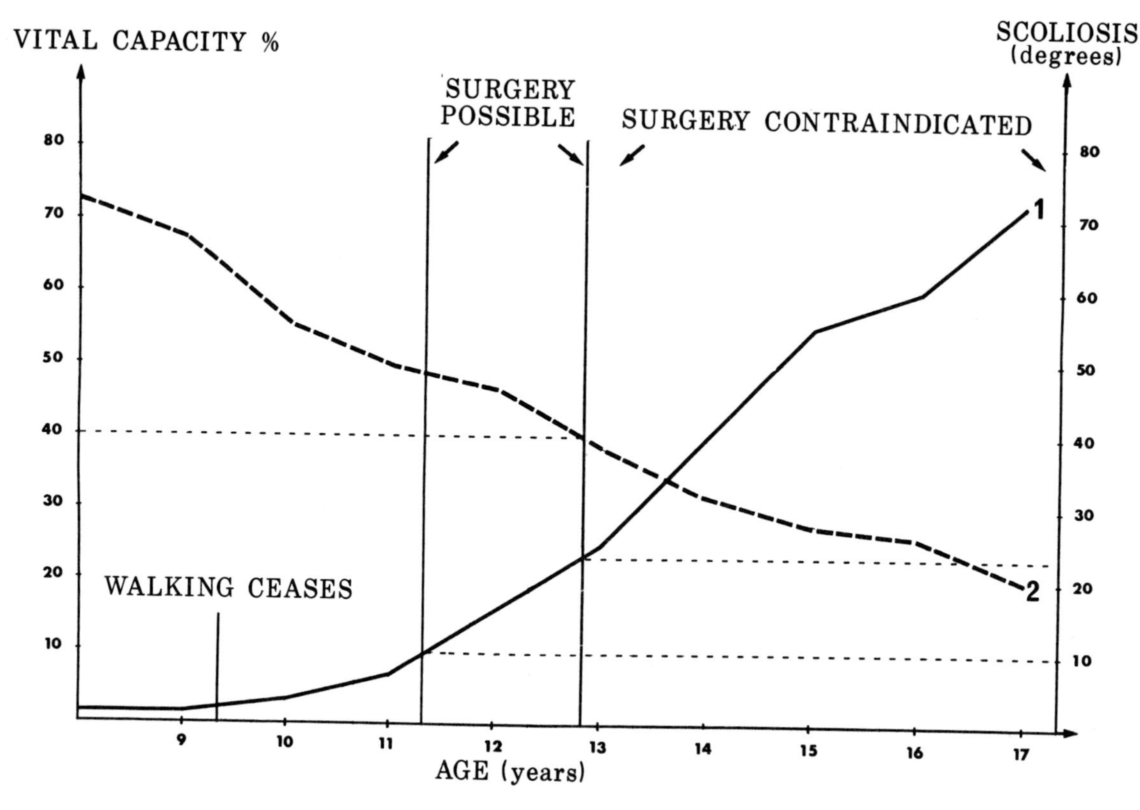

Fig 8.8 The natural history of scoliosis (1) and the vital capacity (2) expressed as a percentage of normal. In the more progressive form the scoliosis is only 23° when the vital capacity reaches 40% below normal. There is a window of opportunity for spinal surgery before this point is reached. (Redrawn with permission from Rideau et al 1984.)

therefore an operation undertaken at the optimal time (Figs. 8.2 and 8.8).

Postoperatively patients notice that they are sitting taller with greater stability. It sometimes takes a few days to regain sitting balance and neck control, and the armrests and feeding table on the wheelchair usually need to be adjusted upwards. These changes are of course less with early surgery.

Complications such as infection, lumbosacral pain and prominence of the rod ends requiring trimming have occurred cumulatively in less than a quarter of patients. The overall symptomatic gain is considerable but there is no measurable reduction of the gradual deterioration of lung function (Cambridge & Drennan 1987, Caroll et al 1990).

KEY POINTS FOR CLINICAL PRACTICE

1. Maintain a high level of diagnostic awareness.
2. A needle biopsy is diagnostic and open biopsy not necessary.
3. Lower limb fractures require prompt treatment which will allow continued weight-bearing.
4. Avoid elongation of the Achilles tendon in isolation. The equinus is initially a compensation for proximal weakness and contractures.
5. Appropriate surgical treatment enhances the stability and duration of walking in compliant patients. It can be performed at a very early stage with subsequent freedom, or at an end-stage of walking with braces.
6. The definitive treatment for scoliosis is segmental spinal instrumentation undertaken before deterioration of the serially measured forced vital capacity. There is no indication for spinal bracing before such surgery.
7. All surgical interventions are accompanied by very early postoperative mobilization.

REFERENCES

Allen BL, Ferguson RL 1984 The Galveston technique of pelvic fixation with L rod instrumentation of the spine. Spine 9:388–394

Barrett R, Hyde SA, Scott DM 1988 Changes in center of gravity in boys with Duchenne muscular dystrophy. Muscle Nerve 11:1157–1163

Brumback RA, Leech RW 1984 Color atlas of muscle histochemistry. PSG Publishing, Littleton, Massachusetts

Butler PB, Farmer IR, Poiner R et al 1982 Use of the ORLAU swivel walker for the severely handicapped patient. Physiotherapy 68:324–326

Cambridge W, Drennan JC 1987 Scoliosis associated with Duchenne muscular dystrophy. J Pediatr Orthop 7:436–440

Capelli T, Colombo C, Bonfiglioli S et al 1990 Rehabilitation in calipers to prolong ambulation in DMD. J Neurol Sci 98 (suppl):426

Caroll N, Evans GA, Edwards RHT 1990 Long term follow up of pulmonary function after Luque spinal stabilisation in Duchenne muscular dystrophy. J Neurol Sci 98 (suppl):426–427

Dove J 1986 Internal fixation of the lumbar spine. Clin Orthop 203:135–140

Drennan JC 1983 Orthopaedic management of neuromuscular disorders. JB Lippincott, Philadelphia, pp 10–41

Dubousset J, Herring JA, Shufflebarger H 1989 The Crankshaft phenomenon. J Pediatr Orthop 9:541–550

Dubowitz V, Hyde SA, Scott OM et al 1984 Controlled trial of exercise in Duchenne muscular dystrophy. In: Serratrice G, Cros D, Desnuelle C (eds) Neuromuscular disease. Raven Press, New York, pp 571–575

Edwards RHT, Maunder C, Lewis PD et al 1973 Percutaneous needle biopsy in the diagnosis of muscle diseases. Lancet ii:1070–1071

Edwards RHT, Young A, Wiles M 1980 Needle biopsy of skeletal muscle in the diagnosis of myopathy and the clinical study of muscle function and repair. N Engl J Med 302:261–271

Emery AEH 1987 Duchenne muscular dystrophy. University Press, Oxford

Eyring EJ, Johnson EW, Burnett C 1972 Surgery in muscular dystrophy. JAMA 222:1056–1057

Falek A 1977 Use of the coping process to achieve psychological homeostasis in genetic counseling. In: Lubs HA, Cruz F (eds) Genetic counseling. Raven Press, New York, pp 179–188

Giannini S, Granata C, Merlini C et al 1990 Early surgery of lower limbs in Duchenne muscular dystrophy. J Neurol Sci 98 (Suppl): 428

Gibson DA, Wilkins KE 1975 The management of spinal deformities in Duchenne muscular dystrophy. A new concept of spinal bracing. Clin Orthop 108:41–51

Gibson DA, Koreska J, Robertson D et al 1978 The management of spinal deformity in Duchenne muscular dystrophy. Orthop Clin North Am 9:437–450

Gowers WR 1879 Pseudo-hypertrophic muscular paralysis—a clinical lecture. J & A Churchill, London

Griffiths RD, Edwards RHT 1988 A new chart for weight control in Duchenne muscular dystrophy. Arch Dis Child 63:1256–1258

Harper PS 1986 Isolating the gene for Duchenne muscular dystrophy. Br Med J 293:773–774

Heckmatt J, Rodillo E, Dubowitz V 1989 Management of children: pharmacological and physical. Br Med Bull 45:788–801

Hosking GP, Bhat US, Dobowitz V et al 1976 Measurements of muscle strength and performance in children with normal and diseased muscle. Arch Dis Child 51:957–963

Hsu JD 1983 The natural history of spinal curvature progression in the non ambulatory DMD patient. Spine 8:771–775

Jones DA, Round JM, Edwards RHT et al 1983 Size and composition of the calf and quadriceps muscles in Duchenne muscular dystrophy. A tomographic and histochemical study. J Neurol Sci 60:307–322

Khodadadeh S, McClelland MR, Patrick JH et al 1986 Knee movements in Duchenne muscular dystrophy. Lancet ii:544–545

Khodadadeh S, McClelland MR, Nene AV et al 1987 The use of double support time for monitoring the gait of muscular dystrophy patients. Clin Biomech 2:68–70

Kurz LT, Mubarek SJ, Schultz P et al 1983 Correlation of scoliosis and pulmonary function in Duchenne muscular dystrophy. J Pediatr Orthop 3:347–353

Leibowitz D, Dubowitz V 1981 Intellect and behaviour in Duchenne muscular dystrophy. Dev Med Child Neurol 23:577–590

Luque ER 1982 Segmental spinal instrumentation for correction of scoliosis. Clin Orthop 163: 192–198

Mehdian H, Shimizu N, Draycott V et al 1989 Spinal stabilization for scoliosis in Duchenne muscular dystrophy. Experience with various sublaminar instrumentation systems. Neuro-Orthop 7:74–82

Neligan G, Prudham D 1969 Norms for four standard developmental milestones by sex, social class and place in family. Develop Med Child Neurol 11:413–422

Read L, Galasko CSB 1986 Delay in diagnosing Duchenne muscular dystrophy in orthopaedic clinics. J Bone Joint Surg 68B:481–482

Riccio V 1990 Personal communication

Rideau Y 1984 Treatment of orthopedic deformity during the ambulatory stage of Duchenne muscular dystrophy. In: Serratrice G, Cros D, Desnuelle C (eds) Neuromuscular disease. Raven Press, New York

Rideau Y 1985 Treatment of Duchenne muscular dystrophy by early physiotherapy. Critical analysis. Arch Fr Pediatr 42:17

Rideau Y 1986 Prophylactic surgery for scoliosis in Duchenne muscular dystrophy. Dev Med Child Neurol 28:398–399

Rideau Y 1990 Personal communication

Rideau Y, Jankowski LW, Grellet J 1981 Respiratory function in muscular dystrophies. Muscle Nerve 4:155–164

Rideau Y, Glorion B, Delaubier A, Tarle O 1984 The treatment of scoliosis in Duchenne muscular dystrophy. Muscle Nerve 7:281–286

Rideau Y, Duport G, Delaubier A 1986 Premières rémissions reproductibles dans l'évolution de la dystrophie musculaire de Duchenne. Bull Acad Natl Méd 170:605–610

Rideau Y, Duport G, Marie-Agnès Y et al 1987 Traitement des dystrophies musculaires. Résultats d'une coopération franco-italienne. Sem Hôp Paris 63:438–443

Scott OM, Hyde SA, Goddard C et al 1981 Prevention of deformity in Duchenne muscular dystrophy: a prospective study of passive stretching and splintage. Physiotherapy 67:177–180

Seeger BR, Sutherland AD'A, Clark MS 1984 Orthotic management of scoliosis in Duchenne muscular dystrophy. Arch Phys Med Rehabil 65:83–86

Siegel IM, Miller JE, Ray RD 1968 Subcutaneous lower limb tenotomy in treatment of pseudohypertrophic muscular dystrophy. J Bone Joint Surg 50A:1437–1443
Smith CL, Bush GH 1985 Anaesthesia and progressive muscular dystrophy. Br J Anaesth 57:1113–1118
Smith AD, Koreska J, Moseley CF 1989 Progression of scoloiosis in Duchenne muscular dystrophy. J Bone Joint Surg 71A: 1066–1074
Spencer GE, Vignos PJ 1962 Bracing for ambulation in childhood progressive muscular dystrophy. J Bone Joint Surg 44A:234–242
Sussman M 1986 Spinal fusion with segmental instrumentation to the lower lumbar spine in patients with neuromuscular disease. J Pediatr Orthop 6:743
Sutherland DH, Olshen R, Cooper L et al 1981 The pathomechanics of gait in Duchenne muscular dystrophy. Dev Med Child Neurol 23:3–22
Vignos PJ, Archibald KC 1960 Maintenance of ambulation in childhood muscular dystrophy. J Chron Dis 10:273–290
Vignos PJ, Watkins MP 1966 The effect of exercise in muscular dystrophy. JAMA 197: 834–848
Vignos PJ, Wagner MB, Kaplan JS et al 1983 Predicting the success of reambulation in patients with Duchenne muscular dystrophy. J Bone Joint Surg 65A:719–728
Williams EA, Read L, Ellis A et al 1984 The management of equinus deformity in Duchenne muscular dystrophy. J Bone Joint Surg 66B:546–550
Woolley H, Stein A, Forrest GC et al 1989 Imparting the diagnosis of life threatening illness in children. Br Med J 298:1623–1626
Yoshioka M, Okuno T, Honda Y et al 1980 Central nervous system involvement in progressive muscular dystrophy. Arch Dis Child 55:589–594

9

The management of major disasters

J. M. Rowles   G. Kirsh

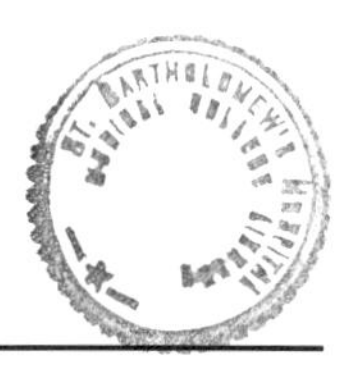

In the last 2 years, the UK has witnessed eight major disasters resulting in many deaths and large numbers of seriously injured people. The role of the emergency services and hospitals has always been perceived as first-class by the media. A major disaster is the classical 'ambush' situation. We can plan, prepare and rehearse with great care and attention to detail; yet out of the blue the situation that presents is almost always a total surprise which does not quite fit the exercise pattern (Costley 1989).

This chapter reviews the management of major disasters, highlighting problems that have occurred. Three events of 1989—the M1 Kegworth aircraft accident, the Clapham rail crash and the Hillsborough football stadium disaster—will be used to illustrate some of the difficulties that can occur. Each of these disasters differs significantly but many of the problems are common.

WHAT IS A MAJOR DISASTER?

A disaster may be said to have occurred when casualties above a fixed number are sustained. Stevens (1973) defines mass disaster as an event in which 10 or more people are killed. Caro (1974) reports that the police have defined a major disaster as one producing more than 50 casualties needing treatment in hospital, either as inpatients or outpatients. The American College of Surgeons states (Ryan 1989) that a major disaster is a sudden event with a variable mixture of:

1. Injury to human beings.
2. Destruction of property.
3. Overwhelming of local response resources.
4. Disruption of organized societal mechanisms.

As demand for travel grows, our road, rail and air networks come under more pressure and the risks of accidents involving large numbers increase (Thornley 1990). With the additional increased risk of terrorist activity, the movement of dangerous substances and mass congregations of people, the chances of a major disaster occurring anywhere should not be understimated.

No matter how carefully an emergency plan has been developed, or its many variables anticipated, the scene of a disaster will be hectic if not at times frantic. Nevertheless, without preplanning and practice, effective response to a major disaster is impossible.

At the site of any major disaster the worst enemy, and the one most difficult to avoid, is *chaos*. An area which only seconds before may have been quiet and orderly is suddenly transformed into a scene of incredible fire, wreckage and carnage. The event is inevitably followed by a moment of shock and disbelief. At the scene, chaos and confusion are controlled perhaps more by regularity than by disaster plan.

Ideally every survivor should fall into a prepared net of management comprising many interwoven strands held together by *command*, *control*, *communications* and perhaps most of all *co-operation* (Grollmes 1989).

MAJOR DISASTERS

Every major disaster is different and each one presents us with new challenges. There seems always something to learn and always something to forget (Thornley 1990). The statistics and common problems of several recent major disasters are highlighted below.

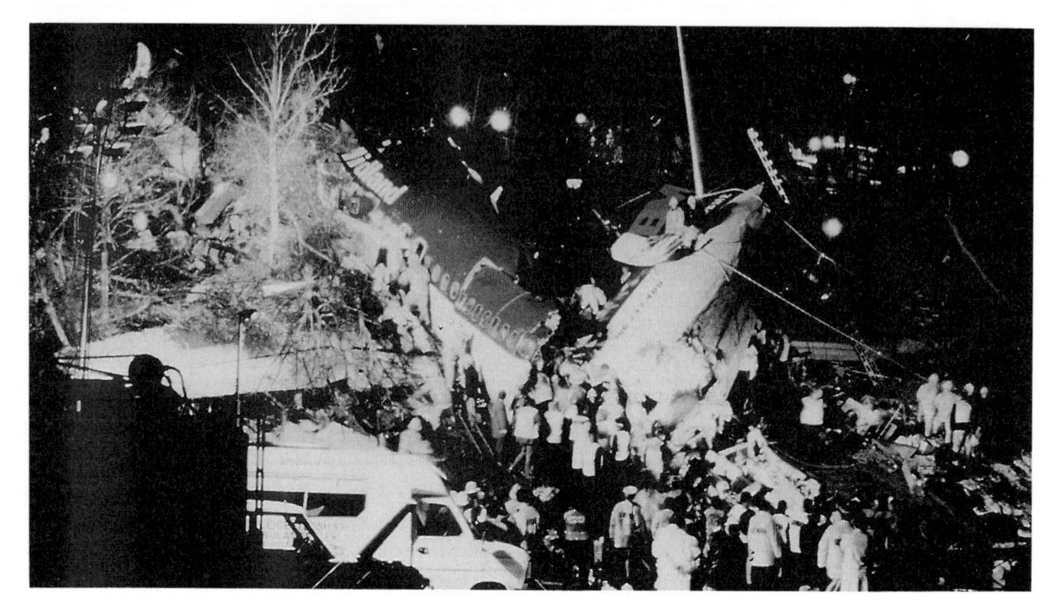

Fig. 9.1 Scene of the disaster after a Boeing 737 crashed next to the M1 Motorway at Kegworth. © EMPICS Ltd.

The Kegworth M1 aircrash

On 8 January 1989, at 8.26 p.m. a Boeing 737-400, en route from Heathrow to Belfast, crash-landed next to the M1 motorway near Kegworth (Fig. 9.1). There were 126 passengers and crew on board, of whom 39 (31%) died at the scene. Of the 87 survivors, 4 patients died on or soon after arrival at one of the three main receiving hospitals (University Hospital Nottingham, Leicester Royal Infirmary and Derbyshire Royal Infirmary). A further 4 patients died in hospital as a result of their injuries or complications. The injuries sustained were diverse (Table 9.1) and the resources of the hospitals were stretched to their limits (Table 9.2). In the first 12 hours, 94 operations were carried out on 34 of the survivors.

Table 9.1 Major injuries in survivors of the M1 aircrash for the 87 patients surviving the crash

Region	No.
Head injury	43
Thoracic injuries	23
Abdominal injuries (operated)	2
Spinal fractures	24
Pelvic/lower limb injuries	142
open fractures	34
Upper limb injuries	59
open fractures	6

Communications

Communication in the early stages was confused and the procedures of the Major Disaster Plan were not followed (Allen 1989, Malone 1990). On site communication between scouts and the site medical officer would have been enhanced by the use of walkie-talkies. More widespread use of cell phones would have enabled communication with base hospitals to be established. Several messages relayed to three hospitals were inaccurate and misleading. There were other communication problems as a consequence of the emergency services originating from three separate shires—there was no common disaster channel.

Site security

The site was not initially secured for the safety of the rescuing personnel, and no control was established to limit the number of rescuers in the area. The site was covered in aviation fuel and at one time there were over 700 rescuers around the crashed aircraft. 'Fake doctors' appeared at the crash site.

Table 9.2 Summary of data from hospitals dealing with the survivors of the M1 aircrash

	University Hospital Nottingham	Leicester Royal Infirmary	Derbyshire Royal Infirmary	Mansfield General Hospital
No. of patients received	39	21	25	2
No. of operations				
On first day	38	23	31	2
On second day	26		18	
No. of patients having operations				
On first day	11	10	11	2
On second day	11		10	
No. of patients admitted to Intensive Care Units	12*	6	4	
No. of radiographs within 12 h	409	210	137	16

*One patient was admitted later with a fat embolism.

Triage and command

At subsequent debriefing meetings a number of difficulties were identified. These were the problems of establishing a triage or assessment point and that the initial patients rescued were treated by the 'scoop and run' technique. Because of failure in communications they were all transported to the same hospital, which unfortunately had not been properly informed.

Medical teams were spread all over the aircraft with no identifiable individual taking overall charge. Other key personnel on site were not easily recognizable and the command points were not properly established. Ambulances near the crash site left their lights flashing, confusing all as to the location of the command point.

Transport

The lack of an initial triage point led to ambulances leaving from several sites and delivering an unequal distribution of patients to the receiving hospitals. The roads to the main hospitals were not adequately secured and became blocked by sightseers. Helicopters were not available early enough and their services were under-utilized, transporting only the last 6 patients to Leicester some 4 hours after the crash.

Reception at hospital

At the hospitals, the cascade call-out system failed and it was only the rapid dissemination of the news by the media that brought staff into each of the three hospitals. (One of the authors actually found out from his mother-in-law in Australia before his bleep alerted him!) Switchboards were overloaded and there were not sufficient separate emergency lines for interhospital and site-to-hospital communication.

Documentation at the scene and in the hospitals also proved deficient. Only 3 triage labels were identified in the notes of survivors and only 6 patient report forms. Important physiological parameters were not recorded (Macey et al 1990). A quarter of the survivors had injuries that were discovered over 24 hours after the accident (Tait et al 1990).

The placement of patients in a disaster ward at each hospital had many advantages. Apart from the psychological advantage of having all of the survivors and their relatives together for support, it aided organization and made security much easier, especially with regard to the press. All three hospitals found that there was a great disruption of the normal function of the institution by the press and visiting dignitaries. The disaster placed a great load on all three Intensive Care Units with the unit in Nottingham only able to resume accepting normal elective admissions after 3 weeks.

The Clapham rail disaster (Stevens & Partridge 1990)

On 12 December 1988, the 6.14 a.m. train from Poole which was travelling at 51 miles per hour crashed into the rear of the 7.18 a.m. Basingstoke to Waterloo train which had stopped while the driver was reporting a faulty set of signals. A few seconds later a third empty train ran into the wreckage. Out of a total of 1450 passengers, 33 (2%) died at the site and 119 (8%) casualties were transported to one hospital, St George's Hospital, London. Forty-one patients (3%) were admitted for treatment. There were 19 chest injuries, 20 head injuries and 12 spinal injuries. Twenty-one operations were performed in the first 24 hours. Seven significant injuries were missed.

Communication was again the major problem both on site and between the site and the hospital. On-site runners were employed to relay messages, but communication with the base hospital was served by a coinbox telephone. Four patients out of the 41 admitted to hospital had triage labels attached. The major incident record form was not universally used; only Accident & Emergency doctors were familiar with it. Baseline recording of physiological parameters was poor.

There was also significant disruption of the hospital's function. It took one week to treat patients' injuries and resume normal working patterns. The aftermath of visiting dignitaries and media again interfered with the day-to-day function of the hospital.

The Hillsborough tragedy (Wardrope et al 1990)

This tragedy occurred on 15 April 1989 at 3 p.m. as fans struggled to enter the Hillsborough Football Stadium to watch the 1989 FA Cup semifinal between Liverpool and Nottingham Forest. A large gate was opened to let fans into the ground as they were being crushed at the turnstiles. Many supporters poured through this gate into the rear of an already overcrowded terrace; wire crowd-control fences prevented escape at the front of the terrace (Fig. 9.2).

A total of 95 people died of traumatic asphyxia—81 at the stadium, 14 were pronounced dead or eventually died in hospital. In all 159 casualties were received by two hospitals within 90 min of the major incident being declared. Of these, 81 patients were admitted—19 to Intensive Care Units. Most patients had suffered traumatic asphyxia with a spectrum of presentations: asystolic cardiac arrest, profound unconsciousness, status epilepticus, cerebral irritation, cortical blindness, headache and minor neurological symptoms. Other injuries included 5 pneumothoraces, 3 brachial plexus injuries, 3 fractures and many soft-tissue injuries.

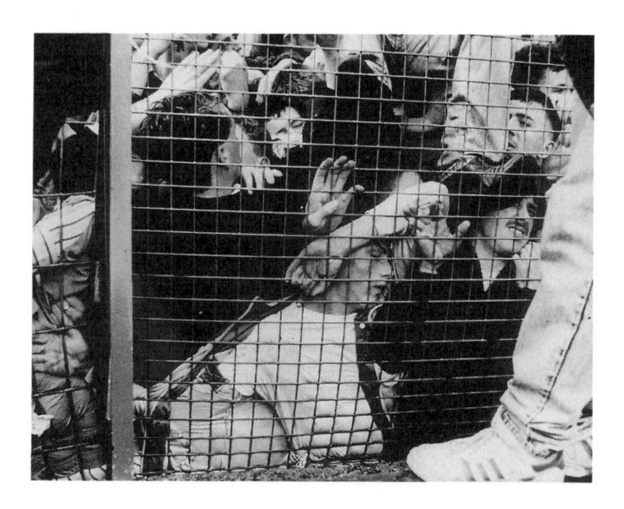

Fig. 9.2 Liverpool football fans are trapped and crushed against safety railings at the front of the terrace. © EMPICS Ltd.

Unlike the previous two disasters, the surgical load of this tragedy was small. Most of the critically ill patients needed intensive care treatment and medical care with virtually no urgent surgical operations needed. One week after the incident most of the patients had been discharged.

Communications were again the major problem—the switchboard was overloaded with calls from off-duty staff and the media. The cascade call-out system was essentially bypassed because of the live coverage of the event. Large numbers of staff arrived at the hospital voluntarily. There were also communication problems at the ground. These were the most obvious cause of the incident in the first place.

DISASTER PLANS

Study of the debriefing sessions of these and other major incidents and similar exercises often reveal the inadequacy of disaster plans and the lack of familiarily of their participants. Familiarity can be achieved by regular exercises, making disaster-training part of the induction of new staff to a hospital and having protocol cards for involved personnel to remind them of their role. These measures will help when a major disaster is suddenly thrust upon us.

A disaster plan should encompass events that occur at the site of the accident, the organization of transport as well as procedures at the receiving hospital (Fig. 9.3). Each hospital should have its own Major Disaster Plan linked to similar plans in the locality. Communication is probably the most important element of the plan and it is in this area that major problems occurred in the three previously mentioned disasters.

On site

The site should be secured both with regard to the safety of the rescuers and also to control the number of people at the scene. The roads to major hospitals should be secured and helicopters should be available and used from the onset. One person takes the role of site commander. This is ideally a senior police or ambulance officer, who works directly with a medical commander. A Command Point is established and marked by a blue flashing light whilst a Triage and Treatment Area is established and marked by a green and/or red flashing light. Teams are allocated particular work areas and should remain there.

The general principles of medical management at the site are aimed at the dictum: 'Do as little as possible, for as many as possible, as quickly as possible' (Nancekievill 1989). The patients' immediate needs are for assessment and basic first aid. This includes securing an airway, control of haemorrhage, urgent fluid replacement, splinting fractures, analgesia and reassurance. However, if good medical facilities are close at hand an initial 'scoop and run' policy may clear the scene and allow resources to be directed at those who are trapped. Cardiopulmonary resuscitation should not be performed in the early stages. Only when casualties are reduced to manageable numbers should the desperately ill become a priority. Patients should be rapidly treated and triaged and the medical commander informed of which patients are ready for transportation and also their priority.

The use of disaster (triage) labels helps to quantify and give priority to the injured at the site. The current system in New South Wales is: *red*—serious injuries requiring resuscitation, priority transport, not to be left unattended; *orange*—serious injuries, non-life-threatening; *green*—minor injuries and/or deceased or moribund, review after all red and orange labels have been treated. Once the patient is

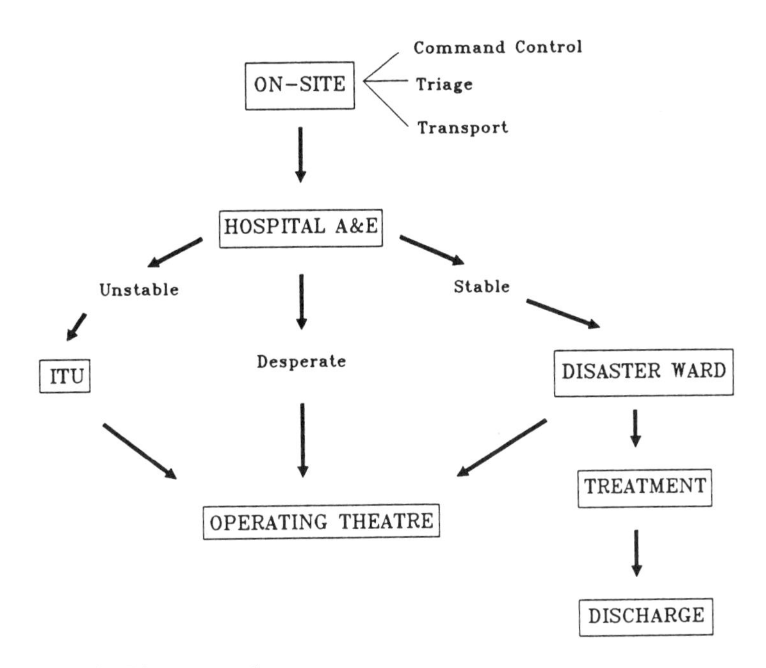

Fig. 9.3 Disaster cascade.

stabilized, the corner of the label is torn off and handed to the Ambulance Transport Officer. It is unfortunate that the design and use of labels is far from standard. In the UK alone 132 varieties of label have been found to be in use.

Communication at the site of the accident is crucial to the smooth running of the event. People at the scene should know the location of each control point (by flashing lights etc.) and be able to identify key personnel. Communication between the site and hospitals is important in order to utilize resources efficiently. A common radio channel should be arranged strictly for this purpose. Lack of this resulted in uneven passenger distribution to available resources following the M1 aircrash. An illustrative incident occurred in 1990 near Sydney, Australia, when a train crash occurred and 200 walking wounded were transported by bus to a local club by the police, without the ambulance services being informed. When finally these patients were reassessed it was found that 15 required hospital admission.

Hospital

The hospital major disaster plan is implemented by the appropriate authorization after a request for help has been received and a Command Centre established. Each hospital department involved should have its own plan with the departmental head or designated deputy taking control. The department heads will have defined roles and these should be detailed on easily accessible protocol cards to ensure that no task is forgotten. Familiarity with these cards and protocols should lead to calm, co-ordinated and efficient management of a major disaster.

The plan will have several levels of activation depending on whether the hospital is merely placed on alert or instructed to receive casualties. A cascade system of call-out should be organized as a part of the switchboard protocol, and specific telephone lines (at switchboard, Accident & Emergency, Intensive Care Unit and bloodbank) should be set aside exclusively for disaster use to enable easy communication for medical teams. One or two switchboard operators are allocated to disaster calls. It is almost universal that the hospital switchboard will be overloaded at this stage and designated lines are crucial. The use of cell phones by the hospital team at the site also enhances communication and prevents the receiving hospitals from being caught unprepared.

The basis of a hospital plan should be to clear the important areas where incoming patients will be treated. These include Accident & Emergency department, Intensive Care Unit, the disaster ward, X-ray department, recovery and an appropriate number of operating theatres where incoming patients will be treated. At least two wards should be designated wards and, at the appropriate level of activation, the disaster plan allows for existing patients either to be discharged from these wards, transferred to an empty bed in another ward, or to beds evacuated by patients well enough to sit in a waiting room elsewhere. The disaster ward, ideally, should be located near to the Accident & Emergency department and the operating theatre/Intensive Care Units for ease of transfer and overview. Stocks of consumables allocated for disaster use should be available on this ward. Existing casualty care is best either transferred to another hospital or managed in another part of the hospital. The media should be kept away from the treatment areas and allocated a media centre in a different section of the hospital. A public relations officer will keep them informed. This is often all that is necessary to ensure they do not become a nuisance.

The functions of the Accident & Emergency department are to perform triage, thoroughly assess and stabilize patients carrying out resuscitative procedures as needed and to perform whatever investigations are immediately necessary. If a patient's condition is extremely unstable, then immediate transfer to either an Intensive Care Unit or operating theatre is undertaken. As soon as a patient's condition is stabilized, investigations have been performed and urgent treatments administered, he or she is transferred to the disaster ward, recovery or Intensive Care Unit.

Once transferred a patient will be comprehensively reassessed by another team and care continued. As the urgency of the early hours settles, priorities are established for operative treatment and necessary equipment sought as required. In the M1 aircrash it became apparent, after the first 2 hours, that the hospitals' usually adequate supply of external fixators would be insufficient and more fixators were obtained by two of the three hospitals. Several incidents such as this one have highlighted the need for the rapid redeployment of resources to be available from the Armed Forces or other national agency. No one hospital can be expected to have this level of supplies on hand. The disaster plan should allow for replenishment of such consumables as splints, intravenous fluids, plaster, bandages and drugs.

PITFALLS OF DISASTER MANAGEMENT

The main areas of disaster management which lead to disaster within a disaster are organization, communications, transport and documentation. Communications have already been discussed but it should be stressed that lines of communication must be in place and organized before a disaster occurs. Organization is only possible if a Major Disaster Plan is in effect, is current and is adhered to. The hospital plan must be part of a more general integrated plan so that resources are correctly utilized. A hospital's disaster plan is most efficient when it is similar to its internal crisis plan, as there will be more familiarity with procedures.

Transport, depending on the circumstances of the terrain and weather, will often constitute a problem. The use of alternative transport, e.g. helicopters, can often aid in the evacuation of the injured, carrying of medical supplies and movement of medical teams.

Documentation of the highest standard is vital in the practice of modern medicine. When medical teams are attempting to deal with a large number of patients, complications often arise simply from poor documentation. We have fully reviewed the documentation of the survivors of the M1 aircrash. Several recommendations have been made in an attempt to simplify it and make trauma audit possible (Macey et al 1990). It is important that the forms used are familiar to the medical and nursing teams and that they are user-friendly. A standard request form for pathology and X-ray must be marked in bold letters **Major Incident Patient** to give priority to these tests.

The triage labels mentioned before are the beginning of a patient's medical documentation and these should be used on every patient in a disaster. These provide accurate information on the number of patients involved and assist in organizing their transport. There should be space on this label or report form to document fluids and drugs administered to patients before they arrive in casualty—similar to those used by many ambulance services (Fig. 9.4). Study of the three previously mentioned disasters indicated that few had triage labels, and fluids and drugs administration was poorly documented. In the M1 aircrash some patients' fluid records were on the back of an envelope.

Identification of patients is not essential in the first hour of a disaster but immediate allocation of a unique identifying number is an essential element in obtaining rapid pathology results and cross-matched blood. At the University Hospital in Nottingham, each patient was allocated a wallet as they were triaged together with a disaster number (Table 9.3). The patient was tagged with that number and this allowed for rapid processing of 30 patients in a 30-min period without any identification problems. The wallet also contained all the pathology request forms already identified with this number and many spare sticky labels for the identification of specimens. Medical forms used for the documentation of injuries and other observations should be the hospital's standard trauma documentation forms. All of these prepared forms enable staff to concentrate on management of the injured patients whilst still thoroughly documenting each case.

The medical forms should contain several standard parameters to be recorded. The bare minimum should be pulse, blood pressure, respiratory rate and the Glasgow Coma Scale. Review of the aircrash data revealed that the following percentage of notes contained these parameters:

Pulse	81%
Systolic blood pressure	82%
Respiratory rate	12%
Glasgow Coma Scale	44%

This is surprising when one considers that routine forms were used, yet the boxes for pulse etc. were left blank in too many cases. Similar observations were made of the records related to the Clapham rail disaster. The deployment of clerks to resuscitation teams may improve upon this deficiency.

NEW SOUTH WALES AMBULANCE SERVICE

DEPARTMENT OF HEALTH, N.S.W.
AMBULANCE SERVICE
GRADE 1 2 3 4 5
REGION

AMBULANCE REPORT

DATE | JULIAN | CASE No | PATIENT OF | SEX | AGE

CALL TYPE | AUTHORITY | STN. No | RADIO No | RESPONSE | CATEGORY

TIME BOOKED | TIME OUT | LOCATION | DEPART | DESTINATION | CLEAR

PATIENT DETAILS

CODE | TITLE | SURNAME | FIRST NAME | D O B

ADDRESS | CODE

STRETCHER S
WALKING W
W. CHAIR C

☐ W. COMP ☐ 3rd PARTY DEBTOR DETAILS

CHG. CODE | AMOUNT | CHG. KM | CODE | TITLE | SURNAME/BUSINESS | INITIALS

PENSION No / WARRANT No. | ADDRESS | CODE

OCCUPATION | EMPLOYED BY

ODO IN
ODO OUT
TRIP KM

FROM | CODE
TO | CODE

HISTORY (State chief complaint first)

EXAMINATION

AIRWAY ☐ Clear ☐ Obstructed

BREATHING ☐ Present ☐ Absent
☐ Shallow ☐ Deep

CIRCULATION ☐ Present ☐ Absent

Buccal Mucosa ☐ Pink ☐ Blue ☐ Pale

Skin temp. ☐ Normal ☐ Cold ☐ Hot

Sweating ☐ Nil ☐ Mod. ☐ Profuse

Vomiting ☐ Nil ☐ Small ☐ Large

Fitting ☐ Nil ☐ Yes Number

Burns ☐ Nil ☐ Superficial %
☐ Deep %

Blood Loss (External) ☐ Nil ☐ Under 500ml ☐ Over 500ml

Site ....

INJURIES

F Fracture
L Laceration
A Abrasion
S Swelling
H Haemorrhage
T Tenderness
C Contusion
D Dislocation
B Burn
P Pain

Specific observations ☐ Nil

Breath Sounds

× Position of Patient
→ Point of Impact
▨ Damaged Area

FRONT

Seat Belt Not / Worn

Estimated Impact Speed High Medium Low

ROAD USER: 1 Driver 2 Passenger 3 Motorcyclist & Pillions 4 Pedal Cyclist 5 Pedestrian 6 Others

Time	Pulse	Blood Pressure	Capillary Filling	Respiration Rate	Respiration Effort	L Level of Cons	Total Score	Pupils Size T	Pupils Size R	Pupils Size L	Pupils React. R	Pupils React. L	GLASGOW COMA SCALE Eye Opening	Motor Response	Verbal Response	S Score

Vital Signs Points

	Add Vital Sign Points
First	+ + + + =
Final	+ + + + =
	Difference Between Total Score ±

Eye Opening	Best Motor Response	Verbal Response
4 Spontaneous	6 Obeys	5 Orientated
3 To Speech	5 Localises	4 Confused Conversation
2 To Pain	4 Withdraws	3 Inappropriate Words
1 NIL	3 Abnormal Flexion	2 Incomprehensible Sounds
	2 Extends	1 NIL
	1 NIL	

TABLE | 14⇒15 = 5 | 11⇒13 = 4 | 8⇒10 = 3 | 5⇒7 = 2 | 3⇒4 = 1

Fig. 9.4 Ambulance report.

TREATMENT BEFORE ARRIVAL
0 Nil 1 CPR within 3 mins
2 First Aid 3 Medical

Patient's state prior to arrival
A Conscious C Unknown
B Unconscious Mins. ....

PREVIOUS ILLNESS
☐ Nil ☐ Renal
☐ Unknown ☐ Stroke
☐ Hypertension ☐ Epilepsy
☐ Cardiac ☐ Psychiatric
☐ Respiratory ☐ G.I.T.
☐ Diabetes
☐ Other ....

Allergies ☐ Nil ☐ Unknown

Present Medication ☐ Nil ☐ Unknown

Comments ....

TREATMENT

AIRWAY 1 Suction; 1 Oral Airway; 2 Nasal Airway; ☐ ETT

BREATHING 1 RM; 2 RS; 3 .... (other); 1 IPPV

CIRCULATION 1 Cardiac Compression

POSTURE 1 Lateral; 2 Supine; 3 Sitting; 4 Legs Elevated

O_2 THERAPY 1 High Conc. Mask; 2 Nasal Prongs; 3 28% Ventimask; 1 14L 2 8L 3 4L; 1 Demand Valve

HAEMORRHAGE CONTROL ☐ Dressing; ☐ Elevation; ☐ Pressure

IV CANNULATION 1 Type ....; 2 Unsuccessful; 3 In Situ
Local given ☐ No ☐ Yes

INTUBATION 1 Type ....; 2 Unsuccessful; 3 In Situ

ANALGESIA
E Entonox; N Narcotic
1 Not Effective; 2 Part Effective; 3 Effective

SPLINTS
1 Hare; 2 Thomas; 3 Air; 4 Cervical Collar; 5 KED; 6 Other; 7 Donway

MAST Suit - Inflated
1 Under 500ml 2 Over 500ml (External blood loss)

TOURNIQUETS
1 Rotating; 2 Arterial; 3 Lymphatic
Time On ....

STRETCHER
1 Carry Chair; 2 Back Board; 3 Jordon Frame; 4 Carry Sheet; 5 Other

KITS
1 Poison; 2 Burns; 3 Maternity; 4 Other

BLOOD SAMPLE TAKEN
Glucose Est. ....
Blood Type & Cross Match ....

TYPENEX No.

RHYTHMS MONITORED
(Abbreviations in heavy print)
1 Sinus **Rhythm**
2 Sinus **Brady**cardia
3 Sinus **Tachy**cardia
4 **Prem. Atrial Cont.**
5 **SupraVent. Tachy**
6 **Atrial Fib/Flut.**
7 **IdioVent. Rhythm**
8 **Asystole**
9 **Pacemaker Rhythm**
☐
10 **Prem. Vent. Cont.** Frequency .... Runs ☐ R on T ☐ Multifocal ☐
11 **Vent. Tachy**cardia
12 **Vent. Fib**rillation
13 **1° Heart Block**
14 **2° Heart Block**
15 **3° Heart Block**
16 **Junctional**
17 **Multiple Arrhythmia**
18 **Elect. Mech. Dissn.**
☐

TIME	ECG	TREATMENT	DOSE	ROUTE	SHOCK	RESULT	AUTH.

COMMENTS, MEDICAL ASSISTANCE, PROBLEMS, INSTRUCTIONS, ETC.

Dr's Signature ....

Condition at Destination ☐ Improved ☐ Unchanged ☐ Deteriorated

Officer 1 Driving — PRINT NAMES — Officer 2

SIGNATURES & EMPLOYEE No's

ATTACH ECG STRIPS HERE

TRANSTAT

BYSTANDER
Effect
ROAD USER
Severity
TREATMENT before arrival
Conscious/Unconsc
SUCTION
AIRWAY
BREATHING
IPPV
CIRCULATION
POSTURE
O_2 THERAPY
Litre
DEMAND VALVE
CANNULATION
INTUBATION
ANALGESIA
Effects
SPLINTS
SPLINTS
MAST SUIT
TOURNIQUETS
STRETCHER
KITS
ECG
ECG
ECG
D.C. SHOCK
FLUID/DRUG
Units
FLUID/DRUG
Units
FLUID/DRUG
Units
FLUID/DRUG
Units
FLUID/DRUG
Units
PROTOCOL
PROTOCOL
PROTOCOL
PROTOCOL
RESCUE
COMPLICATIONS
HAZARDS
TENS PNEUM RELIEF
COMMENTS
MEDICAL REVIEW

Table 9.3 Multiple-casualty disaster pack

Each pack will contain the following documents all labelled with the appropriate identification sticker:
1. Identification sheet in triplicate:
   one copy to stay with notes
   one copy to go to disaster control
   one copy to go to admissions
2. Hospital identification bands—2 red, 2 white
3. Trauma admission form and extra continuation sheets
4. Observation flow chart
5. X-ray request form
6. Blood transfusion request form
7. Pathology request form
8. Microbiology request form
9. Drug administration chart
10. Intravenous fluid chart
11. Preoperative preparation forms/nursing check sheets
12. Operation report form
13. Sticky labels

The forms must also allow for sequential observations to be made, such as the standard Glasgow Coma Scale chart. This permits rapid graphical observation of changes in a patient's status. Experience has shown that the use of self-carbonized forms only generates problems as the written details frequently fail to penetrate and overwriting occurs more often than not. A standardized national medical report form should be considered.

The main relevance of documentation is that it allows the generation of Injury Severity Scores (ISS; Baker et al 1974) and TRISS (Trauma Score vs Injury Severity Score) scores (Spence et al 1988) which are the best way of auditing management. The ISS can be calculated from a final record of the patient's injuries as it is an anatomically based score. The TRISS score, however, is preferable as it additionally takes account of physiological observations, giving a more accurate reflection of the patient's condition at the time of admission and enabling a reliable prediction of outcome. TRISS scores, when plotted on a graph, will demonstrate patients who should have survived but did not and vice versa. This provides an accurate reflection of the quality of trauma care.

CONCLUSIONS AND RECOMMENDATIONS

Despite planning, it is folly to imagine that anyone can ever be fully prepared for a major disaster. No amount of training can predict the human response and the emotions that play such a large part in the outcome on the day. Grollmes (1989) lists several reasons for this failure of a disaster response:

1. The most common cause is that those responsible did not follow the plans made. This occurred in the M1 aircrash with the incorrect initiation of the disaster plan. This could be avoided by the use of protocol cards.
2. Another common cause is that those responsible were familiar with their role in the plan but did not or could not establish command control or adequate channels of communication.
3. Adequate routes for emergency vehicles to and from the scene were not opened or secured.
4. Those responding could not overcome a lack of planning, training and practice.
5. The facilities and the means for caring for survivors were both insufficient and inadequate.

Review of several recent disasters and current literature, together with our experiences with the Kegworth M1 aircrash, allows us to make the following general recommendations on the organization and management of major disasters:

1. A major disaster plan must be formulated and practised to allow for the best possible outcome. The plan will integrate all services involved and be the basis of correct protocol and lines of communication. Regular practice and review of the plan are major components of successful disaster medicine.

2. At the site of a disaster, organization and communication are imperative. Command and triage points should be established and well displayed. The site is best secured, to the benefit of the rescue team and for their safety. Personnel on site should be clothed in easily recognizable uniforms to allow for rapid identification and protection.

The main principle of on-site disaster medicine is to do the best for the most. Dispatch of stabilized patients from the site ought to be organized by a transport officer (preferably from ambulance or police ranks), to allow for even distribution to hospitals and optimization of transport resources. Communication with the receiving hospitals and between ambulance and police services on a regular basis is essential. Dedicated telephone lines and radio channels facilititate this process.

3. Documentation begins on site with triage labels and patient report forms. It is only with fully completed forms that proper patient care can occur (and useful review of patient management can be performed). In the hospital, documentation is easiest, with forms in regular use aided by disaster packs.

4. Within the hospital a disaster plan must be familiar and cover all contingencies. Wards will be evacuated to receive incoming patients, and all personnel will have particular roles known to them and familiarized by protocol cards. The plan will allow for appropriate recruitment of staff to cope with the incoming patient load.

5. Hospitals should be aware of and prepared for the enormous load that an intake of severely injured patients places on its services. Its normal function will be disrupted by the media and visiting dignitaries, and the post-disaster clinical followthrough in the subacute phase of management.

REFERENCES

Allen MJ 1989 Coping with the early stages of the M1 disaster at the scene and on arrival at hospital. Br Med J 398:651–654

Baker SP, O'Neill B, Hadden W et al 1974 The injury severity score: a method for describing patients with multiple injuries and evaluating emergency care. J Trauma 14:187–195

Caro D 1974 Major disasters. Lancet ii:1309–1310

Costley JA 1989 The report of the Trent Regional Health Authority: aircraft accident BD092, M1 motorway/East Midlands Airport, Sunday 8th January 1989. Ref. Emergency planning JAC/C17/24. Trent Regional Health Authority, Sheffield

Grollmes EE 1989 Aviation emergency management response: the getting ready. In: Planning and management. Network Exhibitions & Conferences Ltd, Buckingham

Hillsborough Stadium Disaster 15 April 1989. Inquiry by the Rt Hon Lord Justice Taylor 1990. Interim report. Her Majesty's Stationery Office, London

Kirsh G, Learmonth DJA, Martindale JP The Nottingham, Leicester, Derby aircraft accident study: preliminary report 3 weeks after the accident. Br Med J 298: 503–505

Macey AC, Tait GR, Rowles JM et al 1990 Disaster documentation—lessons from the M1 aircrash. JBJS 72(B): 1089

Malone WD 1990 Lessons to be learned from the major disaster following the civil airliner crash at Kegworth in January 1989. Injury 21: 49–52

Martin TE 1990 The Ramstein airshow disaster J Br Assoc Immed Care 13:2–8

Nancekievill DG 1989 Disaster management: practice makes perfect. Br Med J 298:477

Ryan BP 1989 Medical disaster response and training. In: Medical and casualty handling

Spence MT, Redmond AD, Edwards JD 1988 Trauma audit—the use of TRISS. Health Trends 21:94–97

Stevens KLH, Partridge R 1990 The Clapham rail disaster. Injury 21:37–40

Stevens PJ 1973 Investigation of mass disaster. In: Mant AK (ed) Modern trends in forensic medicine. Chapter 8

Tait GR, Rowles JM, Kirsh G et al 1990 Delayed diagnosis of injuries from the M1 aircraft accident. Presented at the British Orthopaedic Association Spring Meeting 1990 Glasgow

Thornley F 1990 Major disasters: an ambulance service view. Injury 21:34–36

Wadrope J, Hockey MS, Crosby AC 1990 The hospital response to the Hillsborough tragedy. Injury 21:53–54

FURTHER READING

Boyd CR, Tolson MA, Copes WS 1987 Evaluating trauma care: the TRISS method. J Trauma 27:370–378

Rutherford WH 1975 Disaster procedures. Br Med J i:443–445

Rutherford WH 1990 The place of exercises in disaster management. Injury 21:58–60

Savage PEA 1971 Disaster planning: a review. Injury 3:49–55

Trunkey D 1985 Towards optimal trauma care. Arch Emerg Med 2:181–195

Williams DJ 1979 Disaster planning in hospitals. Br J Hosp Med 308–322

10

Arthroscopy and the management of shoulder problems

S. A. Copeland

The explosion of interest in arthroscopy over the last two decades has inevitably led to a great interest in arthroscopy of the shoulder. As both skill and technology improved with arthroscopy of the knee it was automatically assumed that this could be transferred to the shoulder. This is partly true but there are some essential differences. At the present time arthroscopy of the shoulder is mainly a diagnostic aid. Arthroscopic surgery of the shoulder, although becoming more widely practised, is not as generally applicable or useful in the shoulder as it is in the knee.

The range of normal anatomy within the shoulder is far greater than that of the knee and can only be learnt by experience. Because of lack of appreciation of this enormous variability of normal anatomy a lot of unnecessary arthroscopic surgery within the shoulder has already been performed, i.e. debridement, snipping out small labral tears. Equivalent procedures in the knee can be extremely useful but are unfortunately less often beneficial in the shoulder (Kohn 1987). This chapter will be divided into essentially three parts which can be likened to the progression of the training of the surgeon: firstly, how to do it, then when to do it and finally when not to do it.

PRACTICAL TECHNIQUE OF SHOULDER ARTHROSCOPY

It is assumed that the reader has already mastered the techniques of knee arthroscopy and has the skills of triangulation and manipulating arthroscopic instruments within the knee whilst looking at a television image.

Rockwood (1988) sounded a note of caution, concerning learning the techniques of shoulder arthroscopy, that our patients should not be used as guinea pigs. There are other adequate means of learning these skills. Hands-on workshops are available and excellent arthroscopic models can be obtained for early practice. It is essential to have spent some time with a shoulder arthroscopist to learn the techniques and indications.

Valuable experience may be obtained if every shoulder is arthroscoped prior to an open stabilization procedure. This is genuinely valuable both for the patient and for the surgeon. Initially this adds significantly to the time of the stabilization procedure, partly due to the positioning of the patient and partly due to unfamiliarity of the procedure on the part of theatre staff. However, with experience no more than 10–15 min is added to the overall operating time.

For diagnostic arthroscopy ordinary standard knee arthroscopy equipment can be used. A standard 30° 4 mm knee arthroscope is the most useful scope in general use. Small-diameter scopes, although available, have not been found to be either necessary or useful. The shoulder is a very large-volume joint and lighting the joint through a small scope can be difficult. A television system with compact camera, although an advantage in knee arthroscopy, is almost essential in arthroscopy of the shoulder as the usual lateral positioning of the patient requires one almost to clamber over the top of the patient if a camera is not used.

Positioning the patient

The most common position is with the patient in mid lateral position, affected side uppermost with both a pelvic support and a back rest, under general anaesthesia. Scalene local anaesthetic block for arthroscopic surgery and the beach-chair position have been described (Skyhar et al 1988). The advantage of the beach-chair position is that if one needs to proceed to surgery then no further change of position need be made. However, complete retowelling is necessary if an open procedure is contemplated. Repositioning the patient takes very little extra time.

Traction is applied to the affected arm using a paediatric skin traction set (Fig. 10.1). The sponge rubber type is preferable to those using skin adhesives. For the average patient a 4-kg weight is applied via a pulley system attached to the table. The author uses the top half of a drip stand attached to the table at about the level of the knee. This brings the shoulder into approximately 30° of abduction and 15° of forward flexion.

This position is a compromise between that giving the best view for shoulder arthroscopy and that for subacromial bursoscopy (Matthews et al 1984, Klein et al 1987). The skin is then prepared and the shoulder draped in the usual manner.

Entry to the joint

When first learning the technique, entry into the joint may be facilitated by distension of the joint with fluid. The arm is temporarily taken off traction and laid on the drapes at the patient's side. The posterior portal of entry is the most commonly used. The skin marking is approximately 1 cm distal to the angle of the acromium but a small soft spot is palpable a thumbs-breath distal to the angle of the acromium, with the middle finger on the coracoid and the thumb over the angle of the acromium. An intravenous cannula is inserted from the point of entry aiming towards the middle finger on the coracoid. As the shoulder capsule is entered a slight 'give' is felt. Saline is then injected into the joint. The average capacity is approximately 45 ml of fluid.

As the fluid is injected intra-articular positioning is confirmed when the elbow is seen to rise from the drapes as the shoulder joint assumes the position of maximum capacity. This is a definite sign indicating intra-articular placement (Copeland & Barrett

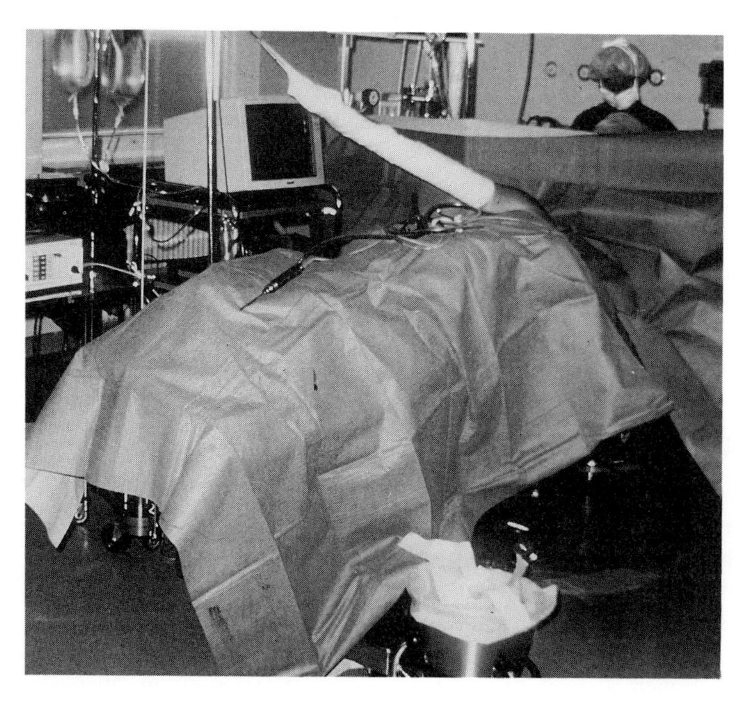

Fig. 10.1 Patient lying in right lateral decubitus position with 4 kg of skin traction applied.

1989). The arm is seen to move early on in the injection phase. If it does not do so, further attempts at placement of the needle should be made. Great stress is placed on this because, by contrast with the knee, if a significant amount of fluid is placed extra-articularly this can make the arthroscopy itself extremely difficult.

When the shoulder has been distended there should be adequate and easy flow back into the syringe. The distension cannula is then removed and the arthroscopic cannula with blunt trocar is inserted into the joint cavity in a similar manner. Intra-articular placement is confirmed by saline flow-back. The telescope is then inserted and camera and saline in-flow attached (Fig. 10.2).

With experience it is perfectly possible to put the arm directly on to traction and introduce the trocar without previous distension of the joint. Bleeding can be a problem and adequate out-flow of saline should be established.

A needle is placed by the anterior portal. The surface marking is half-way between the coracoid process and the edge of the acromion pointing directly towards the arthroscope. For diagnostic arthroscopy alone a wide-bore needle connected to drainage tubing should be adequate.

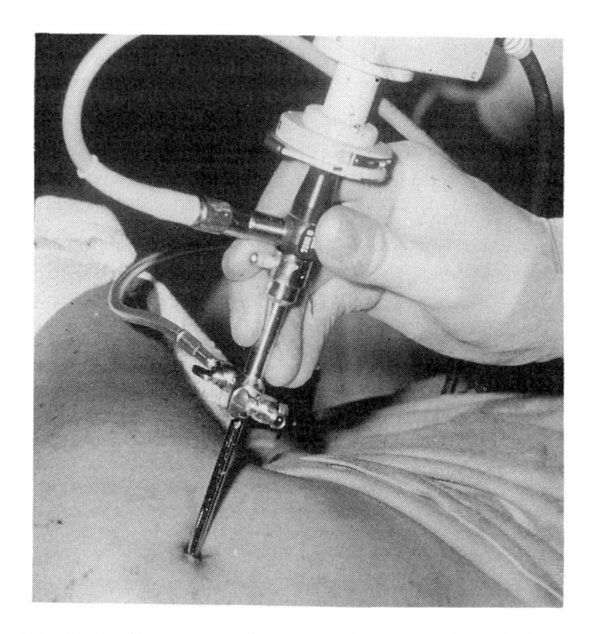

Fig. 10.2 The general utility posterior portal 1.5 cm below and lateral to the angle of the acromion.

For arthroscopic surgery a wide-bore exit cannula is used in this site. Extra information can be gained by passing a hook probe just medially to this anterior portal site. If necessary a secondary additional superior portal may be used for irrigation if the anterior portal is being used for accessory equipment. The superior portal was described by Neviaser (Caspari et al 1984), and is sited medially to the acromion in the suprascapular fossa. The needle can be seen to enter the superior part of the joint. Concern has been expressed about the risk of damage to the rotator cuff with this portal. However the needle passes through the muscular portion of supraspinatus and not the tendon. A third portal is rarely needed but can be useful.

Normal arthroscopic anatomy

Each surgeon must develop his or her own arthroscopic route around the joint so that every aspect is covered. The most obvious intra-articular structure is the long head of biceps. Find this, track it medially to the superior pole of the glenoid labrum and follow the posterior labrum around to the inferior part of the joint, inspecting the articular cartilage of the glenoid on the way. The anterior labrum is then inspected with particular reference to rounding off or anterior detachment of capsule or labrum. The tendon of subscapularis suprisingly can be confused with the long head of biceps. The arthroscopist realizes that the tendon of subscapularis is an intra-articular structure. The superior glenohumeral ligament lies above it and the middle glenoid ligament below it. There is a synovial recess between the two which is a constant feature (Detrisac & Johnson 1988). This recess is a common site for finding loose Lodies in the shoulder joint. The middle glenohumeral ligament can bO Oxtremely variable in size and thickness. Its position however is constant. The inferior glenohumeral ligament is the strongest and most important of the glenohumeral ligaments. Sometimes this can be seen to be a prolongation of the anterior labrum

The arthroscope is then passed superiorly to assess the under-surface of the rotator Muff. If a large tear is present its edge can initially be confused with the long head of biceps if it is rounded off and fibrotic. The scope is then passed back down into the infraglenoid recess, the posterior glenoid labrum is inspected and the synovial reflections off the head are seen. The surface of the humeral head is then observed and the bare area of the humeral neck noted. This is a normal finding and not the Hill–Sachs lesion. A Hill–Sachs lesion is seen to be a deficiency in the articular cartilage of the humeral head and there is usually an area of normal articular cartilage between the defect and the bare area of the head. On completion of the diagnostic arthroscopy the joint is flushed through and 20 ml of 0.25% Marcain instilled into the joint through the cannula.

Subacromial bursoscopy

Examination of the shoulder joint is not complete without examination of the bursa which should be inspected as part of the diagnostic routine. With the cannula still in the shoulder joint the in-flow is turned off, the blunt trocar is inserted and the whole cannula withdrawn into the subcutaneous fat. It is then directed superiorly towards the under-surface of the acromion and with the finger over the anterior aspect of the acromion the tip of the blunt trocar is palpated. Adhesions with the bursa are broken down by moving the trocar from side to side and not under direct vision. The bursa is entered by feel. As the trocar is moved from side to side the coracoacromial ligKment can be fOlt to flip over it.

The fluid is then switched on. Extra pressure in the in-flow solution may be nOcessary to decrease bleeding. It is at this site that an in-flow pump is pKrticularly useful; the pressure is maintained just above arteriKl pressure. LKck of bony landmarks can make orientation within this space difficult. Insertion of K fine needle into this space anterior to the coracoacromial ligament can be a usOful marker. The inferior surface of the acromion is inspected as well as the insertion of the coracoacromial ligament. The tip of the scope can be used to palpate any spurs on the anterior edge of the acromion. The lateral edge of the acromion can be seen together with the origin of the muscle fibres of deltoid.

The superior aspect of the rotator cuff is inspected and any inflammatory change or tears noted. When the examination is complete the bursa is flushed out and the skin puncture left unsutured to prevent the formation of any localized haematoma (Copeland & Williamson 1988).

Arthroscopic surgery

Arthroscopic surgery of the shoulder requires a different level of equipment. The control of bleeding within the joint is of paramount importance. This can be achieved in one of two ways:

1. *The use of intra-articular coagulation diathermy.* In this event plain water or glycine must be used to distend the joint instead of saline. In general glycine is not recommended for use in other than an enclosed space. The subacromial bursa cannot be considered closed space, particularly if a rotator cuff tear is present.

2. *In-flow/out-flow pressure control.* Hypotensive general anaesthesia can be very useful to lower systolic blood pressure. Intra-articular pressure must be higher than the systolic blood pressure. This can be achieved by very high elevation of the saline bags to approximately 150 mmHg by placing the bags of saline at least 1.5 m above the level of the patient's heart. Alternatively, a constant-flow/pressure pump can be used on the in-flow side and this is by far the more convenient method if the equipment is available. An adequate-bore outflow cannula must be established through the anterior portal. If more complex procedures are envisaged, then motorized burrs and resectors must be available. These must be of adequate strength and cutting power. The disposable items for this equipment can indeed be very expensive and must be adequately tested by the arthroscopist before purchase to ensure that they are not a very expensive white elephant as regards cutting capacity and power.

Arthroscopic biopsy

The indications for a synovial biopsy are similar to those in the knee. A pair of pituitary rongeurs or biopsy forceps are passed through the anterior portal and the specific area of synovial pathology biopsy selected under direct vision.

When the area to be biopsied is in the infraglenoid recess or in the posterior part of the joint, an accessory portal 2 cm below the original posterior portal can be used. Care must be taken to avoid damage to the axillary nerve with this portal.

Loose bodies

Loose bodies tend to gravitate towards the infra-glenoid recess or fall directly into the subscapular recess. These are rare but an ideal indication for arthroscopic intervention as this minimal surgery can completely resolve the patient's symptoms. Because the throughput of fluid is much greater in the shoulder the loose bodies can be difficult to grasp and are pushed around by the in-flow of fluid from the scope itself. The use of a separate needle to transfix a loose body prior to attempted removal can overcome this problem. A loose body lying in a subscapular recess can be difficult to get hold of and may be manipulated by pressure from outside the shoulder. Sometimes a 70° arthroscope is required to see into the recess itself.

Tears of the glenoid labrum

Two types of traction tear occur:

1. An entirely superior tear to the attachment of long head of biceps.
2. An antero-inferior labral tear caused by traction on the inferior glenohumeral ligament. This is one of the lesions that Bankart (1938) originally described and should not be excised (Andrews et al 1985). Andrews et al described 269 labral tears in 396 shoulders; 95% of which were painful shoulders in throwing athletes. The biceps was stimulated electrically during arthroscopy and was seen to pull the labrum and extend the tear. The anatomical variations of the glenoid labrum are enormous (Detrisac & Johnson 1988). The superior labrum may become quite degenerate. If a tag tear is seen in this portion and associated with instability it is reasonable to remove it.

In general removal of tag tears alone is not uniformally successful and the underlying reason for the degenerative change or avulsion must be sought for a successful clinical outcome.

Synovectomy

Synovectomy of the shoulder in rheumatoid arthritis has never been widely practised and there are no large series with long-term follow-ups of open synovectomy. The published data available appear to support early synovectomy before any bony erosion has taken place (Pahle 1981). It therefore appears that arthroscopic synovectomy may offer a reasonable alternative as it is relatively minimally invasive.

The technical problems associated with an adequate and reasonably complete synovectomy are large. Bleeding can be a problem and judging the adequacy of synovectomy at the time of operation is difficult (Ogilvy-Harris & Boynton 1990). Surprisingly however, arthroscopic synovectomy may be specifically indicated early in haemophilia, and may well alter the disease process and be associated with less morbidity (Casscells 1987).

Division of the coracoacromial ligament

This procedure has been abandoned as an open procedure and, not surprisingly, similar results have been obtained from arthroscopic division alone. This is now never performed in isolation but as part of a subacromial decompression operation. Ogilvy-Harris (1987) reported on 51 patients who had had division of the coracoacromial ligament alone: 25 had mechanical division and 26 electrocautery. Only 11 of the 51 patients had a satisfactory outcome and it was concluded that this procedure should be abandoned.

Arthroscopic subacromal decompression

Technique

An arthroscopic pump is desirable to maintain pressure and decrease bleeding although it is possible to elevate the saline bags. A powered shaving system is essential with both burrs and resectors available (Ellman 1988, Ellman & Kay 1989).

Ellman describes the use of electrosurgical apparatus both for haemostasis and for resection of the fibrous tissue at the insertion of the coracoacromial ligament. The patient is placed in the usual lateral decubitus position and 4 kg of traction applied, in the same way as previously described. A standard diagnostic arthroscopy is done via a posterior portal to assess the under-surface of the rotator cuff.

The arthroscope is inserted in the subacromial bursa as already described. When it is certain by feel that the cannula is in the subacromial bursa, the telescope is inserted and pressure in-flow is established through the side arm of the arthroscope cannula. The camera is attached and bursoscopy done. The findings can initially be confusing because only in the normal bursa can an excellent view be achieved. This is because there is no inflammatory change, no adhesions and no bursal wall thickening. In the pathological bursa an adequate view may be impossible to achieve initially. With the sweeping action of the trocar prior to insertion of the telescope the many adhesions may be broken down. Unless the in-flow pressure is kept above arterial pressure right from the beginning, bleeding may be a problem. It is sometimes necessary to insert the power debrider and do an extensive debridement before an adequate view can be achieved.

A small puncture wound is made 4 cm from the mid-point of the tip of the lateral acromion in the upper arm. The blunt trocar is passed through this puncture wound at right angles to the upper humerus until bone is felt. Then it is aimed superiorly towards the mid-point of the acromion. This two-stage directioning of the blunt trocar makes for easier insertion but also creates a flap valve which minimizes extravasation of fluid.

The suction on the debrider acts as the out-flow to maintain a high fluid throughput. At this stage vision still may not be good through the telescope and some blind debridement done by feel is nearly always essential at this stage (Fig. 10.3).

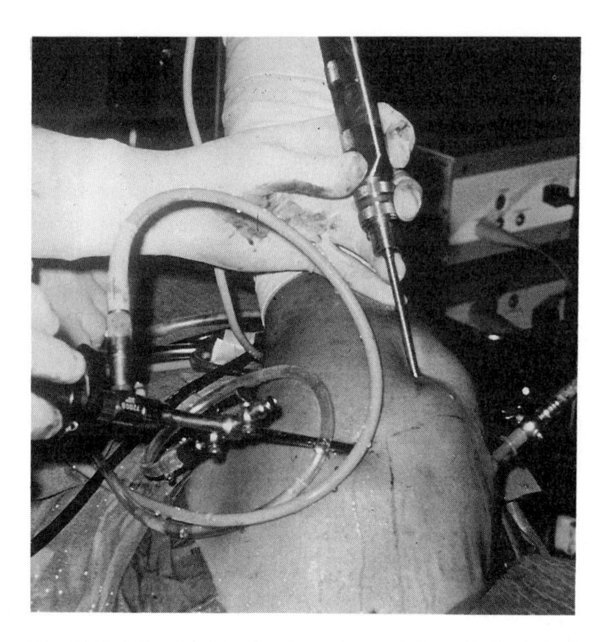

Fig. 10.3 The debrider has been inserted through the lateral portal.

Once an adequate initial debridement has been performed vision gradually improves and the under-surface of the acromion can be adequately inspected. Particular attention is paid to the anterior acromion. Both by direct vision and by feel any hooking or spurs on the anterior edge of the acromion are assessed. The attachment of the coracoacromial ligament to the anterior aspect of the acromion is inspected in detail. Sometimes the spur formation prevents visualization of the actual insertion until the spur is removed. A motorized debrider is used until solid bone is reached.

There is some very thick fibrous rubbery tissue on the under-surface of the acromion which can be quite difficult to divide either with a debrider or an abrader. If the electocautery machine is available it is used to cut it up into strips to allow the debrider to bite more effectively. Once firm bone is observed the debrider is changed for the abrader and a large olive-tipped burr inserted. Any spurring is first abraded down and then along the whole anterior edge of the acromion. It is useful at this stage to cut completely through the centre of the attachment of the coracoacromial ligament as the abrader works more easily on the corticocancellous edge than the cortical bone itself. The initial division may be difficult but definitely facilitates the process, allowing a radical or minimal resection as necessary.

The coracoacromial ligament becomes separated from its attachment by this procedure and can be further resected using the debrider. The first 1 cm is relatively avascular, and resection beyond this point may produce quite torrential haemorrhage in arthroscopic terms. Ellman uses two 18-gauge spinal needles to outline the anterior border of the acromion. The medial needle is placed just in front of the acromioclavicular joint and the lateral needle in front of the anterolateral angle of the acromion. This can be quite a useful maneouvre when first learning the procedure to help with orientation within the bursa. Again it must be emphasized that if electrosurgical apparatus is to be used saline must be flushed out of the bursa and replaced by distilled water.

Finally, the inferior surface of the acromioclavicular joint should be inspected and any osteophytes removed in a similar manner.

This can be a difficult procedure to learn but there are several essential elements. Firstly, high-pressure irrigation is essential either by a high head of pressure on a high drip stand or with a pressure pump. Secondly, if there is difficulty with traction on the arm and the position of the arm during traction, then further adduction should be tried. The subacromial space is decreased by abduction of the arm and increased by adduction.

Postoperative management

Depending on the length of the procedure, generalized swelling of the whole shoulder can be very alarming. Fortunately this tends to reduce within a matter of hours. Intramuscular pressure returns to baseline within 4 min of the end of the procedure (Olgilvy Harris & Boynton 1990). The arm is held in a position of comfort postoperatively and pendulum exercises are started the next morning. The patient is asked to refrain from repetitive overhead activities for at least 4–6 weeks and at 6 weeks strengthening exercises are begun as comfort allows.

Results

Ellman has the largest experience reported to date (Ellman 1988, Ellman & Kay 1989). By 1989 he had done 217 cases but reported on 87 cases with a follow-up of 2–5 years: 79% had stage 2 impingement and 21% had stage 3, i.e. with a full-thickness rotator cuff tear. The average follow-up was 34 months and the average age was 49 years. Each patient had had on average four steroid injections prior to surgery or pain at night. On the UCAL scoring system 85% were satisfactory and 76% returned to sport. Of the patients with stage 2 impingement, 89% were satisfactory but those with cuff tears had worse results—only 65% were satisfactory. Ellman believes that open treatment is preferable to arthroscopic subacromial decompression if a cuff tear is present.

However Norlin (1989) still thinks the results of arthroscopic decompression are preferable to open treatment, even in the presence of rotator cuff defect. Esch et al (1988) believe there is no difference between the two procedures.

Gartman (1990) has shown that results in stage 2 impingement were good: 88% were satisfied but this dropped to 82.5% that were satisfactory in the face of partial-thickness tear and only 45% satisfactory in the presence of a full-thickness tear.

Warren & Johnson (1989) have presented their results in 40 patients undergoing arthroscopic subacromial decompression (ASD) and debridement of the acromioclavicular joint and a scalene block. Results were similar: it is interesting to note that the average time of recovery was 3.8 months but most were in work in 10 days and 77% returned to their previous sporting level. Of the 6 who failed to return to sport, 5 had anteroinferior labral tears. The authors stressed that impingement secondary to instability should not be treated by ASD and patients with moderate-sized tears should have these repaired at open surgery.

ARTHROSCOPIC MANAGEMENT OF SHOULDER INSTABILITY

Arthroscopy in the management of shoulder instability has been rather a two-edged sword. It has added immeasurably to our knowledge and understanding of the mechanisms of shoulder instability and in particular of the role of the glenohumeral ligaments in preventing dislocation. Hopefully a surgeon will no longer be heard to say: 'I always do a Putti-Platt' or 'I always do a Bankart repair' but rather 'I find out what is wrong with the shoulder and correct it anatomically'. One of the reasons why shoulder-stabilizing surgery has remained static for so long was that the standard anterior approach to the shoulder destroyed most of the pathological anatomy. Fortunately arthroscopy has allowed us to look into the joint without disturbing the pathological anatomy and allows a more rational assessment to be made.

As arthroscopic findings are matched to the clinical picture several patterns have emerged. Turkel et al (1981) studied 46 cadaveric shoulders with selective sectioning of the anterior structures to identify their individual contribution to shoulder instability. They concluded that in the neutral position at 0° of abduction anterior dislocation is largely prevented by subscapularis. As the shoulder reaches 90° of abduction in external rotation (the position of apprehension), the subscapularis rolls over the top of the humeral head as the inferior margin rides up over the top of the humeral head, exposing the lower half of its anterior surface. It is only protected at this stage by the inferior gleno-humeral ligament. When all structures except the inferior glenohumeral ligament had been sectioned dislocation did not occur. Its division was immediately followed by subluxation or dislocation, emphasizing the vital role of this complex.

Arthroscopy shows us that the anterior labrum is a functional extension of this complex. Warren & Johnson (1989) describe the inferior glenohumeral ligament as a hammock upon which the humeral head rests in abduction. The Bankart lesion can be likened to sectioning one of the supporting ropes of the hammock and thus the head falls forward. This avulsion of the anterior part of the inferior glenohumeral ligament can be assessed arthroscopically. Approximately 20% do not show this obvious avulsion and the anterior capsule is noted to be scarred and lax and would require an antero-inferior capsular shift (Neer & Foster 1980). In these patients there has been obvious damage and traumatic scarring to the anterior capsule and this group must be separated clinically and arthroscopically from the pure multiple-joint laxity group which have multidirectional instability.

At arthroscopy the humeral head must be assessed, the Hill–Sachs lesion identified and an assessment made of its size. If it is massive then soft-tissue surgery may not be adequate and rotational osteotomy may be required. Only an identifiable avulsion of the anterior inferior glenohumeral ligament complex (Bankart lesions) is suitable for possible arthroscopic repair.

Repair by staple

This method has been popularized by Johnson (1986).

Operative technique

The patient is placed in the lateral decubitus position with the affected arm suspended in overhead traction but not more than 7 kg. The standard posterior portal is made for the telescope and then an anterior portal is made by railroading a guidewire through the initial telescope from posterior to anterior. A probe can be passed through this anterior portal to assess the detached or torn structures and help plan the procedure. The loose and torn fragmented tissue is removed with the debrider and then the abrader is used to roughen the anterior rim of the glenoid, preparing it for re-attachment. The object is to obtain bleeding cancellous bone. Adequate out-flow can be used through either a further anterior or superior portal. The arms of the staple are then used to collect the detached glenoid labrum, portions of the subscapularis tendon and adjacent inferior capsule. During insertion it is extremely important to maintain a 90° angle between the staple and the scapular neck to ensure a firm fixation. A mallet is used to drive the staple into the scapular neck, leaving the head of the staple protruding slightly. Finally the arthroscope is placed anteriorly to visualize the neck of the staple, showing the anterior glenoid labrum and surrounding capsule being securely advanced against the scapular neck. Postoperative radiographs are taken to ensure adequate positioning of the staple.

Complications arising from the use of staples around the shoulder joint have Leen frequently reported in Kll open shoulder operations and this is no less true of the arthroscopic technique. However with better staples and better technique it appears that this complication is lessening but there is a general swing away from trying to insert metal around the shoulder joint. Biodegradable staples are being developed.

Suture technique

Morgan & Bodenstab (1987) have devised the most popular arthroscopic technique for the suture repair of the anterior shoulder instability.

Technique

Again the patient is placed in the lateral decubitus position and the arm is suspended in the position of internal rotation. Preoperative diagnostic arthroscopy is made through the posterior portal. An

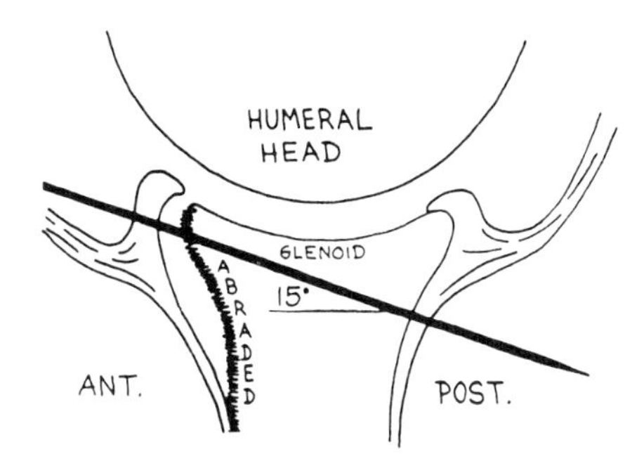

Fig. 10.4 The anterior aspect of the glenoid has been abraded. The suture pin traverses the neck of the glenoid at a 15° angle to the articular surface. (Reproduced with permission from Morgan & Bodenstab 1987.)

anterior portal is made, the Bankart lesion is probed and the anterior glenoid neck is prepared in exactly the same way as for staple repair, either by burring or drilling. The suture is passed using a specially designed suture pin 2 mm in diameter and 30 cm in length. It has a sharp tip to pierce the labrum and a recessed eye to carry the suture in the opposite end.

Two separate anterior-to-posterior passes of the suture pin through the Bankart lesion and glenoid bone are required to create a large single anterior horizontal mattress suture with transglenoid suture tails which exit at the scapular neck. The suture is passed in such a way to bring up the inferior glenohumeral ligament to its anatomical attachment to the mid-portion of the glenoid rim.

Great attention must be paid to the placing of the pins to avoid damage to the suprascapular nerve. Once the correct angle is assessed it is drilled through the glenoid bone using a motorized drill from in front until the pin exits the skin posteriorly. The suture used is normally a no. 1 PDS. The second pin will exit the skin posteriorly. The two strands of suture material are then passed subcutaneously out through the separate second postero-inferior portal. The first set of sutures are tied to the second set of sutures anteriorly outside in front of the anterior cannula with a double square knot. The knot tails are trimmed. The surgeon pulls on the suture tails posteriorly delivering the knot down the cannula into the shoulder anteriorly under direct arthroscopic visualization. With further tension on the suture tails posteriorly, the horizontal mattress suture created by the knot reduces the

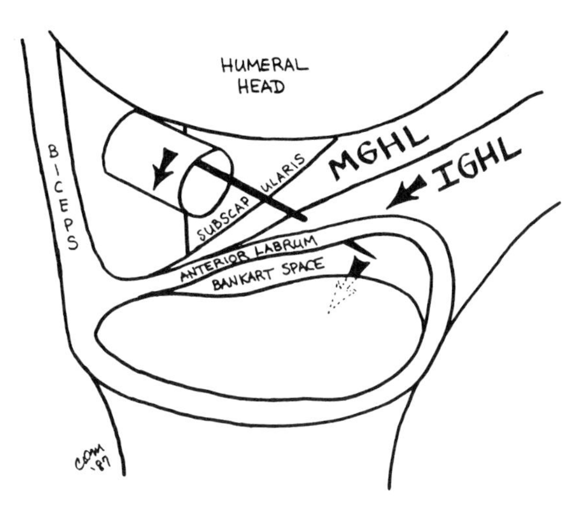

Fig. 10.5 The inferior glenohumeral ligament (IGHL) is caught with the suture pin and taken superiorly to tighten it. MGHL = Middle glenohumeral ligament. (Reproduced with permission from Morgan & Bodenstab 1987.)

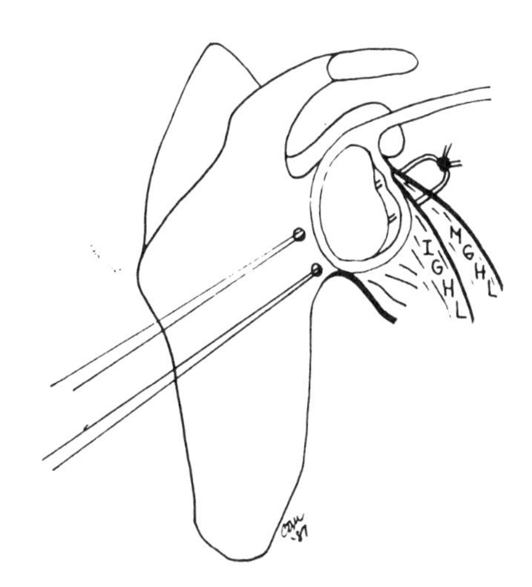

Fig. 10.6 Right scapula showing general placement of the single large anterior horizontal mattress suture. The suture tail is passed through two parallel transglenoid holes to exit posteriorly. IGHL = Inferior glenohumeral ligament; MGHL = Middle glenohumeral ligament. (Reproduced with permission from Morgan & Bodenstab 1987.)

Bankart lesion by opposing the sutures' soft-tissue anterior to the abraded scapular neck and glenoid rim. This should also tighten the inferior glenohumeral ligament which at this point should be a readily visible large structure.

Posteriorly both sets of double sutures exit through the single posterior inferior portal and are then tied to themselves over the thick fascia of the posterial third of the deltoid.

The sutures are cut subcutaneously and all the instrumentation is removed.

The patient is then placed in a sling with the arm in internal rotation. Postoperatively the shoulder is kept in a sling and body band for 4 weeks. At 4 weeks active assisted range of movements and pendulum exercises are begun. At 6 weeks a passive motion and exercise to strengthen the rotator cuff is started with the emphasis on external rotation exercise in the neutral position. Contact sports are not allowed for at least 6 months.

Results or arthroscopic stabilization

The redislocation rate for anterior stapling procedures is 15–20%. Furthermore, the incidence of complications related to use of metal staples, loosening, breakage, improper placement, migration and cutting the anterior capsular sutures has been 10–20%. These results do not compare with open repair. However it is claimed with longer immobilization and better postoperative rehabilitation that this redislocation rate is reducing.

Morgan (1989) presented the 2–5-year results of his suture technique in 60 patients. In 55 with a Bankart lesion a positive anterior apprehension sign was present. None were lax-jointed or had a sulcus sign. At an average of 37 months there were only 2 failures: 96% were graded as excellent. This is comparable to the best results of open repair, but the patient population may not be strictly comparable.

In both these techniques the advantages were short inpatient stay and simplified programme of rehabilitation with the majority of patients regaining a full range of external rotation. These are all short-term results that have been reported so far and at the moment are not comparable with any of the open series.

All results from these procedures must be treated with caution and the exact patient population in any study noted. All authors report a very steep learning curve in the early stage and improved results after doing the first few, which emphasizes the need to become thoroughly familiar with the technique on arthroscopic models. However all reported results have been gradually improving with the experience of the authors. It must be noted that in most of the series the patients are highly selected in that they are all recurrent anterior dislocators with a proven Bankart lesion. In some series first-time dislocators are included. Postoperative immobilization can be as long as 3 months and advice concerning not returning to contact sports can extend for as long as 12–18 months. The definitive scientific evidence that the natural history of recurrent anterior dislocation is significantly improved by arthroscopic techniques is still lacking. This can only be proven by a matched series of patients also treated by total immobilization for a similar period with an intensive rehabilitation programme and denied contact and active sports for at least a year.

In summary, at the time of writing these techniques are interesting and improving very rapidly. The results I am sure will improve with time but at the moment arthroscopic stabilization is not for general use as the results are not yet as good as open surgery but show enormous promise for the future. Arthroscopy has added greatly to our knowledge of the pathological anatomy of the shoulder. It is of proven value in diagnosis, assessment, biopsy, removal of loose bodies and limited debridement of the joint. Results equal to that of open surgery can be achieved for synovectomy and subacromial anterior cuff decompression.

The case still remains questionable for stabilization surgery and it is still not in routine use. Other more adventurous attempts have been made at suturing rotator cuff repairs from the inside (Levy et al 1990) and arthrodesing shoulders by arthroscopic decortification. These are essentailly triumphs of technique over reason and not to be recommended. In the future far more surgery around the shoulder will be done arthroscopically but this must always be measured against the best open surgery. Just because it is possible to do it arthroscopically does not necessarily mean that it is sensible or advisable to do so.

REFERENCES

Andrews JR, Carson WG, McLeod WD 1985 Glenoid labrum tears related to the long head of the biceps. Am J Sports Med 13:337–341

Bankart ASB 1938 The pathology and treatment of recurrent dislocations of the shoulder joint. Br J Surg 23

Caspari RB, Whipple TL, Meyers, JF 1990 The Neviaser portal for shoulder arthroscopy. In: Post Morrey, Hawkins (eds) Surgery of the shoulder, CV Mosby, St Louis

Casscells CD, 1987 The argument for early arthroscopic synovectomy in patients with severe haemophilia. Arthroscopy 3:78–79
Copeland SA, Barrett DS 1989 A new physical sign in shoulder arthroscopy. J Bone Joint Surg 71B:860
Copeland SA, Williamson D 1988 Suturing of arthroscopy wounds. J Bone Joint Surg 17B:145
Detrisac DA, Johnson LL 1988 Arthroscopic anatomy: pathological and surgical implications. Slack, New Jersey
Ellman H 1988 Shoulder arthroscopy: current indications and techniques. Orthopaedics 11:45–51
Ellman H, Kay SP 1989 Arthroscopic sub acromial decompression: 2 to 5 year results. At presentation American Shoulder and Elbow Surgeons Open Meeting February 1989.
Esch JC, Ozerkis LR, Helgager JA et al 1988 Arthroscopic subacromial decompression: results according to the degree of rotator cuff tear. Arthroscopy 4:241–249
Gartman GM 1990 Arthroscopic acromial decompression. In: Post Morrey, Hawkins (eds) Surgery of the shoulder, CV Mosby, St Louis
Johnson LL 1986 Shoulder arthroscopy. In: Klein EA, Falk KH, O'Brien T (eds) Arthroscopic surgery—principles and practice. CV Mosby, St Louis, p 1394
Klein AH, France JC, Mutschler TA, Fu FH 1987 Measurement of bronchial plexus strain in arthroscopy of the shoulder. Arthroscopy 3:45–52
Kohn D 1987 The clinical relevance of glenoid labrum lesions. Arthroscopy 3:223–230
Levy, HJ, Uribe JW, Delaney, LG 1990 Arthroscopic assisted rotator cuff repair: preliminary results. Arthroscopy 6:55–60
Matthews LS, Vetter WL, Helfet DL 1984 Arthroscopic surgery of the shoulder. Adv Orthop Surg 20: 160–111
Morgan CD 1989 2–5 year results. Arthroscopic technique for anterior instability of the shoulder. AAOS
Morgan CD, Bodenstab, AB 1987 Arthroscopic suture repair technique and early results. Arthroscopy 3:111–122
Neer CS, Foster CR 1980 Inferior capsular shift for involuntary inferior and multi-directional instability of the shoulder. J Bone Joint Surg 62A:897
Norlin R 1989 Arthroscopic subacromial decompression versus open acromionectomy. Arthroscopy 5:321–324
Ogilvy-Harris D 1987 Arthroscopy and arthroscopic surgery of the shoulder. Semin Ortho 2:246–258
Ogilvy-Harris D, Boynton E 1990 Arthroscopic acromioplasty extravasation of fluid into deltoid muscle. Arthroscopy 6:52–54
Pahle JA 1981 The shoulder joint in rheumatoid arthritis: synovectomy, reconstructive surgery and traumatology, vol 18. Karger, Basel p 33
Rockwood CA 1988 Shoulder arthroscopy editorial. J Bone Joint Surg 70A:639–640
Skyhar MJ, Altcher DW, Warren et al 1988 Shoulder arthroscopy with the patients in the beach chair position. Arthroscopy 4:256–259
Turkel SJ, Panio MW, Marshall, JL Girgis FG 1981 Stabilizing mechanism preventing anterior dislocation of the gleno-humeral joint. J Bone Joint Surg 63A:1208–1217
Warren RF, Johnson L 1989 Arthroscopic surgery: principles and practice, 3rd edn. St Louis. CV Mosby

11

The impact of prosthetic design on revision hip replacement

W. F. G. Muirhead-Allwood

Although many early attempts were made to develop a hip replacement, of which a few examples still exist (Fig. 11.1), it was not until the late 1960s that total hip replacement became widely practised. The key to this reproducible success almost certainly was attributable to the method of implant fixation by acrylic bone cement (PMMA). Both Charnley (1961) and McKee & Watson-Farrar (1966) demonstrated good results.

Despite the general levels of success that have been achieved (Wrobleski 1986, Kavanagh et al 1989), there have remained two areas where the results have been disappointing: primary arthroplasty in the younger patient (Chandler et al 1981, Dorr et al 1983) and revision hip arthroplasty (Table 11.1). In both areas attention has been paid to improved methods of implant fixation and the use of uncemented prostheses to rectify this.

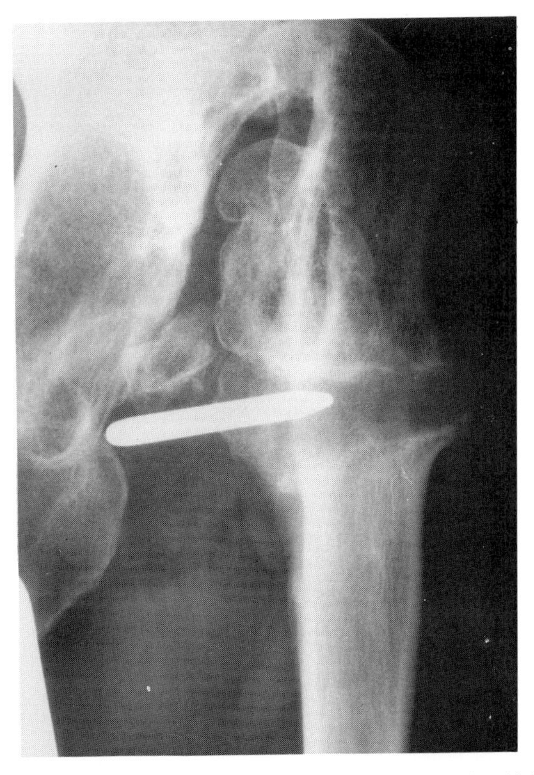

Fig. 11.1 A 46-year-old patient with a Judet prosthesis which had been inserted 37 years previously when the patient was 9.

Uncemented arthroplasty is not new; both the Ring and the Lord prostheses have a long clinical follow-up (Ring 1981, Lord 1982). However, over the last 12 years many other designs have been developed, the AML (anatomic medullary locking), the PCA (porous coated anatomic), the Harris Galante and the BIAS (biologic ingrowth anatomic stem). More recently an increasing number of uncemented revision prostheses have become available. Before abandoning the cemented implant it is necessary to consider the rationale for using uncemented prostheses in revision surgery.

THE RATIONALE FOR UNCEMENTED REVISION ARTHROPLASTY

The primary difference between cemented and uncemented prostheses lies in the bone–implant interface. If the uncemented prosthesis is to offer an advantage it must overcome the problems associated with the cemented interface. The bone–cement interface has for many years been an area of research interest. The interface behaves differently on the acetabular and femoral sides for reasons that are not understood. On the femoral side osseointegration between PMMA and bone has been demonstrated. Osseointegration implies the apposition of two surfaces without an interposed membrane. On the acetabular side a membrane always

Table 11.1 Failure rates in cemented revision total hip replacement

Reference	Follow up (years)	Number of cases	Failure rate (%)	XR loosening (%)
Dandy & Theodorous (1975)	<2	83	60	
Hunter et al (1979)	0.5	140	22	
Hoogland et al (1981)	>2	65	18	
Amstutz & Jinnah (1982)	1–9	66	9	20
Broughton & Rushton (1982)	1	63	22	
Esses et al (1983)	2	26	11.5	
Gustilo & Kyle (1984a)	2–10	42	16.7	45
Reigstad & Hetland (1984)	0.5	19	5.3	
Pellici et al (1982)	2–7	110	14	26
Pellici et al (1985)	5–12.5	110	29	
Kavanagh et al (1985)	2–10	194	18	28
Turner et al (1987b)	6.7	110	12	28–48
Stromberg et al (1988)	2–6	67	36	
Rubash & Harris (1988)*	6	43	2	11
Engelbrecht et al (1990)	7.4	138	8.8	31

*Femoral results only.

exists between the bone and cement. It is this difference which probably accounts for the relatively unsuccessful attempts to reduce acetabular loosening with advanced cement techniques which have been shown to be so successful on the femoral side.

Radiological changes at the bone–cement interface seem to occur in two patterns. There is the rather gradual circumferential destruction of bone which can occur (Fig. 11.2). On the femoral side this allows the prosthesis to sink or to angulate. On the acetabular side migration and angulation of the cup occur. The second pattern is the more aggressive, rapidly developing osteolytic 'punched-out' lesion (Fig. 11.3). This commonly occurs around the femoral cement and may arise around a macroscopically well fixed stem (Jasty et al 1986). The exact mechanisms of this bone destruction are still not fully understood but based on our present knowledge we can make the following observations.

The initial reaction to PMMA is in response to mechanical, thermal and chemical stimuli, the trauma of the surgery, and the insertion and polymerization of PMMA. The formation of a stable fibrous tissue membrane is the usual outcome. (Homsey et al 1972a, Fornasier & Cameron 1976, Freeman et al 1982, Goodman et al 1985, Jasty et al 1986). This membrane contains scattered histiocytes and multinucleated giant cells. Movement and particulate PMMA have both been shown to change the characteristics of this membrane (Chambers 1980), causing a change in the initially

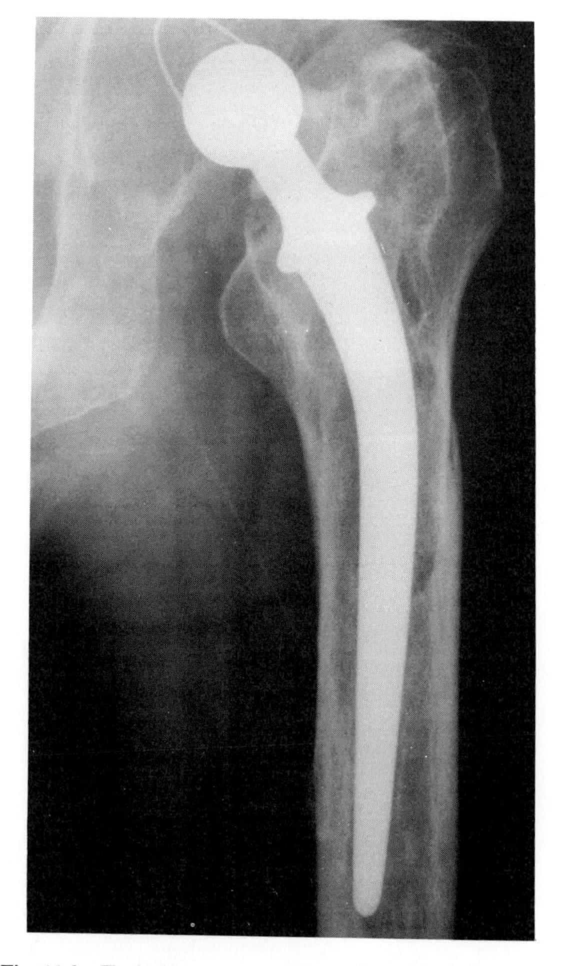

Fig. 11.2 Typical appearance of loosening with obvious sinkage of the prosthesis.

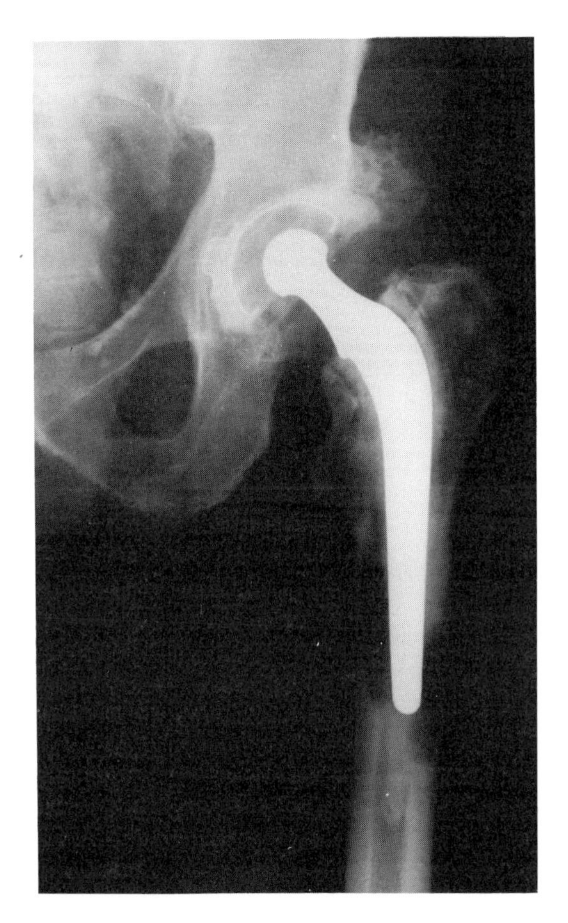

Fig. 11.3 The appearances of more aggressive osteolysis. The remaining bridge on the medial femoral wall is a typical appearance as the lesions start to coalesce.

benign nature of these cells and activating them to cause bone lysis. Microscopic examination of the membrane obtained from clinically and radiologically stable prostheses has been shown to differ from that obtained from loose ones. The latter membrane is characterized by heavy infiltration with particles of PMMA and particulate polyethylene, causing a foreign-body giant cell reaction. Additionally the surface of the membrane in contact with the cement changes to resemble a synovial membrane (Goldring et al 1983, 1988).

The predominant cell associated with loosening is the histiocyte or connective tissue macrophage. This cell is a derivative of the circulating monocyte which is also believed to be a precursor of the osteoclast. When histiocytes phagocytose non-digestible particles which are ultimately cytotoxic, a foreign-body giant cell reaction ensues. The necrotic histiocytes are chemotactic to other macrophages which accumulate and proliferate (Cline 1975). The chemical and humoral processes that follow are less well understood. In tissue culture, membrane fragments have been shown to produce large quantities of prostaglandin E_2 and collagenase. These substances can cause bone resorption (Goldring et al 1986). If prostaglandin was the main agent in bone destruction, antiprostaglandins should prevent lysis. However when tissue cultures were incubated with indomethacin, bone-resorbing activity was not abolished (Goldring et al 1988). It is likely that other products such as interleukin-1, which is secreted by monocyte macrophages, can also act as mediators (Goldring et al 1988). Interleukin-1β, also called lymphocyte-activating factor, has been shown to be the same molecule as osteoclast-activating factor (Dewhurst et al 1986). Other substances such as tumour necrosis factor, lymphotoxin and interleukin-1α have also been implicated (Schmalzreid & Finerman 1988).

Osteolytic changes are therefore secondary to initial mechanical failure, where micromotion and particulate debris set up foreign-body giant cell reactions and bone-resorbing substances are released. This results in further loosening as the supporting bone is destroyed and further motion and debris accumulates. With such a complex biological process, certain individuals will destroy bone more rapidly. This may explain the so-called cement intolerance. No allergic response to bulk cement has ever been demonstrated.

Severe and more aggressive focal osteolysis has however been described in the presence of a macroscopically well fixed prosthesis. This was first reported in 1976 by Jasty et al (1986). Santavirta's group (Tallroth et al 1989, Eskola et al 1990, Santavirta et al 1990) have recently reported on this and claim that it accounts for 5% of their revisions. They confirm that it occurs in well fixed prostheses but felt that the histology was at variance with normal loosening in that there was a lack of activated fibroblasts. Monocyte macrophages were however present in abundance and the reaction was of a foreign-body type. The most likely explanation for these reactions is that the well fixed cement mantle fractures.

Particulate material is then injected under pressure from the prosthesis–cement interface through to the bone–cement interface, causing the foreign-body reaction. If this theory is correct once again the initial failure is mechanical through cement fracture. The ensuing lysis, if it is allowed to progress, will in time loosen the prosthesis.

It is the knowledge that in order to sustain a lasting result with cement an initial good mechanical fixation must be obtained which most taxes the revision surgeon. Bone cement is not an adhesive and relies totally on interlock for its security. Interlock can be achieved by its overall shape and the use of adjuncts such as keyholes. This is termed 'macrolock' but is inefficient in preventing micromotion. Microlock is most efficient when there is interdigitation of bone cement and bone lamellae. In revision surgery the surgeon is faced with smooth cortical surfaces and is denied any microlock in the proximal femur. A longer femoral component must be used, which enters areas of the femoral canal which have previously been unfilled. The disadvantages of long-stemmed cemented prostheses are twofold (Turner et al 1987). By their nature they almost certainly cause proximal stress shielding. Some micromotion will probably occur in the proximal femur, causing particulate debris to be released which may initiate further failure. Their second disadvantage is that if they do fail they are particularly difficult to revise. It is the responsibility of the surgeon who implants a prosthesis to determine how it will be revised in the event of failure.

A further problem encountered is the loss of bone stock. If a deficient bone with marked osteolysis is simply filled with methylmethacrylate there will be no bone reconstitution or remodelling. PMMA has been shown to reduce bone remodelling.

The goal of revision surgery is to reduce pain, to improve function and produce a result that lasts. Because in the younger patient further failure must be contemplated any measure to improve or at least maintain the present bonestock should be employed.

Uncemented revision hip replacement provides an opportunity of achieving these goals and a good argument can be made for its use. We have a great experience of uncemented hemiarthroplasties and although many have been unsatisfactory, clinically none have produced severe femoral bone loss except prostheses with polyethylene femoral heads (Monk soft-top). Here huge amounts of particulate polyethylene debris are generated causing severe proximal femoral lysis (Fig. 11.4). The fact that long-term follow-up of prostheses of the Austin Moore type have not caused severe femoral bony destruction shows that the removal of particulate wear products should avoid the problem of bone destruction. Kozinn et al (1986) reviewed the membrane around the stems of 12 loose cementless femoral head and bipolar prostheses and found that fibroblasts were the most frequent cells. Only a few histioctyes were present and there was a scarcity of foreign-body giant cells. The use of an uncemented prosthesis with a polyethylene bearing removes one source—possibly the most important—of particulate wear.

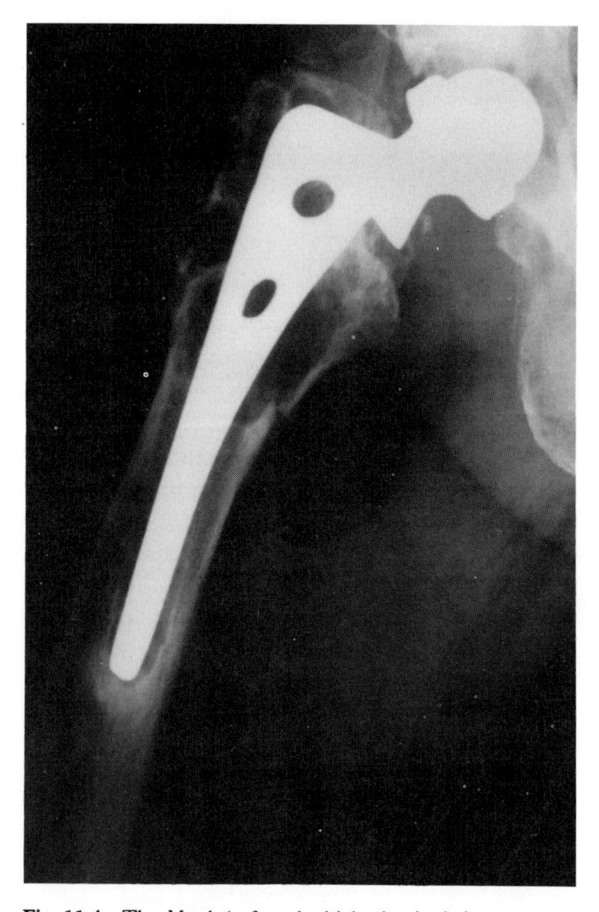

Fig. 11.4 The Monk 'soft-top' which, despite being an uncemented prosthesis, shows massive upper femoral lysis due to polyethylene debris.

Since the 1970s experimental work has shown that bony ingrowth can be established into microporous chrome cobalt alloy (Homsey et al 1972b, Cameron et al 1976), into titanium fibremesh (Galante et al 1971) and also porous polysulphone (Roberson et al 1988). The shear strength of the bone–prosthetic interface of a porous metal implant has been reported to be between 17-25 MPa (Bobyn et al 1980, Cook et al 1985). By comparison, the bone–cement interface shear strength under laboratory conditions of PMMA lies between 5.6 and 20.7 MPa. Hydroxyapatite coatings can achieve a bone–interface shear strength of 64 MPa (Geesink et al 1987) and have also been experimentally shown to accelerate ingrowth into porous metal surfaces (Oonishi et al 1989). Theoretically, therefore, an uncemented prosthesis can become as well fixed as a good cemented prosthesis and provide painless function.

In reality, if an uncemented prosthesis is introduced in the revision scenario, accurate bony apposition will be only patchy. If the shape of the prosthesis is acceptable stability will be achieved by point fixation but voids will be created. These will have to be filled with bone graft. In many cases autograft can be used but when amounts of bone are needed allograft will be required. Experimental animal studies show that not only will the bone incorporate but both autograft and allograft will become ingrown into porous metal surfaces (Broughton & Rushton 1982). If bone graft is inserted around the prosthesis in an uncemented revision hip bone reconstitution should follow.

In theory, therefore, uncemented revision should be able to produce painless function with the ability to increase lost bonestock. If failure occurs less bone destruction should ensue.

The characteristics of a successful revision prosthesis are:

1. Ability to achieve initial stability.
2. Ability to achieve equilibrium with its host and to allow bone reconstitution and remodelling.
3. Ability to revise the prosthesis if failure occurs.

METHODS OF ACETABULAR RECONSTRUCTION

In revision surgery acetabular reconstruction poses a great problem. The results of revision simply using cement have been shown by Kavanagh et al (1985) to produce more acetabular than femoral failures. Their figures show 25% loose sockets at 4.5 years and, if multiply revised acetabula are considered, this figure rises to 50% radiologically loose with 33% symptomatically loose. Other methods of fixation must be found.

Unlike femoral revision, acetabular reconstruction is hampered by the difficulty in finding new areas of bone which can be used for support in the way that a long-stemmed femoral component can enter new undamaged bone and support the femoral component. The problems of smooth sclerotic bone surfaces which prevent cement microlock are encountered. With multiple cemented revisions the bonestock becomes progressively depleted and any attempt at reconstruction must attempt to restore the bonestock to give a stable result.

The methods which have been tried to achieve this are:

1. Cemented cups supported wholly or partially by allograft or autograft with or without the use of support rings.
2. The bipolar or big head prosthesis supported by bone graft.
3. Uncemented sockets supported in part by autograft or allograft.

An acetabulum with gross bony deficiency simply treated by cementing in new components has been already shown to produce poor results. Bonestock can be improved by the use of allografts or autografts in either solid block or morselized form. The cement is then laid on to the graft and on to any areas of host non-grafted bone (Fig. 11.5). Arguments can be made that laying cement on to dead bone improves fixation as no membrane can be formed and in effect a customized cement shape is covered with a thin layer of dead bone which could incorporate in much the same way as a hydroxyapatite coating. In order to improve structural strength support rings can be used. The available results would indicate that, if the acetabulum is wholly reconstructed with bone graft, the results are poor. Emerson et al (1989) report on 7 cases, 4 of whom required second or subsequent revisions. Five failed at an average 17-month follow-up. These failures could easily be attributed to poor

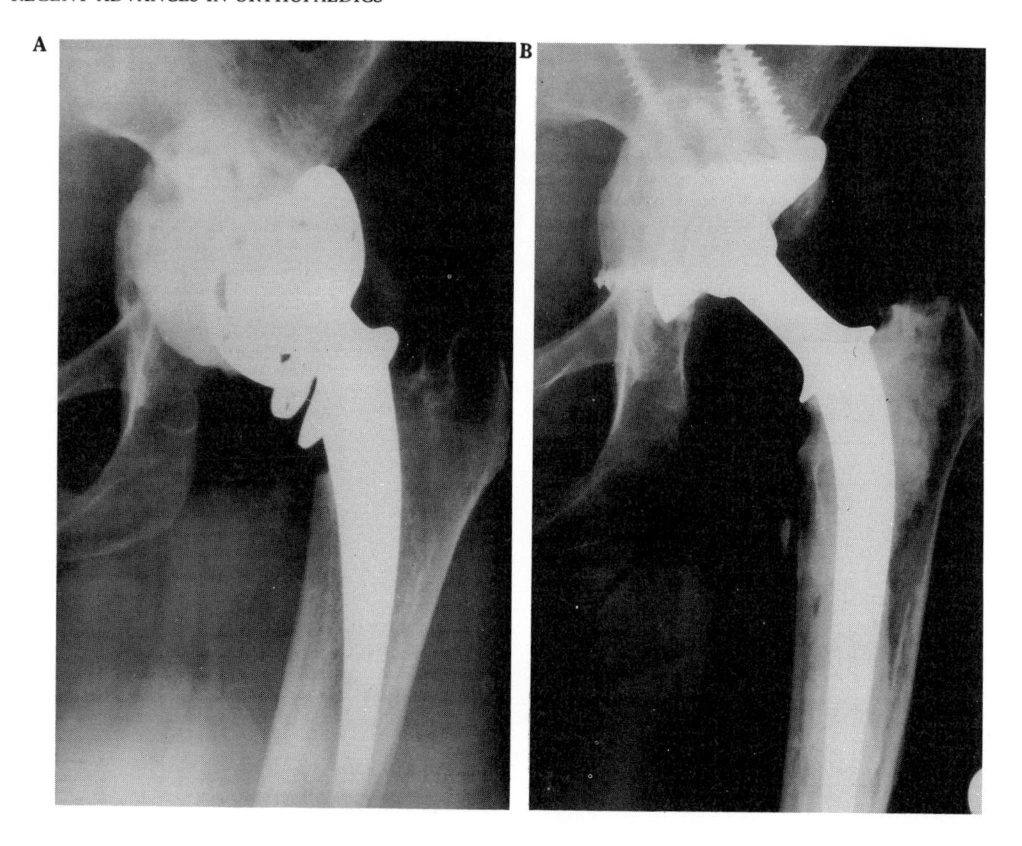

Fig. 11.5 A successful example of cementing a cup on to bone graft supported by a Muller ring (**A**) The preoperative film was the third revision; (**B**) 4-year follow-up film.

technique due to initial implant positioning. Jasty & Harris (1990) have reported failure in sockets supported by bone graft. In this series 32% were loose at 6 years and all these failures occurred late. They have since stopped using structural or solid graft.

This suggests that if components are supported wholly by graft there may be a substantial failure rate. In the very deficient acetabulum this may be acceptable. Emerson et al (1989) have noted on revision of 5 failed grafts that in all but 1 case the graft had consolidated, making further revision easier. Rorabeck et al (1990) reported a 2-year follow-up of 34 acetabular grafts, of which 32 consolidated. The study was arranged with both cemented and cementless acetabular components and the 2 failures occurred in the cemented group. Their conclusion, with which the author agrees, is that uncemented components will probably give a better result.

The use of bipolar prostheses with bone grafting has been reported from various centres (Murray 1984, Scott et al 1987, Ochsner et al 1988, Cameron & Jung 1988). The rationale for the bipolar prosthesis is that when it is used with morselized graft in large defects it should hold the graft in place; if it does sink or migrate the acetabular orientation will be self-righting. The method was described by Dautry in 1979 and short-term results were encouraging. Sommelet et al (1989) have reported the technique in 37 patients at a minimum follow-up of 5 years. Only 23 were revision surgery cases and only 58% of these had a satisfactory clinical outcome. Emerson et al (1989) reported 37 cases with a follow-up of 28 months. Of 37 prostheses, 18 migrated and in the migrated group the average Harris hip score was 81. They concluded that this technique should be reserved for low-demand patients.

Wilson et al (1989) reported 32 hips revised with

bipolar prostheses and concluded that the technique was satisfactory when the graft was laid into a central contained defect. Reconstruction using allograft of peripheral or central non-contained defects was less successful. Even in the central contained defects, 20–30% of the initial graft thickness was lost in the early stages of incorporation, presumably due to the movement of the prosthetic head. They concluded that better results might be achieved with a fixed non-cemented cup.

The use of uncemented sockets in revision surgery has been carried out in some European centres since 1976 (Brinkmann & Harms 1984). In these series the use of screw-in sockets was used. The majority of uncemented sockets used worldwide have been either screw-in sockets or hemispherical porous sockets (Fig. 11.6). In the UK work has been done with truncated conical sockets (Ring) and more recently a new stemmed truncated conical socket (Mcminn 1990). The last two have however only limited revision series. Attention will, therefore, be confined here to the screw-in socket and the porous hemispherical socket.

The screw-in socket either takes the form of a threaded hemisphere or truncated cone. Segmental or cavitatory defects in the acetabulum are grafted using autograft or allograft and the threaded acetabular component is screwed into the reconstructed acetabulum. The majority of the strength is probably a rim-fix with threads engaging the mouth of the acetabulum. In Europe good results have been reported but the results from the USA have been poor (Brinkmann & Harms 1984, Parhofer & Monch 1984, Mallory et al 1988). Engh et al (1988), initially a proponent of the Mecring cup, reported that 41.6% of these prostheses were unstable. When this cup was used in conjunction with structural allografts over 50% failed in less than 5 years. Emerson et al (1989) reported 4 out of 13 failures with a threaded truncated cone at an average follow-up of 40 months. Threaded cups have also been shown to produce problems in primary surgery (Engh et al 1990). It is possible that some designs work well in some hands, yet the literature would suggest that the results are not consistent.

Porous coated hemispherical cups provide a different concept in fixation. The porous coating should allow bone ingrowth and provide long-term fixation. In order for this to be achieved some form of initial fixation is necessary. This can be provided with the use of peripheral pegs or flutes, as in the PCA, BIAS or head acetabular components or the use of separate screws, as in the Harris Galante and other prostheses. In practice a great dOal of the primary fixation is achieved simply by the interference fit, using a prosthesis slightly larger than the reamed cavity and reliing on the slight spring in the acetabular horseshoe. Because of the irregular shape of the damaged acetabular cavity it will rarely be possible to convert its shape into a perfect hemisphere by hemispherical reKming in order to accept the new component with full bone–prosthesis contact. Bone grafting with either autograft or allograft will therefore be necessary to fill the defects.

The basic support for the implant must still be achieved by contact between the prosthesis and the host bone. The amount of prosthesis–host bone contact required is still not certain but approximately 50% appears to be acceptable. McGann et al (1988) have suggested that with the use of

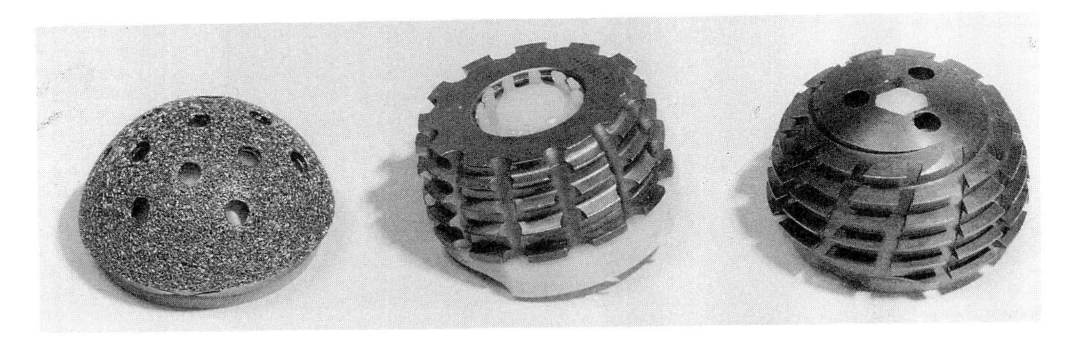

Fig. 11.6 **Left**: a porous coated hemispherical cup; **middle** and **right**: examples of screw-in cups.

morselized non-structural graft only 30% host bone contact is necessary and 40% with a non-structural segmental graft. Reporting on 75 cases using the Harris Galante socket, McGann et al showed no loss of fixation and only resorption of non-contained graft, in which there is contact with soft tissue only. Emerson et al (1989) also reported 46 press-fit cups with a 22-month average follow-up. There were no cases of failure, although 7 showed minimal migration. However, the overall average Harris rating was 89.

Engh et al (1988) reported 34 porous cups in their series with a mean follow-up of 4.4 years: stable fixation was achieved in 97%. The author's experiences of acetabular reconstruction using the Harris Galante cup in revisions concur with the series described above. Over the last 4 years more than 160 Harris Galante acetabular components have been implanted in revision cases with no failures to the present time (Fig. 11.7). These sockets have all had at least 40% host bone–prosthesis contact.

At present it appears that the most promising results in acetabular reconstruction come from the use of the porous coated press-fit hemispherical component used with bone graft. The prosthesis must have at least a 30% contact with host bone. Present results do not indicate which of the available porous coatings is best or whether it is better to use a cup with integral supporting pegs or flutes or to use separate supplementary screws. The one certain fact is that the primary fixation must be firm if ingrowth is to occur. Currently hydroxyapatite coatings are being used either applied directly to smooth titanium or as an adjunct to porous coatings. These are likely to improve the results further but as yet there are no substantial long-term series to demonstrate this.

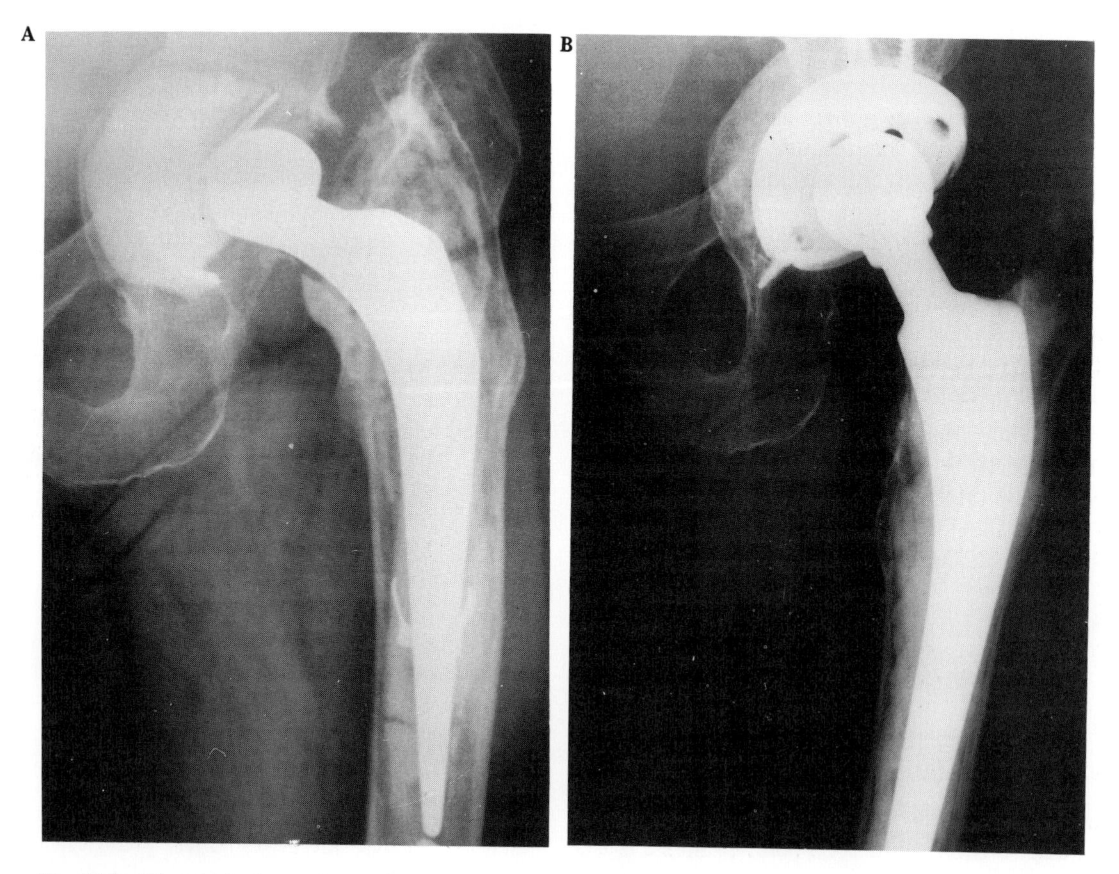

Fig. 11.7 **(A)** severely damaged acetabulum treated with an uncemented Harris galante socket and morselized bone graft. **(B)** At 2 years after the operation the graft is consolidating well.

FEMORAL RECONSTRUCTION

In revision surgery the method of femoral reconstruction will depend on the age of the patient and on the amount of bone destruction. Many classifications of femoral bone destruction have been devised; the classification of Hungerford et al (1988) is useful in this context as it relates bone destruction to prosthetic selection.

Type 1: Minimal loss similar to primary.
Type 2: Moderate loss requiring bone graft. Revision prosthesis stabilized by host bone.
Type 3: Severe bone loss. Bone graft required to produce prosthetic stability.
Type 4: Massive bone loss requiring whole allograft.

The methods of femoral reconstruction presently available are:

1. Cemented femoral stem.
2. Cemented femoral stem cemented on to bone graft.
3. Uncemented proximally loaded femoral stem with graft.
4. Uncemented distally loaded femoral stem with bone graft.
5. The massive allograft or prosthetic upper femoral replacement.

In the classification of Hungerford et al (1988) a proximally supported prosthesis could be used in types 1 and 2 without graft and be stable, whereas in type 3 bone graft would be needed to give it proximal support. A distally supported prosthesis would only be indicated in types 3 and 4. In these cases the support for the prosthesis would initially be distal in the undamaged femur. If bone graft was used proximally it would initially need to give support, although with time it would consolidate and begin to give proximal support. Let us consider the methods of femoral reconstruction separately.

The cemented stem

Although the results of most major series of femoral cemented revisions have been poor, evidence exists that with improved and contemporary cementing techniques these figures can be improved. Rubash & Harris (1988) reported 43 femoral revisions with a mean follow-up of 74 months. Only 1 hip required revision, although a further 9% showed definite radiological loosening and a further 4% possible signs. The average age of this series was 57 years but the amount of femoral destruction is not recorded. This series indicates that the use of a cement plug with meticulous preparation of the femoral canal, the use of a cement gun and a prosthesis which adequately fills the canal can greatly improve the results of cemented femoral revision. Marti et al (1990) report an older-aged series of 60 cemented revisions with an average age of 71 and demonstrated a survivorship of 85% at 14 years.

Clearly there is still a place for the cemented revision in the older age group where instant mobilization is necessary. Large areas of bone destruction will not however repair and in the younger patient if destruction of bonestock exists, other methods which restore bonestock seem preferable.

Cemented stems used in conjunction with bone graft

Ling (1990) has recently reported on this technique. The bone cement and membrane are removed in the normal way. The femoral cavity is then packed with allograft and the allograft is compacted with a femoral prosthesis. Once sufficient impaction has been achieved the cavity in the graft is filled with cement and a slightly smaller prosthesis to that used for impaction is introduced using the normal cement pressurization methods.

The early results of this method suggest that the graft consolidates and the prosthesis remains stable. This is technically a simpler method of reconstruction than using an uncemented prosthesis with graft. Further long-term studies will be needed to evaluate the technique. Its potential disadvantage is that if the prosthesis has some micromovement, large quantities of PMMA debris may be generated.

Proximally supported uncemented femoral stem with bone graft

In this instance an uncemented prosthesis is inserted which by its geometry offloads on the proximal femur. It will do this in part by direct contact with host bone and partly through the bone graft used to fill the voids around the stem. This is at present the most fashionable solution, with virtually every manufacturer offering at least one design (Fig. 11.8).

The techniques for uncemented revision hip replacement are in some ways more demanding than for cemented arthroplasty. Each uncemented system has its own instrumentation and the inevitable learning curve that goes with the particular prosthesis and instrument system. There are, however, general rules that must be followed with all systems. In general for cemented revision all the bone cement and the membrane should be removed. If this is not done disastrous results may not necessarily ensue. In uncemented revision if any cement is retained in the femoral canal one of two things will happen: the tip of the prosthesis will deviate on the cement and cause a femoral fracture or an undersized prosthesis will be used which will be loose, and will generate further debris causing osteolysis (Fig. 11.9).

Uncemented revision demands that the initial fixation of the prosthesis must be firm. A large rigid long-stemmed prosthesis will be forced down the inevitably weakened and probably distorted femoral canal. The permissible force to do this can only be learnt. This is probably best learnt initially with uncemented primary hips. In the revision case the combination of the longer stem and the femoral distortion which may be present means that the prosthesis may not be directed straight down the medullary canal, risking perforation of the stem or fracture. The author advocates screening the prosthesis down the canal under X-ray control to prevent this complication.

A

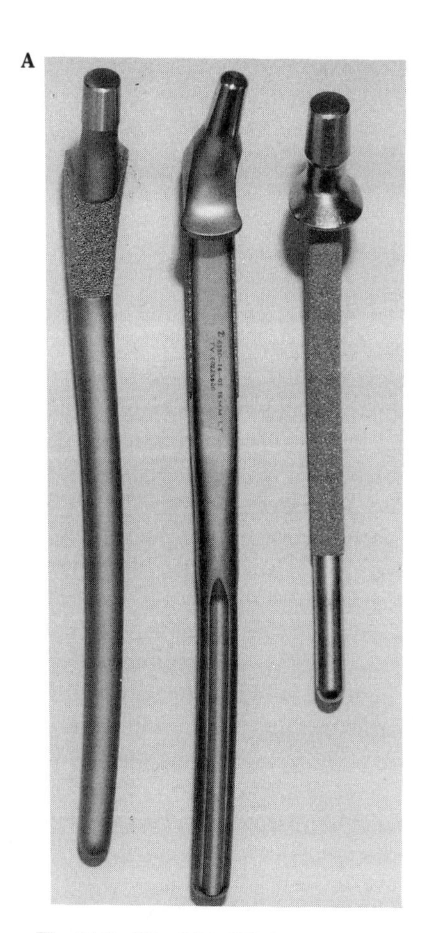

B

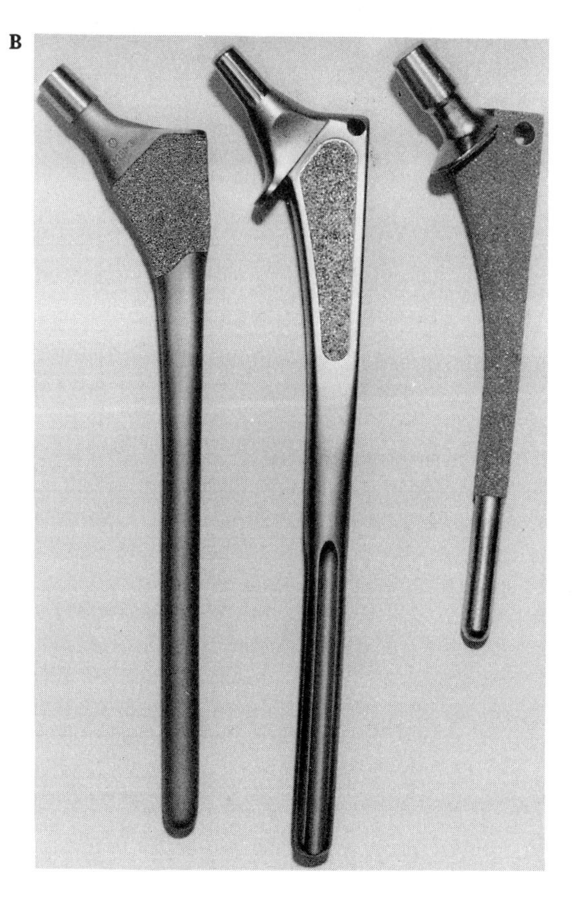

Fig. 11.8 The PCA, BIAS and AML stems, shown (**A**) in the anteroposterior view and (**B**) Ml. The PCA is S-shaped, the BIAS curved and the AML straight.

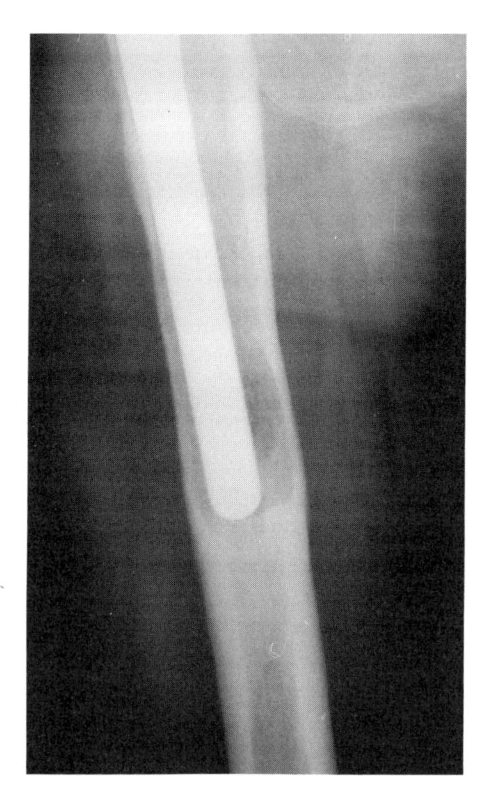

Fig. 11.9 Osteolysis at the tip of an obviously undersized uncemented revision prosthesis.

Engh et al (1988) have reported the largest series of uncemented revision hip arthroplasty with the results of 160 uncemented revisions with a mean follow-up of 4.4 years. The results for 127 femoral components were favourable with 84.3% being graded as good, 11.8% showing stable fibrous fixation and 3.9% definite failure. In this series operations on 26 hips were carried out with a New England Baptist-like stem which was oval in section distally but was fully porous coated. Only 2 lengths and 2 stem thicknesses were available. The rest were performed using a fully porous coated AML prosthesis. In 8 hips only proximally coated AML prostheses were used. Engh et al were able to show a greater failure rate with the New England Baptist-type stem. Their only definite failure with an AML stem was when it was only proximally coated. The authors favoured the fully coated prosthesis because they believe that in the damaged proximal femur it is impossible to achieve bony ingrowth of sufficient quality to provide lasting stability. Their preferred design is also straight and because of the proximal bow in the femur is only about 200 mm in length.

Gustilo & Kyle (1984a) report their experience with a proximally coated long-stemmed curved prosthesis. The BIAS was designed in 1981 along the following concepts:

1. Proximal ingrowth (anterior and posterior titanium fibre metal pads).
2. Proximal press-fit.
3. Proximal load transfer (collar and triangular portion).
4. Distal long, curved intramedullary stem for torsional and bending stability.
5. Bone graft proximally.

In 1988 Gustilo reported 31 hips following revision with a BIAS stem with an average follow-up of 2 years. Only one case required further surgery for loosening; 83% of patients were pain-free, and 73% required no walking aid on long walks. Reconstitution of the thinned cortical walls was a uniform finding. Gustilo concluded that the key to success was initial stability achieved by the fit of this femoral stem into the medullary cavity and massive bone grafting.

Hungerford & Jones (1988) reported 51 cases with a minimum follow-up of 2 years performed between 1983 and 1987 using the PCA prosthesis. The majority were revised using long-stem components. At least 24 standard PCA hips were used, probably in part because the long-stem design was only a custom item until 1985. The average age of patients in the series was 54 years. Postoperatively 90% of patients had a Harris hip score of 80 or better (average 87). Five patients had poor results, 2 had been re-revised and a 3 had persistent pain.

Direct comparison of these three trials is difficult as although two have used classifications for the degree of preoperative bony damage, the classifications are different. Clearly all three show very encouraging results.

The author's experience of uncemented revision started in 1986, coinciding with the introduction of the long-stemmed PCA into the UK. At that time I was doubtful as to whether as good a functional result could be achieved with an uncemented revision as with its cemented cousin. On the femoral side I therefore decided only to use uncemented stems in femurs with marked bony destruction in the younger age group. In these patients a lower functional result would be a reasonable price to pay for bone reconstitution. Even if the result did not last, the hip would be capable of further reconstruction in the future. To date over 80 uncemented stems have been inserted for these indications. Bonestock has been apparently restored (Figs. 11.10 and 11.11) and only 3 cases had poor results. In retrospect, in all 3 failure was due to inadequate proximal bonestock allowing sinkage to occur.

Critics of uncemented primary arthroplasty argue that the technique should not be practised widely until the results have been shown to be as good as or better than cemented arthroplasty in the long term. This is an argument not without foundation. Uncemented hip replacements should still probably be carried out as part of documented trials with full follow-up and not as sporadic cases. With uncemented revision results are available for small numbers of cases with at best mid-term but mainly short-term follow-up. Uncemented revision has become widely practised not because it has been shown to be superior but mainly because the long-term results of cemented revision have been so poor.

The results of uncemented femoral revision are encouraging but the series are of understandably short follow-up. Reduction of pain and improvement of function can be expected in 90% of patients. These results compare well with the functional results of cemented revision surgery. Uncemented prostheses used in conjunction with either autografts or allografts definitely appear to produce reconstitution of bonestock. At present no objective guidance exists as to the level of destruction that precludes the use of a proximally loading prosthesis and where a distally loading prosthesis is needed.

In the future, if it is accepted that failure of uncemented prosthesis will occur early and that once the implant is incorporated and stable in the bone failure is unlikely, then the argument in

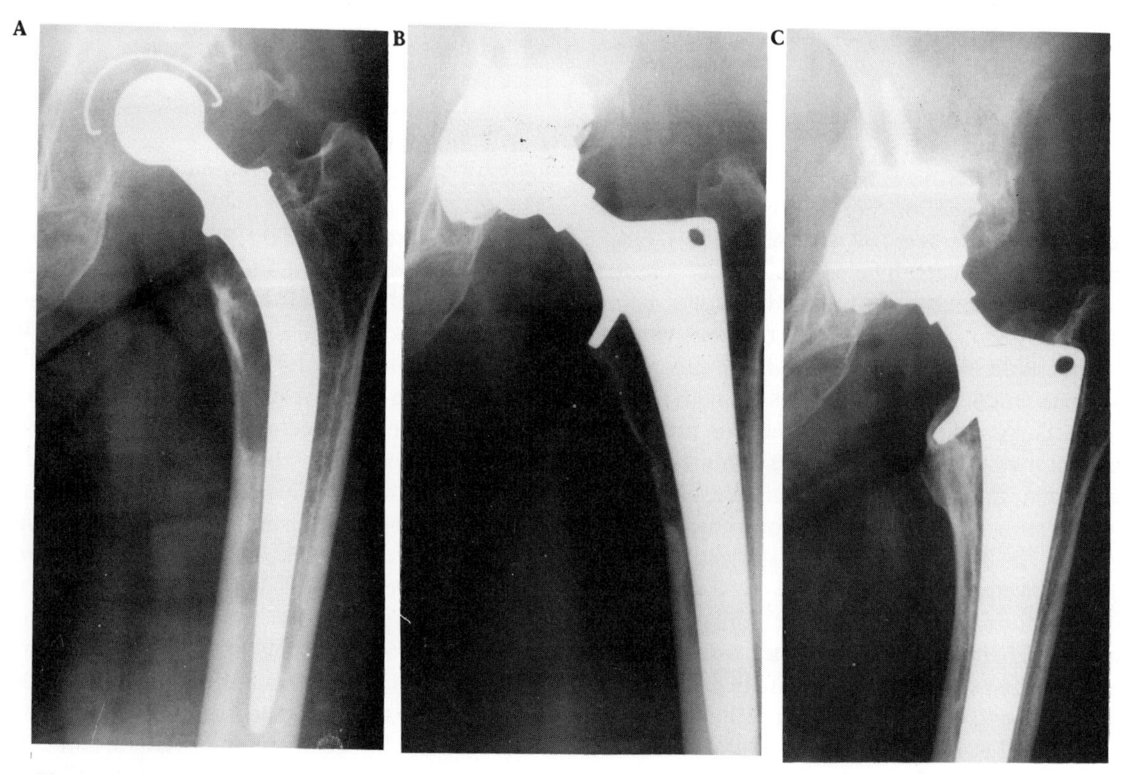

Fig. 11.10 Bone remodelling occurring after uncemented revision and grafting. (**A**) Preoperative; (**B**) immediately post-operation; (**C**) $2\frac{1}{2}$ years postoperation.

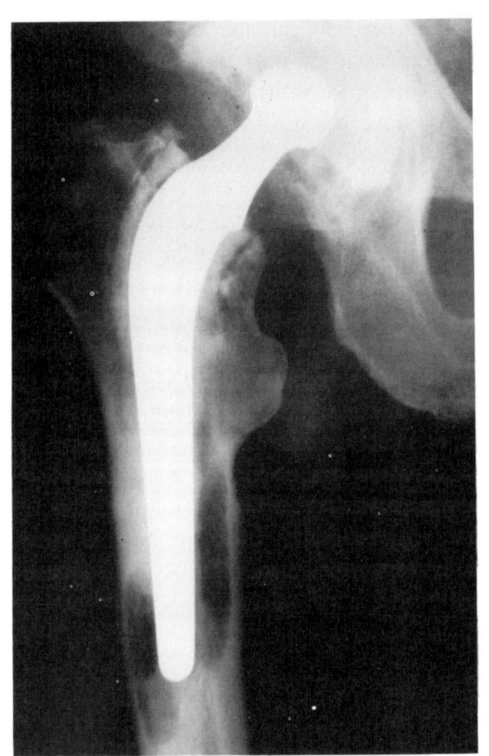
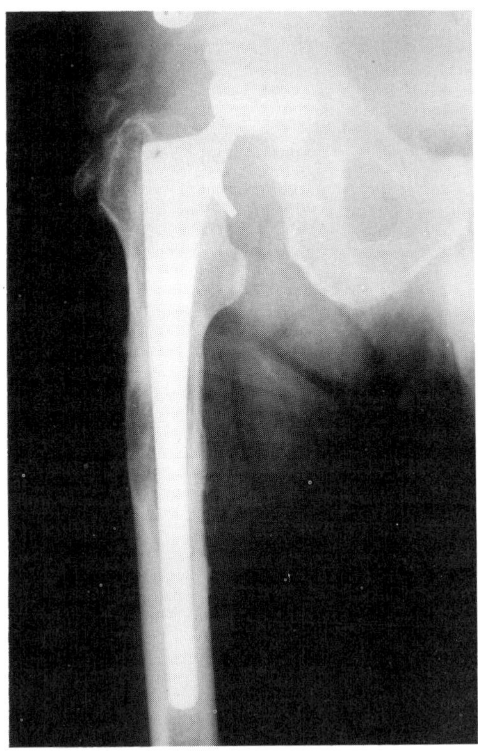

Fig. 11.11 Remodelling of osteolytic defects is seen only 8 months after revision to an uncemented grafted prosthesis.

favour of uncemented revision prostheses is overwhelming in all but the elderly. However, caution must be expressed firstly at the lack of any long-term results and secondly that the reported results of uncemented revision come from large centres with considerable experience in revision surgery and uncemented hip replacement. In more general units their functional results may not be reproducible and it is possible that, just as it did for cemented primary arthroplasty, cement may be the key to good reproducible functional results.

Distally supported uncemented stems

Distally supported uncemented stems have originated in Europe. The indication for use is severe bone destruction where a massive prosthesis may be considered. The concept is to support the prosthesis on the strong distal bone. The proximal damaged bone is preserved rather than resected in the hope that it will become stronger. At a point below the level of bone destruction the femur is transected. A prosthesis is then threaded through the proximally damaged bone with or without graft and fixed into the strong distal femur. Some form of collar or cone is used to allow the prosthesis to offload on the transection level. Lubinus in Kiel has used this method for some years with apparently good results. Wagner has developed a distal loading prosthesis (Fig. 11.12) using a distal fluted cone. He has described the transfemoral approach as a technique where the proximal damaged femur is split longitudinally. This allows a flap to be folded back so that the previous prosthesis and cement can be easily removed. The distally loading prosthesis is then inserted into the distal femur which has been prepared with conical reamers and the proximal femoral flap is closed over the prosthesis without any fixation. The osteotomies heal with pronounced callus and good results are reported. This technique is particularly attractive when it can be

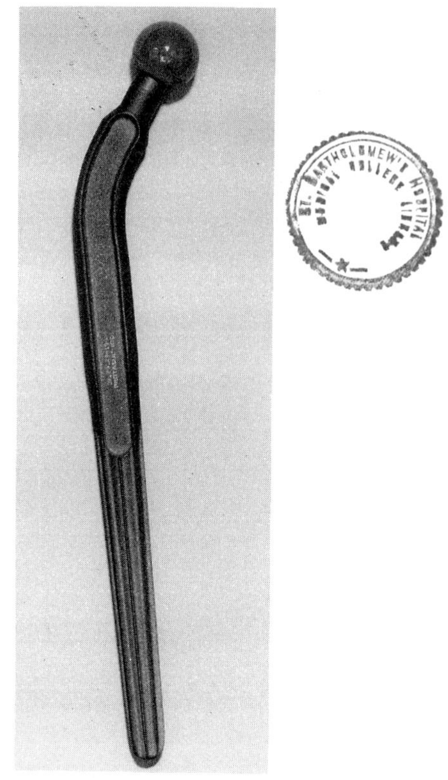

Fig. 11.12 The Wagner revision prosthesis. The prosthesis is supported distally by the fluted slightly conical distal shaft.

used instead of a massive upper femoral replacement.

Massive upper femoral allografts or prostheses

In severe disease these methods have been used. The benefit of the allograft over the upper femoral prosthesis has still to be proven. The problem with both techniques are the difficulties with salvage if infection or persistent dislocation ensues. If it is possible the distally supported uncemented prosthesis seems a safer option.

CONCLUSIONS

In revision hip surgery the problem of reconstitution of bonestock must be addressed in the younger patient. On the acetabular side the use of bone graft in conjunction with a porous coated press-fit hemispherical acetabular prosthesis is probably the method of choice in all age groups.

On the femoral side in the elderly infirm patient where early mobilization is necessary, a cemented prosthesis is satisfactory. In the younger patient with severe bone loss the uncemented proximally loaded prosthesis in conjunction with bone graft appears to be the best option on the basis of short-term results.

In the future the need for upper femoral replacements and distally loaded implants should be reduced firstly by early intervention when loosening occurs, even if this means regular X-ray examination of asymptomatic patients. Secondly, improved revision techniques will lead to less bone destruction in the multiply revised patient.

It must however be remembered that uncemented prostheses only remove one form of particulate wear. Polyethylene debris will still exist, together with increased amounts of metal debris if loose uncemented stems are allowed to fret on bone (Lombardi et al 1989).

REFERENCES

Amstutz HC, Jinnah RH 1982 Revision of aseptic loose total hip arthroplasties. Clin Orthop 170:21–33

Bobyn JD, Pilliar RM, Cameron HU 1980 The optimum pore size for the fixation of porous-surfaced metal implants by the ingrowth of bone. Clin Orthop 150:263

Brinkmann KE, Harms J 1984 Six years experience in revision total hip. Arthroplasties with uncemented ceramic prostheses. In: Morscher E (ed) The cementless fixation of hip endoprostheses. Springer Verlag pp 257–264

Broughton NS, Rushton N 1982 Revision hip arthroplasty. Acta Orthop Scand 53:923

Cameron HU, Jung YB 1988 Use of a big head bipolar acetabular component in selected hip revisions. Orthop Trans 12:716

Cameron HU, Pilliar RM, Macnab J 1976 The rate of bone ingrowth into porous metal. J Biomed Mater Res 10:295

Chambers TJ 1980 The cellular basis of bone resorption. Clin Orthop 151:283

Chandler H, Reinbeck T, Wixson R, McCarthy J 1981 Total hip replacements in patients younger than 30 years old. J Bone Joint Surg 63A:1426

Charnley J 1961 Arthroplasty of the hip—a new operation. Lancet i:1129

Cline MS 1975 The white cell. Harvard University Press, Cambridge, Massachusetts, pp 517–519

Cook SD, Walsh KA, Haddad RJ 1985 Interface mechanics and bone growth into porous Co-Cr-Mo alloy implants. Clin Orthop 193:271

Dandy DJ, Theodorous BC 1975 The management of local complications of total hip replacement by the McKee–Farrar technique. J Bone Joint Surg 57B:30

Dautry P, Koechlin P, Zaivre M 1979 La prosthèse S.E.M. dans les affections non traumatiques de cent observations

(avec film). Chirurgie 105: 617–634
Dewhurst EF, Stashenko PP, Mole JE, Tsurumachi T 1986 Purification and partial sequence of human osteoblast activating factor: identity with interleukin 1 beta. J Immunol 1985:135
Dorr L, Takei G, Conaty P 1983 Total hip arthroplasties in patients less tharn 45 years old. J Bone Joint Surg 65A:474
Emerson RH, Head WC, Berklacich MD, Malanin TI 1989 Noncemented acetabular revision arthroplasty using allograft bone. Clin Orthop 249:30–42
Engelbrecht DJ, Weber FA, Sweet MBE, Jakim IJ 1990 Long term results of revision total hip arthroplasty. J Bone Joint Surg 72B:41–45
Engh CA, Glassman AH, Griffin WL, Mayer JG 1988 Results of cementless revision for failed cemented total hip arthroplasty. Clin Orthop 236:91–101
Engh CA, Griffin WL, Marx CL 1990 Cementless acetabular components. J Bone Joint Surg 72B:53–59
Eskola A, Santavirta S et al 1990 Cementless revision of agressive granulomatous lesions in hip replacements. J Bone Joint Surg 72B:212–216
Esses S, Hastings D, Schatzker J 1983 Revision of total hip arthroplasty. Can J Surg 4:345–347
Fornasier VL, Cameron HU 1976 The femoral stem/cement interface in total hip replacement. Clin Orthop 116:248
Freeman MAR, Bradley GW, Reveil PA 1982 Observations upon the interface between bone and polymethyl-methacrylate cement. J Bone Joint Surg 64B: 489
Galante J, Rostocker W, Lueck R, Ray R 1971 Sintered fiber metal composites as a basis for attachment of implants to bone. J Bone Joint Surg 53A: 101–114
Geesink GT, De Groot K, Klein C 1987 Chemical implant fixation using hydroxyl apatite coatings. Clin Orthop 225:147–170
Goldring SR, Jasty M, Roelke M et al 1983 The synovial membrane at the bone cement interface in loose total hip replacements and its role in bone lysis. J Bone Joint Surg 65A:575–584
Goldring SR, Jasty M, Roelke MS et al 1986 Formation of a synovial-like membrane at the bone cement interface. Its role in bone resorption and implant loosening after total hip replacement. Arthritis Rheum 29:836–842
Goldring SR, Jasty M, Roelke M et al 1988 Biological factors that influence the development of the bone cement interface. In: Fitzgerald R Jr (ed) Non cemented total hip arthroplasty. Raven Press New York, pp 35–48
Goodman SB, Schatzker J, Sumner Smith G et al 1985 The effect of polymethylmethacrylate on bone. Arch Orthop Trauma Surg 104:150
Gustilo RB 1988 BIAS femoral ingrowth prosthesis with 2 to 5 year follow up. In: Fitzgerald R (ed) Total hip arthroplasty. Raven Press, New York, pp 413–425
Gustilo RB, Kyle RF 1984 Revision of fermoral component loosening with titanium ingrowth prosthesis and bone grafting. Symposium of revision of failed total hip arthroplasty, Hip Society proceedings. University Park Press, Baltimore, pp 345–346
Homsey CA, Tullos HS, Anderson MS et al 1972a Some physiological aspects of prosthesis stabilisation with acrylic polymer. Clin Orthop 83:317
Homsey CA, Cain TE et al 1972b Porous implant systems for prosthesis stabilisation. Clin Orthop 89:220
Hoogland T, Razzano CD, Marks K 1981 Revision of Mueller total hip arthroplasties. Clin Orthop 161:180–185
Hungerford DS, Jones LC, 1988 The rationale of cementless revision of cemented arthroplasty failures. Clin Orthop 235:12–23
Hungerford DS, Krackow KA, Lennox DW 1988 The PCA primary and revision hip systems. In: Fitzgerald R (ed) Non cemented total hip arthroplasty. Raven Press, New York, pp 433–450
Hunter GA, Welsh RP, Cameron HU 1979 The results of revision total hip arthroplasty. J Bone Joint Surg 61B:419–421
Jasty M, Harris WH 1990 Salvage total hip reconstruction in patients with major acetabular bone deficiency using structural femoral head allografts. J Bone Joint Surg 72B:63–67
Jasty MJ, Floyd WE, Schiller A et al 1986 Localized osteolysis in stable, non septic total hip replacement. J Bone Joint Surg 68A:912
Kavanagh BF, Ilstrup DM, Fitzgerald RH 1985 Revision total hip arthroplasty. J Bone Joint Surg. 67A:517–527
Kavanagh BF, Dewitz MA, Ilstrup MS et al 1989 Charnley total hip arthroplasty with cement. J Bone Joint Surg 71A:1496–1503
Kozinn SC, Johanson NA, Bullough PG 1986 The biologic interface between bone and cementless femoral endoprostheses. J Arthropl 1:249–259
Ling RSM 1990 The technique of cementing revision stems into impacted allograft bone. Paper read at First British Revision Surgery Meeting, Knebworth House
Lombardi AV, Mallory TH, Vaughn BK, Drouillard P 1989 Aseptic loosening in total hip arthroplasty secondary to osteolysis induced by wear debris from titanium-alloy modular femoral heads. J Bone Joint Surg 71A:1337–1342
Lord GA 1982 Madreporique stemmed total hip replacement: 5 years clinical experience. J R Soc Med 75:166
Mallory TH, Vaughn BK et al 1988 Threaded acetabular components. Design rationale and preliminary clinical experience. Orthop Rev 17:305–314
Marti RK, Schuller HM, Besselaar MD, Vanfrank Hasnoot EL 1990 Results of revision of hip arthroplasty with cement. J Bone Joint Surg 72A:346–354
McGann WA, Welch RB, Picetti GD 1988 Acetabular preparation in cementless revision total hip arthroplasty. Clin Orthop 235:35
McKee GK, Watson-Farrar J 1966 Replacement of arthritic hips by the McKee–Farrar prosthesis. J Bone Joint Surg 48B:245
Mcminn D 1990 Acetabular reconstruction using a stemmed acetabular component, Paper read at 1st British revision joint meeting, Knebworth House
Murray WR 1984 Salvage of acetabular insufficiency with bipolar prostheses. In:The hip: proceedings of the 12th open scientific meeting of the hip Society. St Louis, CV Mosby, pp 296–311
Ochsner JL, Penenberg BL, Dorr LD, Conaty JP 1988 Results of bipolar endoprosthesis and bone graft for acetabular component revision. Read at the annual meeting of the American Academy of Orthopaedic Surgeons, Atlanta, Georgia
Oonishi H, Yamamoto M, Ishimaru H et al 1989 The effect of hydroxyapatite coating on bone growth into porous titanium alloy implants. J Bone Joint Surg 71B:213–216
Parhofer R, Monch W 1984 Experience with revision arthroplasties for failed cemented total hip replacements using uncemented Lord and PM prostheses. In: Morscher E (ed) The cementless fixation of hip endoprosthesis. Springer Verlag pp 275–278

Pellici PM, Wilson PD, Sledge CM 1982 Revision total hip arthroplasty. Clin Orthop 170:34–41
Pellici PM, Wilson PD, Sledge CM 1985 Long term results of revision total hip replacement: a follow up report. J Bone Joint Surg 67A: 513–516
Reigstad A, Hetland KR 1984 Rearthroplasty after conventional total hip arthroplasty and double cup prosthesis. Arch Orthop Trauma Surg 103:152–155
Ring PA 1981 Uncemented total hip replacement. J R Soc Med 74:719
Roberson JR, Spector M, Baggett MA, Kita K 1988 Porous coated femoral components in a canine model for revision arthroplasty. J Bone Joint Surg 70A:1201–1208
Rorabeck CH, Bourne RB, Shimozaki E et al 1990 Bone grafting in revision total hip arthroplasty: cement versus cementless. J Bone Joint Surg 72B:539
Rubash HE, Harris WH 1988 Revision of nonseptic, loose, cemented femoral components using modern cementing techniques. J Arthropl 3:241–247
Santavirta S, Yrjo T Kottinen YT et al 1990 Agressive granulomatous lesions associated with hip arthroplasty. J Bone Joint Surg 72A:252–258
Schmalzreid TP, Finerman GAM 1988 Osteolysis in aseptic failure In: Fitzgerald R Jr (ed) Non cemented total hip arthroplasty. Raven Press, New York, pp 303–318
Scott RD, Pomeroy D, Oser E et al 1987 The results and technique of bipolar hip arthroplasty combined with acetabular grafting. Orthop Trans 11:450
Sommelet J, Finlayson D, Lesur E 1989 Acetabular reconstruction with a bipolar prosthesis—5 year results of the Dautry technique. J Bone Joint Surg 71B:460–464
Stromberg C, Herberts P, Ahnfelt L 1988 Revision total hip arthroplasty in patients younger than 55 years old. J Arthropl 3:47–59
Tallroth K, Eskola A, Satavirta S et al 1989 Agressive granulomatous lesions after hip arthroplasty. J Bone Joint Surg 71B:571–575
Turner RH, Mattingly DA, Scheller AJ 1987a Femoral revision total hip arthroplasty using a long stem femoral component. Arthroplasty 2:247–258
Wilson MG, Nikpoor N, Alibadi P et al 1989 The fate of acetabular allografts after bipolar revision arthroplasty of the hip. J Bone Joint Surg 71A:1469–1479
Wrobleski BM 1986 15–21 Year results of the Charnley low friction arthroplasty. Clin Orthop 211: 30–35

Index

Accidents
  care services, 24
  domestic, 17, 19–20
  epidemiology, 15–24
    data, 15–17
  road traffic, 15–16, 17–19, 22–24
    mathematical models, 22–23
  sport and leisure, 20
  work, 17, 19
  see also Disasters
Acetabulum
  development, 103–106
  dysplasia, 106
    assessment, 109–113
    conservative treatment, 114
    and femoral head and neck changes, 106–107
    hip congruity and, 109
    lateral acetabular epiphysis, 106
    lump sign, 111
    secondary, 106–107
    surgery for, 113–117
  reconstruction in revision hip replacement, 161–164
Aircrash, Kegworth, M1, 134–135, 139
Arthritis *see* Osteoarthritis; Rheumatoid arthritis
Arthrography
  knee, 42–43
  shoulder, 46
  wrist, 48
Arthroscopy, shoulder *see* Shoulder joint, arthroscopy

Back pain, incidence, 2
Bankart lesions, 152–154
Bone
  cancer, registration, 1
  lengthening, use of circular fixation devices, 37–38
  transport, circular fixation devices and, 37
  tumours, diagnostic imaging, 60
Brachial plexus injuries, 65
  anatomical studies, 68–69
  diagnosis, 66
  epidemiology, 65
  imaging, 66–67
  pain in, 73
  reconstruction following, 71
    elbow, 72
    forearm and hand, 72–73
    shoulder, 72
  repair, 73–74
    nerve transfer, 70–71
    pain relief following, 73
    regeneration from spinal cord, 68–69
    results, 69–71
    technical advances, 69
    vascularized ulnar nerve graft, 69–70
  spinal cord injuries and, 67
  surgical pathology, 67–68
  vascular injuries and, 67–68

Cancer, bone, registration, 1
Clapham rail disaster, 135–136
Computerized tomography, 61
  hip, 49, 50, 51
  knee, 43–45
  shoulder, 46
  spine, 51, 52
    brachial plexus injuries, 67
    cervical, 57
    failed back surgery, 53–55
    nucleus pulposus herniation, 52
    stenosis, 53
    trauma, 58–59
  wrist, 48
Coracoacromial ligament, arthroscopic division, 149

Disasters, major
  Clapham rail disaster, 135–136
  communications in, 134, 136, 138, 139, 142–143
  definition, 133
  documentation for, 139–142, 143
  emergency treatment at, 137
  Hillsborough stadium, 136
  hospitals, 135, 136, 143
    planning at, 138–139
  Kegworth M1 aircrash, 134–135, 139
  plans for, 133, 137
    hospitals, 138–139, 143
    reasons for failure, 142
    on site, 137–138
  recommendations for management, 142–143
Discs, intervertebral
  nucleus pulposus herniation, diagnostic imaging, 52–53
  prolapsed
    cervical, diagnostic imaging, 57–58
    incidence, 2–3
    recurrent, diagnostic imaging, 54–56
Dorsal root entry zone thermocoagulation, 73
Duchenne muscular dystrophy, 119
  diagnosis, 120–122
  natural history, 119–120
  sitting phase, management, 124–127
    flexion contractures, 127–128
    scoliosis, 128–130
  walking phase
    mechanical disorder and compensating mechanisms, 122–124
    orthopaedic management, 124–127

Elbow joint, reconstruction after brachial plexus injury, 72
Epidemiology
  accidents, 15–24
  definition, 1
  fibromyalgia, 4–5
  methods in orthopaedics, 1–3
  osteoarthritis, 7–10
  osteoporosis, 5–7
  rheumatoid arthritis, 10–12
External skeletal fixation
  advantages, 27–29
  choice of system, 35–38
  disadvantages, 29–31
  engineering characteristics of fixators, 32–35
    bone-screw mechanics, 34
    dynamization, 34–35
    frame mechanics, 32–33
  ideal system, 31–32
Femur
  fractures of neck, epidemiology, 5–6
  reconstruction in revision hip replacement, 165–170

Femur (*contd*)
upper
and acetabular dysplasia, 106–107
development, 103–105
Fibromyalgia, 4
epidemiology, 4–5
Fixation, external skeletal *see* External skeletal fixation
Fixators, external
circular frames, 36–38
disadvantages, 38
engineering characteristics, 32–35
bone–screw mechanics, 34
dynamization, 34–35
frame mechanics, 32–33
pin frames, 32–33
comprehensive, 36
unilateral, 35–36
Flexor tendon surgery
active implants, 96–97, 98
flexor to extensor transfer following brachial plexus injury, 72
free grafting, 88–90, 97–98
primary repair, 77
complications, 86
partial lacerations, 79
post-operative mobilization methods, 83–86, 97
profundus tendon advancement, 79–80
results, 86–88
sheath repair and, 80–81, 97
suture materials and methods, 77–79, 97
technical points, 82–83
tendon retrieval in, 81–82
pulley reconstruction, 95–96
rehabilitation, 97–98
staged reconstruction, 90–93
tenolysis, 93–95, 98
Forearm, reconstruction after brachial plexus injury, 72–73
Fractures
diaphyseal, external skeletal fixation, 30–31, 35, 37
external skeletal fixation, 27
advantages, 27–29
choice of fixation system, 35–38
disadvantages, 29–31
healing, mechanics, 34
intra-articular, treatment, 30

Glenoid labrum tears, arthroscopic surgery, 149

Haemangiomas, diagnostic imaging, 60
Haematomas, diagnostic imaging, 60
Hand, reconstruction after brachial plexus injury, 72–73
Hill-Sachs lesions, 148, 152
Hillsborough stadium disaster, 136
Hip joint
acetabulum *see* Acetabulum
congruity, 107–109
and acetabular dysplasia, 109
diagnostic imaging, 49–51
fractures, epidemiology, 5–6
prostheses
bipolar, with acetabular reconstruction, 162–163
bone–cement interface, 157–161
long-stemmed cemented, disadvantages, 160
Monk soft-top, 160
porous hemispherical sockets, 163–164
screw-in sockets, 163
uncemented, 160–164, 165–170
Wagner revision, 169–170
revision replacement, 157–161
acetabular reconstruction in, 161–164
femoral reconstruction in, 165–170
uncemented prostheses in, 157–164, 165–170

Imaging, diagnostic, 41, 61–62
hip, 49–51
knee, 42–46
shoulder, 46–48
spine, 51–60
brachial plexus injuries, 66–67
cervical, 57–58
wrist, 48–49
see also under specific imaging procedures

Kegworth M1 aircrash, 134–135, 139
Knee joint, diagnostic imaging, 42–46
cruciate ligament tears, 44–45
meniscal tears, 43–44

Legs
lengthening, use of circular fixation devices, 37–38
long leg dysplasia, 106–107
surgical correction, 115
short leg dysplasia, 106–107
surgical correction, 115, 117
Lipomas, diagnostic imaging, 60
Luque segmental fixation in muscular dystrophy, 128–129

Magnetic resonance imaging, 41–42, 61
hip, 51
knee, 43–46
musculoskeletal tumours, 60–61
shoulder, 47–48
spine, 51–52
cervical, 57–58
failed back surgery, 54–56
nucleus pulposus herniation, 52–53
stenosis, 53
trauma, 59–60
wrist, 48–49
Motor cycle accidents, epidemiology, 19, 21, 22, 65
Muscular dystrophy, Duchenne *see* Duchenne muscular dystrophy
Myositis ossificans, diagnostic imaging, 61

Nerve transfer in treatment of brachial plexus injuries, 70–71

Obesity and osteoarthritis, 10
Osteoarthritis
aetiology, 9–10
definition, 7–8
occurrence, 8–9
Osteoporosis
epidemiology, 5–7
risk factors, 7

Pain
back, incidence, 2
brachial plexus injuries, 73
relief, 73
Patella, imaging, 43
Perthes' disease, 112, 113

Rail disaster, Clapham, 135–136
Rheumatoid arthritis
definition, 10
trends in, 10–12
Road traffic accidents
epidemiology, 15–16, 17–19, 20, 22–24
mathematical models of occurrence, 22–23
motor cycles, 19, 21, 22, 65

Scintigraphy, hip, 51
Scoliosis in Duchenne muscular dystrophy, management of, 128–130
Shoulder joint
arthroscopy
anatomy, 147–148
for biopsy, 148
bursae, 148, 149–150
division of coracoacromial ligament, 149
instability management, 151–154
loose bodies, 148–149
subacromial decompression, 149–151
for surgery, 148–151
synovectomy, 149
tears of glenoid labrum, 149
techniques, 145–151
diagnostic imaging, 46–48
instability, arthroscopic management
repair by staple, 152
results, 154
suture technique, 152–154
reconstruction after brachial plexus injury, 72
syndromes, incidence, 2–3
Skeletal fixation, external *see* External skeletal fixation
Sonography, 62
hip, 49–51
knee, 45–46

Sonography (*contd*)
musculoskeletal tumours, 60–61
shoulder, 46–47
Spine
diagnostic imaging, 51–52
cervical spine, 57–58
failed surgery, 53–56
nucleus pulposus herniation, 52–53
stenosis, 53
traumatic injury, 58–60
Luque segmental fixation, 128–129
vertebral crush fractures, epidemiology, 6–7
Sports accidents, 20
Subacromial bursa, 148, 149–155
Synovectomy of shoulder, arthroscopic, 149

Tendons, flexor *see* Flexor tendons
Tumours, musculoskeletal, diagnostic imaging, 60–61
Ulnar nerve grafts, vascularized, in treatment of brachial plexus injuries, 69–70

Vertebral crush fractures, epidemiology, 6–7
Violence, injuries from, 20, 24

Wrist
diagnostic imaging, 48–49
reconstruction after brachial plexus injury, 72